GN00836199

OXFORD MEDICAL PUBLICATIONS

Paediatric
Radiology

General Oxford Specialist Handbooks
A Resuscitation Room Guide
Addiction Medicine
Perioperative Medicine, Second Edition
Post-Operative Complications, Second Edition

Oxford Specialist Handbooks in Anaesthesia
Cardiac Anaesthesia
General Thoracic Anaesthesia
Neuroanaesthesia
Obstetric Anaesthesia
Paediatric Anaesthesia
Regional Anaesthesia, Stimulation and Ultrasound Techniques

Oxford Specialist Handbooks in Cardiology
Adult Congenital Heart Disease
Cardiac Catheterization and Coronary Intervention
Echocardiography
Fetal Cardiology
Heart Failure
Hypertension
Nuclear Cardiology
Pacemakers and ICDs

Oxford Specialist Handbooks in Critical Care
Advanced Respiratory Critical Care

Oxford Specialist Handbooks in End of Life Care
End of Life Care in Cardiology
End of Life Care in Dementia
End of Life Care in Nephrology
End of Life Care in Respiratory Disease
End of Life in the Intensive Care Unit

Oxford Specialist Handbooks in Neurology
Epilepsy
Parkinson's Disease and Other Movement Disorders
Stroke Medicine

Oxford Specialist Handbooks in Paediatrics
Paediatric Endocrinology and Diabetes
Paediatric Dermatology
Paediatric Gastroenterology, Hepatology, and Nutrition
Paediatric Haematology and Oncology
Paediatric Nephrology
Paediatric Neurology
Paediatric Respiratory Medicine

Oxford Specialist Handbooks in Psychiatry
Child and Adolescent Psychiatry
Old Age Psychiatry

Oxford Specialist Handbooks in Radiology
Interventional Radiology
Musculoskeletal Imaging

Oxford Specialist Handbooks in Surgery
Cardiothoracic Surgery
Hand Surgery
Hepato-pancreatobiliary Surgery
Oral Maxillo Facial Surgery
Neurosurgery
Operative Surgery, Second Edition
Otolaryngology and Head and Neck Surgery
Plastic and Reconstructive Surgery
Surgical Oncology
Urological Surgery
Vascular Surgery

Oxford Specialist
Handbooks in
Paediatrics
Paediatric
Radiology

Karl Johnson
Consultant Paediatric Radiologist,
Birmingham Children's Hospital, UK

Helen Williams
Consultant Paediatric Radiologist,
Birmingham Children's Hospital, UK

Katharine Foster
Consultant Paediatric Radiologist,
Birmingham Children's Hospital, UK

Claire Miller
Consultant Paediatric Radiologist,
Birmingham Children's Hospital, UK

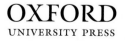

OXFORD
UNIVERSITY PRESS

OXFORD

UNIVERSITY PRESS

Great Clarendon Street, Oxford OX2 6DP

Oxford University Press is a department of the University of Oxford.
It furthers the University's objective of excellence in research, scholarship,
and education by publishing worldwide in

Oxford New York

Auckland Cape Town Dar es Salaam Hong Kong Karachi
Kuala Lumpur Madrid Melbourne Mexico City Nairobi
New Delhi Shanghai Taipei Toronto

With offices in

Argentina Austria Brazil Chile Czech Republic France Greece
Guatemala Hungary Italy Japan Poland Portugal Singapore
South Korea Switzerland Thailand Turkey Ukraine Vietnam

Oxford is a registered trade mark of Oxford University Press
in the UK and in certain other countries

Published in the United States
by Oxford University Press Inc., New York

British Library Cataloguing in Publication Data
Data available

Library of Congress Cataloging-in-Publication-Data
Data available

Typeset by Cepha Imaging Private Ltd., Bangalore, India
Printed in China
on acid-free paper
by Asia Pacific Offset

ISBN 978–0–19–920479–3

10 9 8 7 6 5 4 3 2 1

Preface

Paediatric imaging is unique within the many radiology sub-specialities, as it is the only one which defines its patient group by age, namely birth to 18 years. As a consequence, paediatric radiology covers all the different anatomical and organ system groups. This book is written using this system-based approach. For each system, there are three separate sections. The first deals with common presenting symptoms in childhood, listing the most likely diagnoses in different age groups. There is then a review of the imaging approach to each of these presenting conditions and the value of each modality. The second section lists the common radiological findings which may be encountered when imaging children and the differential diagnoses which need to be considered. The final section discusses in detail a number of common conditions which anybody doing paediatric radiology may be expected to see. Using this approach, the authors hope that this book will be useful both to the radiologist and the referring clinician.

With a book of this size, it is impossible to include all known paediatric conditions. The authors have concentrated on those conditions which are either common, unique to paediatrics or of such importance that any delay in diagnosis may be significant.

In preparing the text, the authors are aware that many of the lists, statistics used and radiological signs described have previously been published. Acknowledgement is made to the following texts: *Diagnostic Imaging Paediatrics* (Donnelly *et al.*), *Imaging Children* (Carty *et al.*), *Aids to Radiological Differential Diagnosis* (Chapman and Nakielny), *Radiology Review Manual* (Dähnert), *Paediatric Neuroimaging* (Barkovich).

The authors would value feedback on the text as there may well be omissions, errors and improvements which could be made.

Contents

ix

Detailed contents

2c Chest and cardiac: disorders

Gastrointestinal (GI)

3a Gastrointestinal (GI): clinical presentations and role of imaging

3b Gastrointestinal (GI): differential diagnosis

3c Gastrointestinal (GI): disorders

Hepatobiliary

5a Hepatobiliary: clinical presentations and role of imaging

5b Hepatobiliary: differential diagnosis

Neurology

8a Neurology: clinical presentations and role of imaging

8b Neurology: differential diagnosis

Symbols and abbreviations

📖	Cross reference
❶	Warning
⚠	Warning
♂	Male
♀	Female
▶	Important
↑	Increased
↓	Decreased
↔	Normal
~	Approx
≈	Equal to
1°	Primary
2°	Secondary
AA	aortic arch
AARF	atlanto-axial rotatory fixation
ACL	anterior cruciate ligament
ACTH	adrenocorticotropic hormone
AD	autosomal dominant
ADC	apparent diffusion coefficient
ADEM	acute demyelinating encephalomyelitis
ADPKD	autosomal dominant polycystic kidney disease
AF	anterior fontanelle
AFP	alpha-fetoprotein
AIDS	acquired immune deficiency syndrome
AKA	also known as
AP	anterior posterior
AR	autosomal recessive
ARDS	acute respiratory distress syndrome
ARM	anorectal malformation
ARPKD	autosomal recessive polycystic kidney disease
ASD	atrioseptal defect
AV	arteriovenous
AVM	arteriovenous malformation
AVSD	atrioventricular septal defect
AXR	abdominal radiograph

BA	branchial anomaly
BIH	benign intracranial hypertension
BPD	bronchopulmonary dysplasia
C+	addition of contrast
C1, C2	cervical vertebrae
Ca	calcium
CAH	congenital adrenal hyperplasia
CAII	carbonic anhydrase type II deficiency
CBD	common bile duct
CDH	congenital dislocation of the hip
CF	cystic fibrosis
CHARGE	coloboma, heart disease, atresia of nasal choana, mental or growth retardation, genital and ear abnormalities
CHD	congenital heart disease
CHL	conductive hearing loss
CI	cochlear implantation
CK	creatine kinase
CMV	cytomegalovirus
CN	cranial nerve
CNS	central nervous system
CO_2	carbon dioxide
CP	cerebral palsy
CPAM	congenital pulmonary airway malformation
CPAP	continuous positive airway pressure
CRITOL	capitellum, radial head, internal (medial) humeral epicondyle, trochlea, olecranon and lateral (external) humeral epicondyle
CSF	cerebrospinal fluid
CT	computerized tomography
CXR	chest radiograph
DDH	developmental dysplasia of the hip
DIOS	distal intestinal obstruction syndrome
DIP	distal interphalangeal joint
DISIDA	diisopropyl iminodiacetic acid
DJF	duodeno–jejunal flexure
DKA	diabetic ketoacidosis
DMSA	Tc-2,3 dimercaptosuccinic acid
DNET	dysembryoplastic neuroepithelial tumour
DWI	diffusion weighted imaging
EAC	external auditory canal
EBV	Epstein–Barr virus

ECA	external carotid artery
ECG	electrocardiogram
ET	endotracheal
FASI	focal areas of signal intensity
FB	foreign body
FDG	fluorodeoxyglucose
FLAIR	fluid attenuated inversion recovery
FNA	fine needle aspiration
FS	fat saturated
FTT	failure to thrive
GA	general anaesthesia
Gd-DTPA	gadolinium diethylenetriaminepentaacetic acid
GI	gastrointestinal
GOR	gastro-oesophageal reflux
GRE	gradient echo
GU	genitourinary
GVHD	graft versus host disease
HB	haemoglobin
HD	Hirschprung's disease
HbF	fetal haemoglobin
HIE	hypoxic ischaemic encephalopathy
HIV	human immunodeficiency virus
HLHS	hypoplastic left heart syndrome
HRCT	high- resolution computerized tomography
HSP	Henoch–Schönlein purpura
HSV	herpes simplex virus
HU	Hounsfield units
HUS	haemolytic uraemic syndrome
IAC	internal auditory canal
IBD	inflammatory bowel disease
ICA	internal carotid artery
ICP	intracranial pressure
IDA	iminodiacetic acid
IJV	internal jugular vein
iv	intravenous
IVC	inferior vena cava
IVU	intravenous urogram
JDMS	juvenile dermatomyositis
JIA	juvenile idiopathic arthritis
kV	kilovoltage

L1, L2	lumbar vertebrae
LCH	Langerhans' cell histiocytosis
LDH	lactic dehydrogenase
LESA	large endolymphatic sac anomaly
LL	lymphoid leukaemia
LM	lymphatic malformation
LVAS	large vestibular aqueduct syndrome
MAG3	Tc mercaptoacetyltriglycine
mAs	milliampseconds
MCDK	multicystic dysplastic kidney
MCP	metacarpal phalangeal joint
MCUG	micturating cystourethrogram
MIBG	metaiodobenzylguanidine
ML	myeloid leukaemia
MPNST	malignant peripheral nerve sheath tumour
MPS	mucopolysaccharidoses
MRA	magnetic resonance angiography
MRCP	magnetic resonance cholangiopancreatography
MRI	magnetic resonance imaging
NAA	N-acetylaspartate
NAI	non-accidental injury
NEC	necrotizing enterocolitis
NF-1	neurofibromatosis type 1
NG	nasogastric
NGT	nasogastric tube
NSAID	non-steroidal anti-inflammatory drug
OA	oesophageal atresia
OCD	osteochondral defect
OI	osteogenesis imperfecta
OSD	Osgood–Schlatter disease
p.r.	per rectum
PAN	polyarteritis nodosa
PCL	posterior cruciate ligament
PCR	polymerase chain reaction
PD	proton density
PDA	patent ductus arteriosus
PDFSE	proton density fast-spin echo imaging
PET	positron emission tomography
PHACE	posterior fossa malformations, haemangiomas, arterial abnormalities, coarctation of the aorta, eye abnormalities

PID	pelvic inflammatory disease
PIE	pulmonary interstitial emphysema
PIP	proximal interphalangeal joint
PN	parenteral nutrition
PNET	primitive neuroectodermal tumour
PRES	posterior reversible encephalopathy syndrome
PUJ	pelvi-ureteric junction
PUV	posterior urethral valves
PV	portal vein
PVL	periventricular leukomalacia
PVNS	pigmented villonodular synovitis
RhF	rheumatoid factor
RIF	right iliac fossa
RLQ	right lower quadrant
RMS	rhabdomyosarcoma
RSV	respiratory syncitial virus
RUQ	right upper quadrant
SB	small bowel
SCFE	slipped capital femoral epiphysis
SCIWORA	spinal cord injury without radiological abnormality
SCM	sternocleidomastoid
SH	Salter–Harris
SLE	systemic lupus erythematosus
SMA	superior mesenteric artery
SMV	superior mesenteric vein
SNHL	sensorineural hearing loss
SNR	signal to noise ratio
STIR	short tau inversion recovery
SUFE	slipped upper femoral epiphysis
SVC	superior vena cava
T1, T2	thoracic vertebrae
T1WI	T1-weighted imaging
T2WI	T2-weighted imaging
TAPVR	Total anomalous pulmonary venous return
TB	tuberculosis
TBIDA	Tc trimethylbromo-iminodiacetic acid
Tc	technetium
TE	echo time
TGDC	thyroglossal duct cyst
TI	terminal ileum

TM	tympanic membrane
ToF	tetralogy of Fallot
TOF	tracheo-oesophageal fistula
TORCH	toxoplasmosis, rubella, CMV, herpes
TPN	total parenteral nutrition
TR	repetition time
TS	tuberous sclerosis
UAC	umbilical arterial catheter
UC	ulcerative colitis
URTI	upper respiratory tract infection
US	ultrasound
UTI	urinary tract infection
UVC	umbilical vein catheter
VA	visual acuity
VACTERL	vertebral, anorectal, cardiac, tracheal, oesophageal, renal, limb abnormalities (usually radial)
VATER	vertebral, anorectal, tracheal, esophageal, renal abnormalities
VIP	vasoactive intestinal peptide
VM	venous malformations
VMA	vanillylmandelic acid
VSD	ventricular septal defect
VUJ	vesico-ureteric junction
VUR	vesico-ureteric reflux
WAGR	wilms' tumor, aniridia, genitourinary abnormalities, mental retardation
WCC	white cell count
XPGN	xanthogranulomatous pyelonephritis

Imaging procedures

Karl Johnson

Paediatric imaging

When imaging children it is important to consider the age and development of the child under investigation. This is vital when considering the differential diagnosis of the any particular clinical symptom and assessing the appropriateness of any imaging investigation. Procedures and processes need to take account of the expected changes that occur within the growing child. For example, in younger children there is a greater amount of unossified cartilage within the skeleton and a different body fat composition, so exposure parameters for radiographs need to be altered: additionally the faster respiratory and heart rate should be taken into consideration when performing chest radiography. As a child is more sensitive to radiation than an adult, repeat X-rays should be avoided. Similarly magnetic resonance imaging (MRI) sequence selection in the neonatal brain (which contains more water and less myelinated tissue) is different from that in the older child.

Environment

Imaging departments should be as child-friendly as possible, though consideration must be given to the different requirements of the older child and adolescent compared to that of the young infant. Decorations and signing should ideally be at a lower level to help the orientation of the child. Explanation of any procedure should be aimed predominantly at the child wherever possible. Children should not be lied to and obtaining the child's cooperation, while a more time-consuming process, is ultimately more productive than forcing them into situations against their will.

Sedation and general anaesthesia

For some investigations, primarily MR imaging (but also angiography, nuclear medicine and computerized tomography [CT]) achieving a suitable level of cooperation in the younger or developmentally delayed child, so that they remain stationary for the procedure, may not be possible. In this instance sedation or general anesthesia may be required to ensure the child remains stationary.

Sedation is an artificially induced level of decreased consciousness. Increasing the amount of sedation and thus lowering the level of consciousness will lead first to a reduction of muscle tone of the oropharynx, and then to a loss of the glottic reflex. This has the risk of aspiration and respiratory compromise. The level of sedation should be aimed at keeping the child asleep but does not result in the loss of vital reflexes and the child is still rousable if necessary. Any sedated child should be closely monitored, particularly their respiration rate and blood oxygen saturation, and appropriate resuscitation facilities should be available. A variety of different sedation regimes have been described.

Anaesthesia is an unrousable state with loss of normal airway reflexes. The method of anaesthesia and monitoring of the child will vary but must be closely supervised by an appropriately trained paediatric anaesthetist. If used within a MR scanner then suitably compatible machinery is required.

Radiographs (X-rays)

Standard radiographs are the commonest imaging investigation undertaken. X-rays are part of the electromagnetic spectrum: they are a form of ionizing radiation and as such can damage any tissue they pass through. The use of X-rays should be carefully scrutinized and inappropriate and unnecessary examinations avoided. Children are particularly sensitive to ionizing radiation and have a greater risk of developing malignancy, following exposure to any ionizing radiation. ▶ Radiographs should only be performed if they will have an alteration on the child's clinical management.

Image viewing

Conventional X-ray films (radiographs) should be viewed on a light box, and digital images on high-quality monitor screens. The appearance of digital images can be adjusted by altering the windowing, contrast, brightness and magnification of the images.

Fluoroscopy

The basic principle of fluoroscopy is similar to conventional radiographs: the image is produced following the passage of an X-ray beam through the body. However, instead of producing a static image, an instantaneous image is generated on a fluorescent screen, allowing visualization of a real time moving image. Fluoroscopy is used for dynamic investigations and is often used with contrast agents to improve the visualization of organs and viscera. In paediatric practice common fluoroscopic examinations are barium swallows and meals, micturating cystograms and air enemas.

Advantages
- Readily available.
- Relatively cheap.
- Very good anatomical detail.
- Good detail of bone injuries.

Disadvantages
- Two-dimensional representation of a three-dimensional body part
- Ionizing radiation
- Limited soft tissue contrast

Terminology
- Side marker. By convention when viewing radiographs, the patient's right side is on the left side of the radiographic image (as if the patient were present).
- Radiographs are described in the manner in which the X-rays pass through the body. For example a posterior anterior (PA) chest radiograph indicates that the X-rays initially pass through the posterior surface of the patient and then expose the detector, which is against the anterior surface of the chest.
- Radiographic exposure. This is a measure of the amount of radiation that passes through the patient to produce the image. The two major variable factors are the kV and mAs which are settings on the X-ray tube.

- Radiographic (image) contrast. The difference in contrast between separate parts of the image is what forms the image: the greater the contrast, the more visible features become. Image contrast is dependent on subject contrast and film contrast. Subject contrast is the difference in physical/chemical properties of two structures which allows different intensities of radiation to be transmitted. Film contrast is related to the way the image is produced, processed and viewed.
- Radio-opaque. This refers to structures that absorb X-rays and appear white on the image. Typical radio-opaque structures are metallic objects, the bones, calcification, lung consolidation/contusion/fluid.
- Radiolucent. These are typically areas that allow X-rays to pass through them and appear either dark grey or black on X-ray, such as the lungs. Structures such as fat and muscle are predominately radiolucent but do absorb some X-rays and therefore appear relatively grey.

Contrast agents

These can be used with radiographs, ultrasound , MR imaging and CT. They improve the visualization of structures and can assess the vascularity and permeability of tissues. Contrast agents can either be instilled into body cavities or injected into the bloodstream. The type and use of a contrast agent will depend on the imaging modality, the anatomical and the clinical indication.

Air

On radiographs or CT will appear dark. It is typically introduced either per rectum or into the stomach to cause distension and improved visualization of the bowel. Water that has been aerated is easier to detect on ultrasound.

Barium sulphate

This compound is radiopaque on X-rays and CT. It is used for both upper (swallows, meals, small bowel studies) and lower (enemas) GI contrast studies. The concentration of barium is altered depending on the type of investigation (very low for CT). Air can be instilled at the same time to produce a double contrast effect. ►Contraindicated for suspected perforation or when there is a risk of aspiration as it can cause a fibrotic reaction in the peritoneum and lungs.

Organic iodide preparations

Iodine based compounds are radio-opaque. They can be used orally or per rectum (as a substitute for barium sulphate) or can be administered into the urinary tract (micturating cystourethrogram MCUG). They are formulated such that they can be administered for intravascular studies (venography, angiography, cardiac studies).

In CT post-contrast imaging will demonstrate the vascularity and cell wall permeability of tissues. In general inflammation within a tissue will result in increased contrast uptake and higher attenuation on CT.

Contrast reaction

An unwanted side-effect of intravascular administered iodinated contrast is allergic reactions. These range from mild symptoms such as flushing, urticaria and headache to severe anaphylactic shock. ►Children who have suffered a previous contrast reaction should not have repeat doses.

Iodinated contrast can also exacerbate renal failure and should be avoided in children with known or suspected renal failure.

Contrast procedures

Micturating cystogram

Indications
- ▶The examination can be stressful and is not routinely indicated in children >1yr. The examination must be appropriate and justifiable.
- Detection of vescio-ureteric reflux (VUR).
- Suspected posterior urethral valves (PUV).
- Possible urethral stricture/narrowing.
- Bladder abnormalities.

Technique
Aseptic catherization of the bladder, in some institutions prophylactic antibiotics are given. Under fluoroscopic screening iodinated contrast is slowly instilled into the bladder. Oblique views of the bladder when it is partially filled to detect early VUR or small ureterocoeles are required. Images of any reflux are stored. The examination should be continued until the child micturates. In boys sagittal images of the whole urethra need to be obtained in micturition (▶to exclude the presence of PUV). A post-micturition cross-kidney image should be taken to demonstrate any reflux into the kidneys that may not have been noticed during any dynamic screening.

Contrast swallow and/or meal

Indications
- In children the aim is to depict the anatomical orientation of the oesophagus, stomach and duodenum.
- To detect any congenital abnormality of the oesophagus, trachea and vasculature of the adjacent vessels.

Technique
Either barium or iodinated contrast can be used. ⚠ If there risk of aspiration, a tracheo-oesophageal fistula (TOF) or perforation then iodinated contrast is indicated.

Depending on the child's cooperation, contrast is given orally with a cup, straw or bottle. In the uncooperative child it may be necessary to inject slowly into the mouth with a syringe or use a nasogastric tube (NGT).

▶Regardless of the age of the child, after they have initially taken a small amount of contrast it is important this is allowed to reach the duodenal–jejunal flexure (DJF) and its position confirmed with a correctly centred AP image of the upper abdomen to exclude a malrotated gut. If a large amount of contrast is used this can opacify the stomach and it may obscure the DJF. The inability to confirm the presence of a normal DJF indicates an inadequate examination.

AP and lateral images of the oesophagus should then be obtained and the presence of reflux determined. If a TOF is suspected this may not be visualized unless there is sufficient distension of the oesophagus so an NGT should be introduced into the oesophagus and iodinated contrast injected, whilst withdrawing the tube and simultaneously imaging in the lateral plane. Some institutions image the child prone.

Ultrasound

Ultrasound uses high frequency sound (region 1-15MHz) and their resultant echoes to create an image. Different structures and tissues have different acoustic properties, and therefore reflect varying amounts of sound energy which creates a structure and contrast between tissues and allows a image to be formed. For good contact and to allow sound to pass from the ultrasound probe to the skin surface a viscous gel is used.

Advantages
- No ionizing radiation.
- Relatively quick.
- Portable.
- Good anatomical detail.
- Dynamic so can be used to assess function and useful for guided procedures such as biopsies and aspirations.

Disadvantages
- In small children compliance may be difficult.
- Relatively poor for air-filled and bony structures as these do not transmit sound.
- Deep structures can be difficult to visualize.

Terminology
- When images are acquired, the transducer should be held such that the right or cranial portion of the body is viewed on the left side of the image.
- Depth indicates the distance from the transducer surface to the body part in question.
- Those structures that reflect a large amount of sound waves back are termed *hyperechoic* and appear bright on an image. Structures which reflect a small amount of sound waves are dark on the image and are *hypoechoic*.
- Hyperechoic structures:
  - Vessel walls.
  - Acute haemorrhage.
  - Calcification or stones.
  - Fatty lesions.
- Hypoechoic structures:
  - Water/fluid.
- Fluid will allow easy passage of sound waves through it so more sound is reflected back from behind a fluid-filled structure. Consequently, behind the fluid-filled structure will be relatively bright. This is termed posterior acoustic enhancement and is a typical feature of cystic fluid-filled structures.
- Some dense structures will not allow any sound to pass through them, so there is no reflected sound from behind them. This creates an acoustic shadow. This is a feature of stones and metallic fragments within organs.
- Resolution is the ability to discriminate between two separate points. The higher the resolution of an image, the nearer two points can be within the body before they can not be distinguished as separate

identities on the image. There are a variety of different frequency probes available: the higher the frequency of the probe the better the resolution, but the less depth of tissue that can be imaged.

- Doppler effect this utilizes the change in frequency of sound that occurs when it interfaces with a moving object (typically blood). This enables an assessment of both direction and speed of flow of blood within tissues.
  - Colour flow Doppler will determine the direction of flow of blood. Arbitrarily red is towards the transducer and blue is away.
  - Pulsed Doppler can provide an estimation of velocity of flow.

Computerized tomography

Computerized tomography (CT) utilizes X-ray radiation to produce an image. As opposed to conventional radiographs where a single X-ray beam is passed through the body, with CT multiple beams are passed through the patient and are absorbed by a number of detectors. ⚠ A CT examination involves a considerably higher radiation dose when compared with radiographs. The body is imaged in a number of slices but the use of computer software allows the data to be manipulated and images produced in any plane or three-dimensional (3D) reconstructions.

Advantages
- Relatively quick and easily available.
- Good anatomical detail.
- Good bony detail.
- High-quality imaging.
- Multiple planar reconstruction.

Disadvantages
- Ionizing radiation.
- Limited intra-articular pathology.

Terminology
- By convention, the images are viewed as if looking from the foot of the patient up towards the head, so the left side of the patient is on the right side of the image.
- **Spatial resolution** is the ability to discriminate between two separate points or a structure against its background. The higher the resolution of an image, the nearer two points can be within the body, before they are unable to be distinguished as separate identities on the image. Typically the resolution of CT is in the region of 0.5–1mm.
- **Attenuation** refers to how many X-rays are absorbed by a piece of tissue. Dense tissue such as bone will absorb a large amount of the X-ray beam: they are of a high attenuation and appear relatively bright on the CT image. Low attenuation tissues (e.g. air) will appear relatively darker. The attenuation value of a tissue is measured in Hounsfield units (HU). Water has a value of 0 HU.
- High attenuation:
  - Bone/calcium.
  - Intravenous contrast.
  - Metallic objects.
- Intermediate attenuation:
  - Muscle.
  - Water.
  - Solid abdominal organs.
- Low attenuation:
  - Air.
  - Fat.

Data presentation/windowing
- CT images are produced in greyscale in which the more radio-opaque (higher attenuation tissue) appears relatively bright compared with

lower attenuation tissue. The human eye is only able to resolve a limited number of levels of grey, far less than the computer images can produce. Windowing is the method used to optimize the level at which the images are viewed. The two adjustable parameters are the window level and the window width.

- The *window level* is the attenuation value of the the midpoint of the window width. Window width is the difference between the highest and lowest attenuation values that will appear grey on an image. Tissue with attenuation values outside the window width will appear either black (low attenuation value) or white (higher attenuation value).

- It is only possible to visualize subject contrast between the structures and tissues whose image attenuation values lie within the window width.

- Altering the window level and width ('windowing the image') allows the contrast and brightness of the image to be optimized within the tissues of interest. For example, when reviewing bone structures the window level will be set at higher values than when reviewing fat and soft tissues.

- Slice thickness. The thickness of the slices can be varied; thinner slices provide a better resolution (ability to distinguish two separate points) but the signal to noise ratio (the amount of signal forming the image compared to the background) appears less.

Contrast agents

- These can be used orally or intravenously.
- Iodinated contrast and barium are of high attenuation.
- Oral contrast agents include iodinated compounds and barium sulphate. They are used to opacify bowel to aid discrimination between lymphadenopathy and masses within the abdomen.
- Intravenous contrast is used to improve visualization of the vascularity of different tissues.
- In cases of inflammation and infection there is an increase in uptake of involved tissue. An abscess will show peripheral rim enhancement.

Magnetic resonance imaging

Magnetic resonance imaging (MRI) does not use ionizing radiation, but utilizes the interaction of magnetic fields and radio waves to create an image. MRI scanners use very strong magnets, that can vary in strength from 0.25 to 3 Teslas. A Tesla is a measurement of magnetic strength. The earth's magnetic strength is 25 gauss and 1 gauss is 1/1000 of a Tesla.

Advantages
- Excellent image contrast.
- No ionizing radiation.
- Excellent anatomical detail.

Disadvantages
- Time.
- Claustrophobia.
- Relatively expensive.
- There may be a need for sedation or general anaesthesia.
- Cannot put pacing wires or patients with metallic fragments near the magnet.

Terminology

Imaging sequences
There are an immense number of sequences that can used and their use depends on the body part under examination and the suspected pathological process.

The commonest sequences are spin echo (SE) sequences. There are essentially three basic SE sequences; T1-weighted, T2-weighted and proton density (or intermediate weighted). They vary in their repetition time (TR) and echo time (TE). Fast-spin echo (FSE) sequences are an adaptation of SE sequences.

Gradient echo (GRE) sequences decrease acquisition time and reduce movement artefact, but there is reduced signal to noise ratio.

Signal intensity and Imaging sequences
Tissue that returns a lot of signal will appear bright on an image (high signal intensity). The signal intensity of tissue is partly a reflection of its physical properties but dependent on the imaging sequence used. Some tissue will be of high signal intensity on one sequence but of low signal intensity on another.

Signal intensity of tissue on SE sequences
- Low signal (dark) on T1-weighted images:
  - Increased free water (oedema, tumour, infarction, inflammation, infection.
  - Haemorrhage (hyperacute or chronic).
  - Low density of protons (calcification, fibrous tissue, bone cortex).
  - Flow void.
- High signal (bright) on T1-weighted images:
  - Fat.
  - Subacute haemorrhage.

- Melanin.
- Protein-rich fluid.
- Slowly flowing blood.
- Paramagnetic substances: gadolinium, manganese, copper.
- Calcification (rarely).
- Low signal (dark) on T2-weighted image:
  - Low density of protons (calcification, fibrous tissue).
  - Paramagnetic substances: deoxyhaemoglobin, methaemoglobin (intracellular), iron, ferritin, haemosiderin, melanin.
  - Protein-rich fluid.
  - Flow void.
- High signal (bright) on T2-weighted image:
  - increased water (oedema, CSF, tumour, infarction, inflammation, infection).
  - Methaemoglobin (extracellular) in subacute hemorrhage.
  - Fat.

Signal to noise ratio (SNR)

The signal is the image pattern produced by the structures in the body. The noise is the random information produced as result of quantum mottle (the inherent random nature of molecules within the body). The higher the signal to noise ratio the better the quality of the images.

MRI contrast agents

In MR imaging, gadolinium diethylenetriaminepentaacetic acid (Gd-DTPA) is the commonest used contrast agent. This is a paramagnetic agent that appears bright on T1 weighted image (T1WI). It is water-soluble and can increase the contrast between normal and pathological tissue. It does not cross the normal blood–brain barrier and so can be used to detect a breakdown in this barrier.

MRI sequence selection

Sequence selection will depend on the body part under investigation and its tissue characteristics, the clinical condition, presentation and the pathological changes suspected. MR machine availability and experience will also be determining factors.

Suggested MR imaging sequences

Brain

Routine
- Sagittal T1WI (SE).
- Axial T1WI (SE).
- Axial T2 WI(SE).
- Coronal T2WI (SE).
- Axial fluid-attenuated inversion recovery (FLAIR) for children over 3 months of age.

Additional sequences as necessary
- Neonates: inversion recovery.
- Acute changes in neurological status: diffusion imaging.
- Developmental delay: T1 volume.
- Suspected haemorrhage: gradient echo imaging.
- Epilepsy: fine coronal T2 slices through the hippocampus.
- Tumour: post-gadolinium and spinal imaging.

Spine
- Sagittal SE T1 and T2 WI.
- Axial SE T1WI through the conus to the coccyx.
- Coronal SE T2.

Hip
- Axial turbo SE T2 WI (with fat saturation).
- Coronal SE T1WI.
- Sagittal short tau inversion recovery (STIR).
- Coronal turbo SE PD-weighted (with fat saturation).
- Coronal STIR.
- Post-contrast if needed.
- Coronal and sagittal SE T1WI (with fat saturation).

Knee
- Axial turbo SE T2WI (with fat saturation).
- Coronal SE T1WI.
- Sagittal SE Proton density (PD) WI.
- Sagittal turbo T2WI (with fat saturation).
- Coronal turbo SE PD weighted.
- Coronal turbo SE T2WI (with fat saturation).

Abdominal MRI

The choice of sequences used depends on the indication. The upper abdominal organs are susceptible to respiratory artefact and either breath-hold techniques or respiratory gating is used to minimize this effect.

When imaging the biliary tree with magnetic resonance cholangiopancreatography (MRCP) T2 weighted sequences are used which show fluid as very bright signal, making it easier to distinguish any filling defects such as stones or areas of stricture formation.

For oncology staging or follow-up a combination of pre-contrast T1 and T2 sequences are used with at least 2 planes performed as post-contrast T1 fat saturated images.

There are a variety of liver-specific contrast agents which can be used to classify intra-hepatic lesions but more detailed description is beyond the scope of this text.

Nuclear medicine (scintigraphy)

Images are created from the gamma radiation emitted from radioactive nucleotides (or radioisotopes) which are attached to different protein labels. It is these labels that enable the isotope to be taken up by the specific tissue under investigation and allow an assessment of both anatomy and physiological activity. The labelled isotope is usually administered intravenously: after a variable time it is taken up by the tissue/organ under examination and the patient is then imaged using a Gamma camera.

A Gamma camera detects the emitted radiation, converts it into light signal using NaI crystals, this emitted light is then subsequently converted into a digital image. This conversion process creates images of relatively low resolution compared with all other imaging modalities.

Nuclear scintigraphy does involve a significant radiation burden and its use in paediatric medicine should be closely monitored and investigations appropriately indicated.

The most commonly used radioisotope in paediatric nuclear medicine is Technetium (^{99m}Tc). This is 140keV gamma-emitting radioisotope with a half-life of 6hrs.

Indications and labels

Renal scintigraphy

Static renal imaging

The radiopharmaceutical is ^{99m}Tc 2,3 dimercaptosuccinic acid (DMSA), which binds to plasma proteins, that are cleared by tubular excretion and retained in the renal cortex, with no excretion into the renal collecting system during the imaging period.

Indications

- Good assessment of renal function.
- Demonstration of ectopic renal tissue.
- Demonstration of renal scars.
- Acute UTIs.

Dynamic renal imaging

The radiopharmaceutical commonly used is ^{99m}Tc-MAG 3 (mercapto-acetyltriglycine), which is cleared by tubular secretion. Often a diuretic is administered at the same time as the isotope to aid excretion.

Indications

- Assess the degree of obstruction in a dilated renal collecting system.
- Assessment of bladder function.
- PUJ obstruction.
- VUR (diuretic should be omitted if reflux is being investigated).

Bone imaging

^{99m}Tc-methylene diphosphonate (MDP) or other diphosphonate compounds. These are phosphate analogues and will assess bone turnover.

Indications

- Staging and assessment of malignant metastatic disease.
- Detection of primary bone tumours.
- Trauma (occult fractures and NAI).

- Infection: three phase studies. The initial blood flow to an area , the blood pooling in an area of interest and uptake within the bone on delayed images (all increased in acute infection).

The use of bone scintigraphy is becoming less common with the increased use of MR imaging, which does not involve radiation and is often more specific. The use of bone scintigraphy should be closely monitored.

Neuroblastoma imaging

- The radiopharmaceutical is 123 I Metaiodobenzylguandine (MIBG), taken up by neuroblastoma, phaeochromocytomas, for metastases, response to treatment.
- This uses iodine as the radioisotope which will be taken up by the thyroid gland; it is important children given are given iodine prior to study to block thyroid uptake.

Advantages
- Information about organ function.
- Useful whole body screening investigation.

Disadvantages
- Radiation dose.
- Poor anatomical detail.
- Less specific that some other modalities.

SPECT (single photoemission computed tomography)

These are tomographic images which are acquired in multiple planes to allow improved anatomical localization and resolution.

Positron emission tomography

Positron emission tomography (PET) uses isotopes of basic biological elements that are positive β emitters (positrons). As the isotopes decay, energy is released as β and α radiation. This radiation is detected, magnified and converted to electrical signals, which are then processed to generate images. A commonly used isotope is Fluorine 18 (F-18) with a label fluorodeoxyglucose (FDG), so called FDG-PET. This tracer is a glucose analogue and is taken up by glucose-using cells. Uptake is often elevated in rapidly growing malignant tumours and can be used to detect malignant disease.

Chest and cardiac
Clinical presentations and role of imaging

Katharine Foster
Karl Johnson

Acute chest infection

Chest infections are one of the most common causes of admission to hospital in children. The causative organism varies with the age of the child.

Common causes of pneumonia

Neonates
- Viral:
  - Respiratory syncitial virus (RSV).
  - Cytomegalovirus.
- Bacterial:
  - *E. Coli.*
  - Group B haemolytic Streptococcus.
  - Haemophilus influenzae (now rare).

Infants and toddlers
- Viral:
  - RSV.
  - Adenovirus.
  - Rhinovirus.
  - Influenza.
- Bacterial:
  - *Staphlococcus Aureus.*
  - *Streptococcus Pneumoniae.*

School age (4 years and above)
- Viral:
  - Adenovirus.
  - Influenza.
  - Cytomegalovirus.
- Bacterial:
  - *Streptococcus Pneumoniae.*
  - Mycoplasma pneumonia.

Role of imaging

The majority of respiratory illness in children affects the upper respiratory tract, presents with typical features (colds, rhinitis, sore throat) and does not require further tests.
- Many lower tract infections also do not require imaging.
- Chest radiograph (CXR) may be helpful if bacterial infection is suspected. There are often surprisingly few clinical signs of pneumonia, particularly in young children, and for this reason a chest radiograph is often performed as part of a 'septic screen' to try and determine the cause of fever.

Radiographs
Viral infections
- Perihilar bronchial wall thickening, hyperinflation.
- Air space opacity may also be seen, this is typically in the perihilar regions. (📖 p. 58)
- Areas of collapse, or atelectasis may be seen due to plugging of the airways with mucus.
- Asthma can have the same appearance.

Bacterial infections
- Usually unilateral, lobar, segmental, or rounded area of airspace opacity with air bronchograms.
- Can affect the whole of one lung, or be bilateral.
- Staphylococcal pneumonia can cavitate. Cavities are typically thick-walled, and may contain fluid levels.
- Streptococcal pneumoniae infection may form pneumatoceles (usually thin-walled).

CT/Ultrasound
May be useful when bacterial infection is complicated by formation of an empyema (📖 p. 36).

Wheeze

Wheeze is produced by the partial obstruction of the lower airways, and is heard on expiration. It should not be confused with stridor, which is heard on inspiration, and is due to partial obstruction of the upper airway.

Causes of wheeze

- Reactive airways:
  - Asthma.
  - Bronchiolitis (📖 p. 58).
- Mechanical:
  - Foreign body.
- Aspiration:
  - Gastric contents.
  - Foreign body.
- Cardiac:
  - Left to right shunts, e.g. atrioseptal defect (ASD).
  - Cardiac failure (📖 p. 27).
- Hypersensitivity reactions, e.g. allergic Aspergillosis.
- Inhalation or smoke injury.
- Genetic:
  - Cystic fibrosis (📖 p. 66).
  - Alpha-1 antitrypsin deficiency.
  - Kartagener's syndrome.
  - Immunodeficiencies.
- Congenital lung abnormalities:
  - Bronchogenic cyst (📖 p. 56).
  - Congenital lobar hyperinflation p. 48.
  - Sequestration (📖 p. 52).
  - Congenital pulmonary airway malformation (📖 p. 50).
- After pertussis infection (Loeffler's syndrome: rare).

Role of imaging

A child who is known to have reactive airway disease does not require a CXR for each episode of wheeze. CXR can be helpful in those who have significant respiratory distress, localizing signs or history of aspiration.

Chronic infection (or cough)

- Repeated coryzal illness
- Asthma (cough may be the only symptom)
- Infection:
  - Viruses, causing tracheitis, partial lung collapse.
  - TB.
  - Mycoplasma.
  - Post-pertussis.
- Aspiration:
  - Gastro-oesophageal reflux (📖 p. 186).
  - Cerebral palsy.
  - Foreign body.
  - H-type tracheo-oesophageal fistula (📖 p. 168).
- Inherited:
  - Cystic fibrosis (📖 p. 66).
  - Kartagener's syndrome (immotile cilia).
- Extrinsic compression of the trachea or bronchi:
  - Enlarged heart.
  - Enlarged lymph nodes.
  - Bronchogenic cyst.
- Extrinsic allergic alveolitis.
- Smokers cough, in adolescence.
- Congenital lung lesions:
  - Pulmonary sequestration (📖 p. 52).
  - Congenital pulmonary airway malformation (📖 p. 50).
- Immunosuppression:
  - White cell and immunoglobulin deficiencies.

Role of imaging

Radiographs
CXR often helpful.

Fluoroscopy
If aspiration thought to be the cause.

CT
Indicated if extrinsic compression, or a congenital lung lesion is suspected. If the cough is suppurative then bronchiectasis should be considered. If very severe, bronchial dilatation may be visible on the CXR. These children will often require a sweat test to exclude cystic fibrosis. If this is normal, and bronchiectasis is suspected high-resolution CT (HRCT) can be helpful.

Chest pain

There are a large number of causes of chest pain in children. A good history and examination is required before imaging is requested.

Pulmonary

- Pneumonia.
- Pneumothorax (📖 p. 37).
- Empyema (📖 p. 37).
- Pulmonary infarction (e.g. in sickle cell disease).

Musculoskeletal

- Trauma.
- Musculoskeletal pain (e.g. from lifting or coughing).
- Costochondritis (Tietze syndrome).
- Tumour (e.g. Ewings' arising from the chest wall).
- Herpes zoster (cutaneous).

Gastrointestinal

- Gastro-oesophageal reflux (📖 p. 186).

Cardiac

- Pericarditis.
- Kawasaki's disease.
- Cardiac ischaemia (very rare in children).

Role of imaging

Radiographs

These are useful to show pulmonary pathology, and can be helpful in some cardiac conditions. For example, the heart may be enlarged in cardiomyopathy. If a cardiac cause is suspected, then a cardiologist should be contacted, as echocardiography would be the most useful investigation. Plain radiographs of the chest should not be requested when pain is thought to be musculoskeletal, for example due to a sport or lifting injury.

Fluoroscopy

Upper GI contrast studies can be used to demonstrate gastro-oesophageal reflux. However, the gold standard is a pH study.

CT

A CT scan may be requested when more detailed imaging is required to help guide treatment. For example, if a child had a chest wall tumour, a CT scan would help to show the extent of the lesion, and also evaluate the lungs for possible metastases. CT angiography can be used to diagnose pulmonary emboli, but these are very rare in children.

MRI

MRI is excellent to demonstrate soft tissue pathology, and is often used in oncology imaging to determine the extent of tumour involvement.

Haemoptysis

Blood-stained sputum is an uncommon symptom in childhood.
- Infection:
  - Bacterial pneumonia.
  - Tuberculosis.
  - Aspergillosis.
- Sickle cell crisis.
- Coagulopathy.
- Inflammatory:
  - Goodpasture's disease.
  - Wegener's granulomatosis.
  - Haemosiderosis.
- Cardiac failure can produce pink-tinged sputum.
- Pulmonary emboli are rare in children.

Role of imaging

Radiographs
- CXR would be indicated in most cases.
- Consolidation may be due to pneumonia.
- Hilar lymphadenopathy and consolidatation may be seen in TB.
- CXR is often normal in patients who have pulmonary emboli; often the only radiological sign is a tiny pleural effusion.
- Pulmonary nodules may be seen in Wegener's granulomatosis.

CT
- Nodules can be seen in fungal disease, aspergillosis and Wegener's granulomatosis.
- Cavitating nodules can be seen in aspergillosis and Wegener's granulomatosis.
- Lymph nodes with central necrosis seen in TB.
- CT pulmonary angiography can diagnose pulmonary emboli.

Nuclear scintigraphy
- Pulmonary emboli: mismatched ventilation and perfusion defect.

Apnoea

- Causes specific to neonates:
  - Hyaline membrane disease.
  - Meconium aspiration.
  - Diaphragmatic hernia (📖 p. 54).
  - Choanal atresia.
  - Hypoplastic jaw (Pierre Robin).
  - Tracheo and laryngomalacia.
  - Persistent fetal circulation.
- In all children consider:
- Respiratory:
  - Pneumonia.
  - Asthma.
  - Pneumothorax (📖 p. 37).
  - Acute respiratory distress syndrome (ARDS).
  - Aspiration.
- Cardiac:
  - Congenital heart disease.
  - Cardiomyopathy.
- Gastro-intestinal:
  - Gastro-oesophageal reflux.
- Neurological:
  - Acute intracranial haemorrhage.
  - Venous sinus thrombosis.
  - Epilepsy.
  - Meningitis/encephalitis (📖 p. 544).
  - Guillain Barre (severe).
  - Acute demyelinating encephalomyelitis (ADEM) (📖 p. 546).
- Accidents:
  - Trauma.
  - Burns.
  - Drowning.
  - Poisoning.
- Metabolic:
  - Hypoglycaemia.
  - Urea cycle disorders.
- Neuromuscular disorders:
  - Iatrogenic.
  - Opiate overdose.

Role of imaging

This will depend on the clinical setting. CXR will be indicated in many cases. CT of the brain is often helpful in the acute setting to exclude a neurological cause that would require neurosurgical intervention.

Cardiac failure

- Stress:
  - Hypoxia.
  - Fever.
  - Overwhelming sepsis.
- Anaemia.
- Fluid overload.
- Cardiac:
  Neonates
  - Patent ductus arteriosus (PDA).
  - Ventricular septal defect (VSD).
  - Hypoplastic left heart.
  - Coarctation of the aorta.
  - Total anomalous pulmonary venous drainage.
  - Large arteriovenous malformation causing shunting.
  Infant
  - Cardiomyopathy.
  - Pulmonary stenosis.
  - Anomalous left coronary artery.
  Older children
  - Myocarditis.
  - Systemic hypertension.
  - Endocarditis.
  - Kawasaki's disease.
  - Pericardial effusion.
- Endocrine:
  - Thyrotoxicosis (rare).

Role of imaging

Radiographs

- Cardiomegaly: this can be difficult to detect as many X-rays in small children are taken AP, and in the unwell patient, they are often supine.
- The central vascular markings are more prominent in children with a left to right shunt.
- Pulmonary vessels become indistinct in pulmonary interstitial oedema.
- Pleural effusions.

Ultrasound

Echocardiography is the best initial test if congenital heart disease or poor cardiac function is suspected.

Cyanosis

Respiratory

- Infection:
  - Bacterial.
  - Viral.
  - Mycobacterial.
  - Fungal in immunosuppressed patients.
- Inflammatory:
  - Systemic lupus erythematosis.
  - Goodpasture's.
  - Haemosiderosis.
- Pneumothorax.
- Congenital:
  - Cystic fibrosis.

Central

- Traumatic head injury.
- Intracranial haemorrhage (📖 p. 502).
- Meningitis/encephalitis.
- Venous sinus thrombosis (📖 p. 552).
- Stroke (📖 p. 550).

Cardiac

- Transposition of the great arteries.
- Fallot's tetralogy.
- Truncus arteriosus.
- Total anomalous pulmonary venous drainage.
- Pulmonary stenosis.
- Ebstein's anomaly.
- Pulmonary atresia.
- Tricuspid atresia.
- Cardiomyopathy.
- Pericardial effusion.
- Eisenmenger's syndrome: due to chronic left to right shunt causing irreversible pulmonary hypertension.

Neonatal cyanosis

With increased pulmonary blood flow

- Transposition.
- Truncus arteriosus.
- TAPVD.
- Single ventricle.

Where cyanosis is not a constant feature:

- Hypoplastic left ventricle.
- Interrupted aortic arch.

With oligaemia and cardiomegaly

- Pulmonary stenosis.
- Ebstein's anomaly.
- Pulmonary atresia with an intact ventricular septum.
- Tricuspid atresia.

With oligaemia but no cardiomegaly

- Tetralogy of Fallot.
- Pulmonary atresia with a VSD.
- Tricuspid atresia.

Categorization of congenital heart disease

Cyanotic heart disease

Increased pulmonary blood flow
- Truncus arteriosus.
- TAPVD.

Decreased pulmonary blood flow
- Fallot's tetralogy.
- Ebstein's anomaly.
- Pulmonary atresia with an intact ventricular septum.

Variable flow
- D-transposition of the great arteries.
- Tricuspid atresia.

Acyanotic heart disease

Normal pulmonary flow
- Obstructive lesions:
  - Coarctation of the aorta.
  - Aortic stenosis.
  - Pulmonary artery stenosis.

With increased pulmonary arterial flow (due to left to right shunting)
- VSD.
- ASD.
- Atrioventricular septal defect (AVSD).
- PDA.

With increased pulmonary venous flow (congestive cardiac failure in the newborn)
- Left-sided anatomic obstruction:
  - Coarctation of the aorta.
  - Aortic stenosis.
- Left ventricular dysfunction:
  - Abnormal origin of the left coronary artery.
  - Myocarditis.
  - Shock.
  - Birth asphyxia.
  - Hypoplastic left heart.
  - Pulmonary venous atresia/stenosis.
- General systemic illness:
  - Anaemia.
  - Polycythaemia.
  - Hypoglycaemia.
  - Sepsis.
  - Arteriovenous malformations (e.g. haemangioendothelioma of the liver, Vein of Galen malformation).

Role of imaging

Radiographs

CXR will be required in the majority of patients. This is helpful to eluci-date whether pneumonia is the cause of cyanosis. An abnormal cardiac outline would suggest a cardiac cause. Lungs are often oligaemic in cya-notic patients. Interstitial opacity obscuring vessels, pleural effusions and cardiomegaly are signs of cardiac failure, which can complicate congenital cardiac disease.

Ultrasound

If a cardiac cause is suspected, a cardiology opinion and echocardiography is indicated.

Chest and cardiac
Differential diagnosis

Katharine Foster
Karl Johnson

Air space shadowing

Air space shadowing (or consolidation) is due to replacement of air in the alveoli. This may be due to fluid, pus or blood. It can be very difficult to distinguish these causes by looking at the plain radiograph in isolation without knowing the clinical history and examination findings.

Infection

Bacterial infection often involves one lobe, causing a large area of increased opacity. The pattern on the plain radiograph depends on which lobe is affected, the same as adult patients. Pneumonia can be more widespread, involving the whole of one or both lungs, or may be bilateral and patchy in appearance. Air bronchograms (branching patterns of low density) may be seen due to air in the larger airways. Young children sometimes develop 'round pneumonias', so called because of their circular appearance. They can reach up to several cm in diameter, and are commonly due to *Streptococcus Pneumoniae* infection.

Pulmonary oedema

Pulmonary interstitial oedema usually causes ill-defined perihilar opacity. The pulmonary lung markings are often indistinct , giving a hazy appearance to the lungs. Other signs of fluid overload or cardiac failure include pleural effusions and cardiomegaly. 'Kerley B' lines are rarely seen in children. Causes of pulmonary oedema include:

- Heart failure.
- Fluid overload.
- Severe head injury or cerebral event.
- Near drowning.
- Aspiration.
- Radiotherapy (usually several weeks after treatment).
- Hypoproteinaemia, e.g. nephrotic syndrome, liver disease.
- Smoke inhalation.
- Mediastinal tumours causing impaired venous return.

Pulmonary haemorrhage

The plain radiograph appearance of pulmonary haemorrhage is non-specific. There is often a history of trauma, bleeding diathesis, haemoptysis, or blood from the endotracheal (ET) tube.

Aspiration

Children who have poor swallowing, for example due to cerebral palsy, or have depressed consciousness are at risk of aspiration. This can cause consolidation, and can be difficult to differentiate from bacterial pneumonia.

Other causes

There are other rarer causes of air space disease. These include:

- Shock lung (respiratory distress syndrome).
- Lymphoma.
- Eosinophilic lung disease.
- Fat emboli (following major trauma).

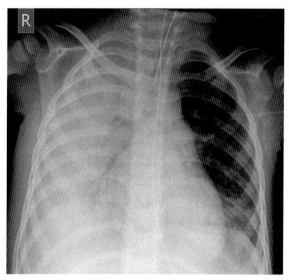

Fig. 2.1 CXR of a child with extensive right-sided pneumonia. There is a prominent air bronchogram.

Pleural effusion

The appearance of a pleural effusion in a child depends on the position of the child when the film is taken. When the child is erect, fluid can be seen in the inferior aspect of the chest, often with a clear meniscus. However, particularly in unwell children, the film is taken when the child is lying on their back, causing a hazy opacity throughout the hemithorax. Small effusions may be seen at the lung apices in supine patients.

Infection

Empyemas can complicate pneumonia. These often require drainage, either with a catheter, or open debridement and drain placement. In these cases ultrasound can help to demonstrate whether the effusion is loculated and demonstrate pleural thickening. CT is sometimes used to demonstrate the appearance of the underlying lung (which may be necrotic in severe pneumonia), the presence of lymphadenopathy, and the exact location of loculated effusions.

Cardiac failure

Effusions are often seen in cardiac failure, most frequently due to fluid overload. They are usually small.

Pulmonary emboli

Pulmonary emboli are rare in children, but are seen; for example patients with complex cardiac disease, and those with sickle cell disease. Often the only sign on the CXR is a small effusion. Pulmonary embolus can be confirmed with a ventilation perfusion scan, or with contrast-enhanced CT.

Tumour

Neoplastic causes of pleural effusions are uncommon, but can be seen in lymphoma, and in primary lung/pleural tumours (very rare).

Pneumothorax

Pneumothorax is an important cause of chest pain, breathlessness, and hypoxia in children. Those particularly at risk are those with asthma, and also tall teenagers, and patients with necrotic pneumonia. Necrotic pneumonia can cause a bronchopleural fistula; this type of pneumothorax can be particularly difficult to treat. Pneumothoraces can be iatrogenic, particularly after central line insertion. It is important to consider a pneumothorax in trauma patients. These may be difficult to detect on the routine trauma films, as they are nearly always taken with the patient supine. Rarer causes include osteosarcoma lung metastases.

Radiographic signs

- Paucity of normal lung markings.
- The lung edge is usually seen.
- 'Deep sulcus sign' in supine patients: the costophrenic angle is wider and more inferior than normally seen, as it is splayed by air in the anterior aspect of the pleural space.
- ⚠ Mediastinal and tracheal shift are signs of a tension pneumothorax that requires immediate treatment.

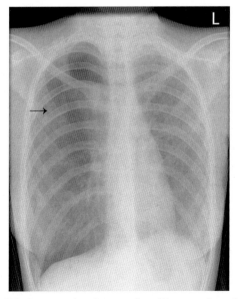

Fig. 2.2 CXR of a patient with a right pneumothorax. The arrow indicates the edge of the right lung.

Pneumomediastinum

This can be seen in combination with surgical emphysema and subcutaneous emphysema. The heart border is crisper than normally seen. Air is often seen to track superiorly into the soft tissue of the neck. They are usually managed conservatively.

- Pneumomediastinum is usually due to sudden rise in intra-alveolar pressure. Air tracks though a 'burst' alveolus, along the interstitium to the hilum and then the mediastinum. Causes include:
  - Spontaneous
  - Asthma
  - Severe and protracted vomiting
  - Trauma
  - Foreign body aspiration
- Perforated oesophagus:
  - Often associated with a hydropneumothorax.
- Abdominal perforation, with extension of air into the chest via retroperitoneal tissues.

Pneumopericardium

This is similar in appearance to a pneumomediastinum, except that air is seen all round the heart, resulting in a 'continuous diaphragm sign'. They are less common than pneumomediastinum. The causes are the same as above. They are usually small and hence are usually managed conservatively.

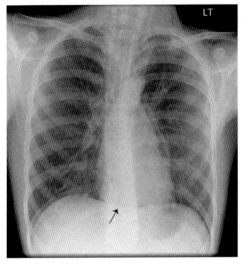

Fig. 2.3 CXR of a patient with a pneumomediastinum and pneumopericardium. There is a 'continuous diaphragm' sign (arrow), and surgical emphysema tracking into the neck.

Thymus

Normal thymus

The thymus is normally seen in children up to the age of 5. Its appearance can be very variable; lobular or sail-shaped. The thymus is a very soft homogeneous organ so is often indented by the anterior ribs, causing its edge to appear scalloped or wavy. Abnormal thymic masses tend to displace surrounding structures.

▶A normal thymus NEVER displaces the trachea, and this feature should prompt further investigation.

Thymic hyperplasia

The thymus can show 'rebound hyperplasia' following severe illness or chemotherapy. This can be pronounced: the thymus can grow by 40% after chemotherapy. Rebound hyperplasia does not require further investigation or treatment. Its features are of the normal thymus listed above, as the thymus remains a soft and malleable structure that does not cause compression or displacement of surrounding structures.

Abnormal thymus

Superior vena cava (SVC) compression, tracheal compression or shift are features of an abnormal thymus.

- Lymphoma is the most common cause of an anterior mediastinal mass in children. It can be associated with pleural effusions, hilar and peri-cardial involvement. These children can be critically unwell, and may be unable to lie flat without becoming severely breathless. It is important to consider this when planning investigations: particularly staging CT. It can be very dangerous to anaesthetize these patients.
- Germ cell tumours (teratoma).
- Thymic cysts

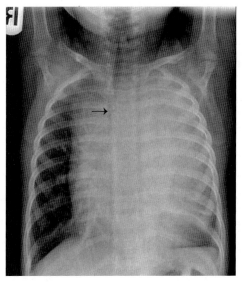

Fig. 2.4 CXR of a patient with lymphoma. Notice that the trachea is displaced to the right by the large anterior mediastinal mass (black arrow).

Mediastinal masses

Anterior mediastinal mass

- Normal thymus.
- Thymic tumour:
  - Lymphoma.
  - Leukaemia.
  - Germ cell tumours.
  - Thymoma.
- Lymphatic malformation.
- Grossly enlarged thyroid gland extending into the chest (rare).

Middle mediastinal mass

- Neoplastic: mass extending from anterior mediastinum.
- Lymphoma.
- Lymphadenopathy secondary to infection, e.g. TB.
- Foregut duplication cyst:
  - Includes bronchogenic cysts, oesophageal duplication cysts and neuroenteric cysts.
  - Usually round, homogenous, well defined.
- Lymphatic malformation.
- Achalasia.
- Hiatus hernia.

Posterior mediastinal mass

- Neuroblastoma and other ganglion cell tumours (95% of posterior mediastinal masses in children):
  - Ribs often separated or thinned by the mass.
  - CT often shows calcification.
  - CT and MRI often required to stage the tumour, and to demonstrate extension through the vertebral foraminae into the spinal canal.
- Bochdalek hernia.

Hilar lymphadenopathy

Hilar lymphadenopathy is frequently overdiagnosed on CXR. It is important to recognize the normal appearances of the hilar regions. The left hilum is higher than the right, because the left pulmonary artery loops over the top of the left main bronchus. The hilar regions often appear asymmetrical on films when the patient is slighty rotated to the left or right.

Infection
- Viral.
- Bacteria.
- Mycoplasma.
- TB.

Neoplastic
- Lymphoma.
- Neuroblastoma.
- Germ cell tumours.

Inflammatory (rare)
- Acquired immune deficiency syndrome (AIDS).
- Sarcoidosis.
- Systemic lupus erythematosus (SLE).

Other causes of an enlarged hilar region include:
- Perihilar pneumonia.
- Bronchogenic cyst.
- Asymmetry of the pulmonary arteries:
  - Pulmonary stenosis.
  - Bronchiolitis obliterans or congenital lung hypoplasia result in reduced pulmonary blood flow, and a relatively small pulmonary artery.

Pulmonary nodules

Large pulmonary nodules

- Metastatic lung disease: eg: Wilm's tumour.
- Single large nodule: consider round pneumonia.
- Wegener's granulomatosis.
- Aspergillosis.
- Multiple haemangiomas.

Small pulmonary nodules

- Miliary TB.
- Septic emboli (e.g. from central line infection).
- Fungal/candida disease in immunosuppressed patients.
- Metastatic disease: e.g. rhabdomyosarcomas, osteosarcoma.
- Past history of chickenpox pneumonia (calcified).
- Tuberous sclerosis and histiocytosis (usually cysts are also present).
- Sarcoid.

Pulmonary nodules are a relatively unusual finding on a CXR in children. Large 'cannon ball'-type lung nodules are often due to Wilm's tumour. These renal tumours are often very large by the time they present, and may be palpable on clinical examination. These patients warrant further investigation, first with ultrasound.

The clinical history is very important in determining the cause of lung nodules. For example, patients with a known tumour are more likely to have metastatic lesions. Those that are immunosuppressed are more prone to fungal, aspergillus or candida infections. Patients with miliary TB are usually systemically very unwell; these patients are at risk of developing TB meningitis.

Sometimes CT is useful to further characterize lung nodules; particularly in rarer causes such as Langerhan's cell histiocyotosis and sarcoidosis. This is because other lung change such as cysts or interstitial thickening are better demonstrated. CT may also demonstrate small areas of cavitation, which are more commonly seen in aspergillus infection, septic emboli and Wegener's granulomatosis. CT is also helpful to guide the best place for lung biopsy.

Interstitial lung disease

This is often difficult to appreciate on a CXR, until lung disease is quite advanced. It may be easier to appreciate on high resolution CT. This is different from a normal 'spiral' CT in that very thin 'slices' of the lungs are imaged, but there are 'gaps' between each slice. This technique is excellent at defining the appearance of the lung parenchyma. It is poor in other circumstances, however, for example, if you were looking for lung metastases they may be missed as they were in the 'gaps', not in the area of imaged lung. Interstitial lung disease can be split into three imaging findings: nodular (covered in the previous section), reticular (linear opacities) and reticular nodular (linear and nodular opacities present).

Reticular

- Heart failure causing interstitial oedema.
- Idiopathic interstitial lung disease.
- Alveolar proteinosis (ground-glass alveolar opacity also present).
- Radiation therapy.
- Sarcoidosis (rare in children) nodules usually also present.
- Lymphoma (rarely involves the lung parenchyma).
- Secondary to treatment, e.g. immunosuppressants such as tacrolimus.

Reticular nodular

- Histiocytosis (irregular cysts and nodules usually present).
- Sarcoidosis.
- Tuberous sclerosis and neurofibromatosis.

Hyperlucent lung

▶ Make sure that you are sure that it is the lungs that are hyperlucent: do not miss a pneumothorax! (📖 p. 37)

Bilateral hyperexpanded hyperlucent lungs

- Asthma.
- Bronchiolitis.

Bilateral normal size or small hyperlucent lungs

- Congenital cyanotic heart disease causing oligaemia.

Unilateral hyperlucent lungs

▶ Be sure that it is not the contralateral more opaque hemithorax that is abnormal, e.g. due to a pleural effusion in a supine patient

- Aspirated foreign body in a major airway causing air trapping. The air trapping can be difficult to see on a normal CXR. If a foreign body is suspected an expiratory film should also be taken. If the foreign body is in the trachea, both lungs will be hyperinflated.
- Macleod's syndrome or bronchiolitis obliterans: most commonly due to childhood viral infection resulting in damage and poor development. The affected areas appear hyperlucent due to air trapping. It is commonly asymmetrical, which is why one lung usually appears hyperlucent.
- Congenital lobar hyperinflation (previously called congenital lobar emphysema).
- Scoliosis.
- Rotation due to poor radiographic technique.
- Poland syndrome: unilateral absence of pectoralis muscle.

It can be difficult when lungs are asymmetrical in appearance to establish which side is abnormal. The side with increased or normal vascularity is usually the normal side.

Chest and cardiac
Disorders

Katharine Foster
Karl Johnson

Congenital lobar hyperinflation

This was previously called congenital lobar emphysema, which is a poor term as there is no alveolar destruction. It is due to progressive over-distension of a pulmonary lobe due to antenatal airway obstruction. The alveoli are dilated; the walls are thinned but intact. Patients usually present with respiratory distress in the neonatal period, but increasingly it is being diagnosed with antenatal ultrasound.

Imaging findings

Radiographs

▶The most useful diagnostic feature is a radiodense lobe that becomes radiolucent and hyperexpanded as fetal fluid is replaced with air.
- Lobar predelicion:
  - Left upper lobe 42%.
  - Right middle lobe 35%.
  - Right upper lobe.
- Compression of ipsilateral lung.
- Mediastinal shift to contralateral side.

CT
- Useful for surgeon to be certain which lobe is affected.
- Hyperlucent area of lung with attenuated vessels.

Nuclear scintigraphy
- Matched ventilation perfusion defect.

Differential diagnosis
- Congenital pulmonary airway malformation (CPAM).
- Bronchial atresia.
- Pulmonary artery hypoplasia (affected lung is small).
- Pulmonary hypoplasia (affected lung is small).
- Congenital diaphragmatic hernia.

Management
- Bronchoscopy to exclude an endobronchial lesion.
- Surgical lobectomy.
- Conservative treatment may be considered for patients with minimal symptoms.

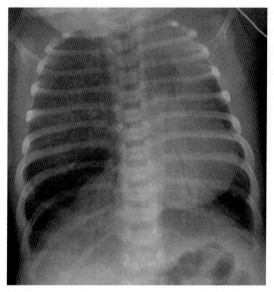

Fig. 2.5 CXR of a newborn baby with congenital lobar hyperinflation of the right upper lobe of the lung. The lobe will become more hyperlucent over time as fluid from the lung is absorbed.

Congenital pulmonary airway malformation

This entity was previously called congenital cystic adenomatoid malformation. It is an uncommon cause of respiratory distress in neonates and infants characterized by a multicystic mass of pulmonary tissue with an abnormal proliferation of bronchial structures. The etiology is unknown. This malformation was originally classified by Stocker et al.[1] into three histologic types.

- Type I is composed of variable-size cysts, with at least one dominant cyst (>2cm in diameter). This type is the most common.
- Type 2 and contain smaller cysts (0.5–2cm).
- Type 3 appear solid, but contain multiple small cysts (0.3–0.5cm).

Imaging findings

Radiographs
- Solid/multicystic mass depending on cyst size and amount of fluid.
- May cause mass effect: mediastinal shift, compression of adjacent lung.
- If the lesion is very large and causes cardiac compromise heart failure (hydrops) may occur.

CT
- Solid or multicystic mass depending on cyst size.
- Contrast enhancement is useful to demonstrate NO systemic arterial supply (seen in sequestrations).
- Cyst walls and solid components may enhance.

MR
- Lesion hyperintense on T2 images.

US
- Increasingly, CPAMs are diagnosed by antenatal ultrasound, as an echogenic mass. Lesions may not be visible on the neonatal CXR. CT should be performed to demonstrate the lesions.

Differential diagnosis
- Sequestration: usually do contain air, and have a systemic blood supply.
- Congenital lobar hyperinflation.
- Congenital diaphragmatic hernia.
- Cavitating pneumonia.

Management and prognosis
- Most advocate that the lesion is resected to avoid risk of infection. There have been multiple case reports associating CPAMs with malignancy.
- Lesions are easier to resect electively rather than after infection.

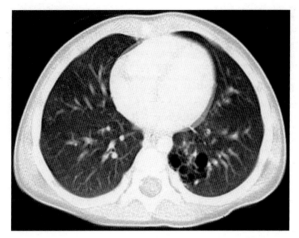

Fig. 2.6 CT of a cystic pulmonary airway malformation. Notice the small cysts in the medial aspect of the left lower lobe.

References

[1] Stocker JT, Madewell JE, Drake RM. Congenital cystic adenomatoid malformation of the lung. Classification and morphological spectrum. *Human Pathology*. 1997 Mar; **8**(2): 155–71.

Sequestration

Pulmonary sequestration is a congenital abnormal area of lung that does not connect to the bronchial tree or pulmonary arteries. This area of lung is dysplastic and does not function, and is prone to infection. The most common symptomatic presentation is with repeated infection, but increasingly they are diagnosed antenatally. It has a systemic arterial supply, usually from the aorta. There are two main types:

Intrapulmonary
- Lies within the pleura of the lung.
- Venous drainage is to an inferior pulmonary vein.
- Previously thought to be secondary to infection, but increasingly described antenatally.

Extrapulmonary
- Has its own pleural covering (the pleura cannot be seen on imaging- this is a pathological finding).
- Venous drainage variable, often systemic.
- Associated with other abnormalities, such as congenital cardiac malformations.
- May be located below the diaphragm.

Imaging findings
Radiographs
- Persistent lower lobe opacity, usually left-sided.
- If infected may appear multicystic.

Ultrasound
- Antenatal ultrasound—hyperechoic mass.
- Hyperechoic mass may be seen postnatally.
- Feeding artery can be visualized. This feature can help differentiate from other masses, particularly if infradiaphragmatic.

CT
- Opaque lower lobe parenchyma.
- Systemic and venous supply demonstrated with intravenous (iv) contrast.

MRI
- Hyperintense on T2 images.
- Can be used to demonstrate arterial supply.

Differential diagnosis
- CPAM
- Chronic pneumonia
- Diaphragmatic hernia
- Infradiaphragmatic lesions:
  - Neuroblastoma
  - Adrenal haemorrhage
- Pulmonary blastema (rare)

Management
- Most advocate surgical resection, to avoid risk of infection.

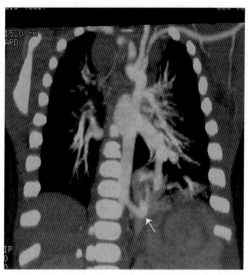

Fig. 2.7 CT coronal reconstruction of a patient with a sequestration in the left lower lobe. It was supplied by a vessel from the thoracic aorta (white arrow) and drained via a pulmonary vein (black arrow).

Congenital diaphragmatic hernia

A congenital defect in the diaphragm results in herniation of abdominal contents into the chest. There are two main types:
- Bochdalek hernia. Posterior defect: most common
- Morgagni hernia. Anterior: rare

The hernia can cause significant compression of the lungs *in utero*, and associated pulmonary hypoplasia. Clinical presentation is usually at birth with severe respiratory distress. Most are now diagnosed by antenatal ultrasound. There are often associated abnormalities: congenital heart disease is reported in up to 50%.

Imaging findings

Radiographs
- Most commonly left-sided.
- Rounded lucencies within the chest that look like bowel.
- Appearance depends on the contents of the hernia and whether bowel is air-filled.
- Right-sided hernias may contain liver.
- Poorly visualized diaphragm.
- Hernia may cause mediastinal shift to contralateral side.
- Lungs often small due to hypoplasia.
- Abnormal position of NG tube tip.

Ultrasound
- Antenatal: mass within the thorax of mixed echogenicity.
- Postnatal: can be helpful to exclude a paralysed diaphragm (particularly right-sided lesions which can mimic this).

Fluoroscopy
- May be required to confirm abnormal lucencies are due to bowel loops.

CT
- Not usually necessary, but may be useful in patients who are more complex to define anatomy.

MRI
- Antenatal MRI useful to confirm US findings: loops of bowel are high signal.
- Antenatal MRI: assess degree of mediastinal shift, which can cause hydrops if severe. Can also be used to assess lung volumes. Presence of the liver in the chest has a worse prognosis.

Differential diagnosis
- CPAM.
- Congenital lobar hyperinflation.
- Cavitating pneumonia.
- Diaphragmatic eventration.

Management and prognosis
- Surgical repair.
- Morbidity and mortality usually relates to lung hypoplasia.

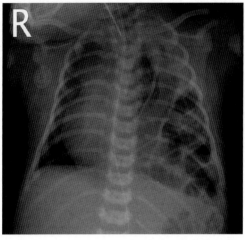

Fig. 2.8 CXR of a neonate with a left diaphragmatic hernia. Multiple loops of bowel herniated into the left hemithorax.

Bronchogenic cyst

Bronchogenic cysts are congenital abnormalities. The bronchial tree develops from a bud from the foregut in early gestation. Abnormal budding results in bronchogenic cyst (hence also called foregut duplication cysts). Lesions do not communicate with the bronchial tree. They can cause symptoms from compression (respiratory distress, dysphagia). The true incidence is unknown, as probably most are incidental.

Imaging findings

Radiographs
- Well-defined round mass.
- May not be visible.
- Usually requires further cross-sectional imaging.

US
- Increasingly being diagnosed on antenatal ultrasound, well-defined hypoechoic lesion.

CT
- Round homogenous lesion.
- Attenuation value depends on cyst content which can range from water to proteinaceous fluid.
- Do not enhance, but the rim may enhance, and the cyst may contain air if complicated by infection.
- Most common location is close to the carina, but they can occur in the lung parenchyma.

MRI
- Well-defined round lesion.
- High signal on T2WI.
- Variable signal on T1WI, depending on cyst contents.
- Post-contrast may show rim enhancement if infected.

Differential diagnosis
- Round pneumonia.
- CPAM (usually not unilocular).
- Neurogenic tumours (more solid in appearance, often calcified).
- Lymphadenopathy.
- Pulmonary sequestration (usually lower lobe, with feeding artery).
- Pulmonary blastema (rare).

Management and prognosis
- Surgical resection to avoid infection.
- There have been some case reports of associated malignancy.

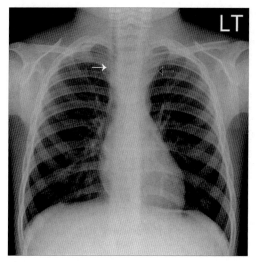

Fig. 2.9 CXR of a patient with a bronchogenic cyst. (a) The trachea (white arrow) is displaced to the left by (b) the cyst (black arrow).

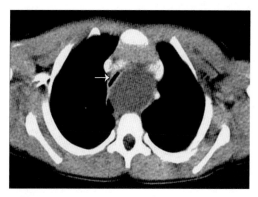

Fig. 2.10 CT of the same patient. The trachea (white arrow) is deviated to the right by the bronchogenic cyst.

Bronchiolitis

Bronchiolitis is a viral infection of the lower respiratory tract. It is very common in young children. Not all children with bronchiolitis require a chest radiograph, particularly if the child has typical features of a viral infection (cough, wheeze, runny nose). CXR is indicated in children when a bacterial infection is suspected.

Imaging findings

Plain radiographs
- Increased peribronchial markings.
- Hyperinflation:
  - Flattening and depression of the diaphragms to more than 6 anterior ribs.
- Subsegmental atelectasis:
  - Wedge-shaped areas, or linear areas of increased density can be confused with consolidation.

Differential diagnosis
- Asthma:
  - The radiographic appearances are almost identical, as both viral infections and asthma cause inflammation of the small airways.
- Left to right shunts:
  - Pulmonary plethora can have a similar appearance, there is usually associated cardiomegaly.

Management and prognosis
- Supportive treatment only.
- Symptoms resolve over time.
- Antibiotics are not required.

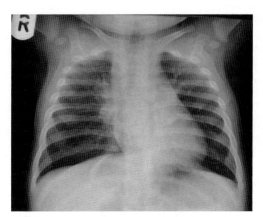

Fig. 2.11 Plain radiograph of a child with a viral chest infection, demonstrating peri-hilar bronchial wall thickening and hyperinflated lungs.

Pneumonia

Lower respiratory tract infections are one of the most common causes of hospital attendances.

Imaging findings

Plain radiographs

- Viral lower respiratory tract infection: perihilar bronchial wall thickening, hyperinflated lungs. There may be areas of focal opacity, and subsegmental atelectasis due to bronchial plugging.
- Bacterial pneumonia usually manifests as an area of consolidation; segmental to lobar opacity with air bronchograms.
- Bacterial pneumonia can be complicated by the formation of:
  - Empyemas: these may require surgical intervention or drainage
  - Cavities: which may result in the formation of bronchopleural fistulas and recurrent pneumothoraces.
- Mycoplasma pneumonia is a common cause of pneumonia in older children and typically causes bilateral perihilar opacity.
- 'Round' pneumonias, which appear as solitary large round masses on the CXR, are more common in children.

In the majority of cases, a plain film is the only investigation that is required, and in the majority 'follow up films' are not required. A minority of patients will require further investigation with CT. Bronchoscopy may be indicated, for example if a 'forgotten' inhaled foreign body is suspected, or atypical infection, such as pneumocystis pneumonia in patients with AIDS.

Ultrasound

- Helpful to demonstrate effusions and whether they are simple (anechoic) or are complex (containing septae and debris).

Fluoroscopy

Recurrent aspiration due to gastro-oesophageal reflux may cause repeated pneumonia. This can usually be demonstrated by a barium meal examination. Very rarely, an H-type tracheo-oesophageal fistula may be the cause of recurrent pneumonia.

CT

CT may be required to exclude an underlying cause of repeated chest infections in children, for example:

- Sequestration or CPAM.
- Bronchiectasis.
- CT may be requested if surgical intervention is necessary to treat complications of pneumonia. CT demonstrates loculated collections, lung cavitation and abscess formation or purulent pericarditis.

Differential diagnosis

- Normal thymus.
- Sequestration or CPAM.
- Bronchogenic cyst.

Management and prognosis

- Antibiotics.
- Prognosis is usually good.

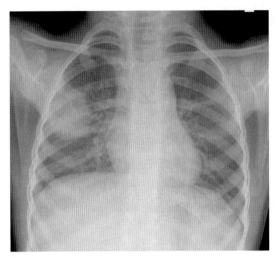

Fig. 2.12 CXR of a child with a right-sided round pneumonia.

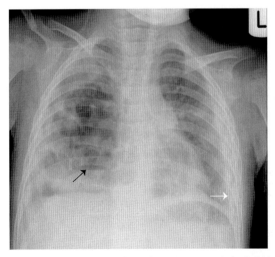

Fig. 2.13 CXR of a child with severe, bilateral cavitating pneumonia. An air–fluid level is seen within one cavity on the right (black arrow). There are associated bilateral pleural effusions (white arrow).

Tuberculosis

Tuberculosis (TB) is increasing in frequency throughout the world. It is more common in poorer, crowded communities. Infection in children is due to close contact with a person with active, cavitating, sputum-positive disease.

Spectrum of disease

Primary complex
- Usually asymptomatic, may cause malaise, fever, erythema nodosum.
- Consolidation in lower or middle lobe, and enlarged draining lymph node.

Ghon focus
- Calcified lesions seen in the lung 1-2yrs after primary infection.

Progressive primary TB
- Lobar or bronchopneumonia, associated with haemoptysis, weight loss and cavitation.

Reactivation TB
- Uncommon in children.
- Apical fibrosis, cavitation and endobronchial spread.

Pleural effusions
- Usually reactive, but can be due to bacilli that have ruptured into the pleural space.

Lymphadenopathy
- Most common extrathoracic site is the neck (scrofula).
- Nodes are typically non-tender.
- Imaging (ultrasound of neck nodes, or CT of chest or abdominal disease) often shows central necrosis.

Miliary TB
- Widespread blood-borne dissemination.
- Multiple small nodules (the size of millet seed) scattered throughout the chest. These are usually visible on CXR.

Meningitis
- Insidious disease.
- Seen in 30% of patients with military TB.
- Thickened basal meninges (best seen on post-contrast MRI).
- Associated perivascular inflammation can result in strokes. Acute infarction best demonstrated with diffusion MRI.

Abdominal TB
- Lymphadenopathy.
- Ascites.
- Bowel wall thickening; particularly the caecum.
- Features can be shown on ultrasound, CT or MRI.

Osteomyelitis
- Ill-defined lucent areas due to bone destruction and periosteal reaction, can be seen on radiographs. Skeletal lesions are usually delayed 2–3yrs after the primary infection.
- The spine is the most common site (Pott's disease).

- Other common sites include the hips and fingers (dactylitis).
- Bone scans are more sensitive.
- MRI is the gold standard investigation as it will give information about surrounding tissue and joint inflammation, sinus tracts and sequestrae (areas of dead bone).

Septic arthritis
- Synovial thickening and effusions. Can be detected with ultrasound or MRI.

Diagnosis
Mantoux skin test:
- 10mm induration 48hrs after injection indicates disease.
- False negative results can occur in patients early in the disease, in patients who are immunosuppressed, with AIDs, malnutrition, overwhelming disease, or patients with atypical TB.

Histology
- Caseating granulomas.

Microbiology
- Sputum or gastric washings, or tissue samples show acid-fast bacilli. Culture can take 3–6 weeks.

Other
- DNA probes and antigen detection can help, particularly in central nervous system (CNS) disease.

Management and prognosis
- Prognosis is usually good with correct antituberculous therapy.
- Prognosis is worse for CNS disease.

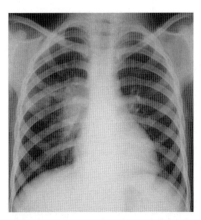

Fig. 2.14 CXR of a child with TB. There is right-sided consolidation and associated right perihilar lymphadenopathy.

Hyaline membrane disease

Surfactant deficiency is common in premature infants. Surfactant lowers surface tension, and allows the lungs to expand, and stay open. Without surfactant, the lungs remain of low volume. Proteinaceous exudates line the alveoli, forming hyaline membranes. Patients often need ventilatory support. Complications are common.

Acute
- Pneumothorax, pneumomediastinum.
- Pulmonary interstitial emphysema.
- Infection.
- Intracranial haemorrhage.
- Patent ductus arteriosus.

Chronic
- Bronchopulmonary dysplasia (chronic lung disease): continued oxygen requirement after 36 weeks gestation.
- Retinopathy of prematurity.
- Neurological impairment.

Imaging findings
Radiographs
- Diffuse reticular granular opacity.
- Air bronchograms.

Differential diagnosis
- Group B Streptococcal pneumonia.
- Congenital heart disease causing interstitial oedema.
- Transient tachypnoea of the newborn (retained fetal lung fluid) usually term infants.
- Meconium aspiration: usually term infants, lungs are hyperinflated.

Management
- Prevention. Delay delivery, maternal steroids.
- Surfactant.
- Artificial ventilatory support.

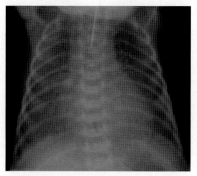

Fig. 2.15 CXR of a newborn premature baby with surfactant deficiency. There is ground-glass opacity thoughout both lungs.

Pulmonary interstitial emphysema (PIE)

Air within the interstitium and lymphatics can occur in neonates on ventilatory support secondary to barotrauma. This is usually transient, but unless ventilatory pressures are altered, complications may include pneumothorax and pneumomediastinum. PIE usually develops in the first week of life.

Imaging findings

Radiographs

- Linear and small bubbly lucencies.
- Lucencies often radiate from the hila.
- Can be focal (most commonly left upper lobe).

Differential diagnosis

- Bronchopulmonary dysplasia (BPD) or chronic lung disease, is very similar in appearance: BPD usually occurs later, and changes are more gradual in onset.
- Treated surfactant deficiency: it can be difficult to deliver surfactant uniformly to all areas of the lung, which can result in partial clearing of alveoli.
- Congenital lobar hyperinflation, usually involves a whole lobe.

Management

- Reduction in ventilatory pressures.
- High-frequency ventilation.

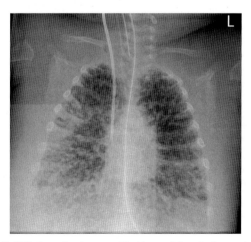

Fig. 2.16 CXR of a ventilated neonate with widespread bilateral pulmonary interstitial emphysema.

Cystic fibrosis

Cystic fibrosis (CF) is an autosomal recessive condition, most common in the Caucasian northern European population, causing abnormal exocrine function. Abnormal chloride transport results in thick sticky secretions, resulting in recurrent chest infections, and bronchiectasis. Thickened gastrointestinal secretions can cause obstruction. Neonates may present with meconium ileus. Pancreatic dysfunction causes steatorrhoea, diabetes and diabetes mellitus. Other symptoms include cirrhosis and portal hypertension, and failure to thrive. Diagnosis is made by a positive sweat test, and genotyping is important.

Imaging findings

Bronchiectasis

Radiographs

- Perihilar interstitial opacity, ring and tramline in shape (📖 Fig. 2.17) due to bronchial wall thickening.
- Plugging of airways results in small opacities, and areas of atelectasis.

HRCT

- Signet ring sign: the airway is dilated, and is larger than the adjacent artery.
- Mosaic pattern: airway trapping, most marked on expiration.
- Bronchiolitis, or 'tree in bud': small airways plugged with mucus gives small V- or Y-shaped opacities.

Complications

Radiographs

- Persistent areas of collapse (small segmental areas to lobar).
- Pneumonia, often recurrent.
- Lymphadenopathy due to recurrent infection.
- Allergic bronchopulmonary aspergillosis: fleeting opacities on CXR.

Differential diagnosis

- Asthma.
- Recurrent aspiration: can cause bronchiectasis.
- Chronic foreign body: can cause bronchiectasis.
- Allergic bronchopulmonary aspergillosis.
- Immotile cilia syndrome: may have situs inversus.
- Immunodeficiency resulting in chronic lung infections.
- Bronchopulmonary dysplasia: usually history of prematurity and prolonged ventilation.

Management and prognosis

- Physiotherapy.
- Enzyme replacement.
- Bronchodilators, antibiotics.
- Bronchial artery embolization for massive haemoptysis.
- End-stage disease may require lung transplant.

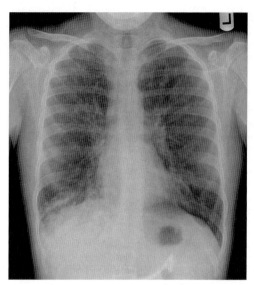

Fig. 2.17 CXR of a teenager with cystic fibrosis. The lungs are hyperexpanded, and there are multiple ring and tramlining opacities due to dilated, thickened bronchi, This patient also has pneumonia in the right lower lobe.

Lymphoma

Lymphoma is one of the more common malignancies seen in children in the second decade of life. It commonly involves lymph nodes. There are three main types:
- Hodgkin's: often involves the chest.
- Non Hodgkin: commonly involves abdominal solid organs and bowel.
- Lymphoproliferative disorder: can complicate organ transplantation.

Imaging findings

Radiographs
- Anterior mediastinal mass: widened superior mediastinum.
- Tracheal shift or compression.
- Enlarged, rounded hilar regions due to lymphadenopathy.
- Pericardial effusion: enlarged cardiac contour.
- Pleural effusion.

CT
- Mediastinal and hilar lymphadenopathy, usually not calcified.
- Pericardial thickening and effusion.
- Pleural effusion.
- Lung involvement: pulmonary nodules and consolidation.
- Airway compression.
- Vascular compression (e.g. SVC) associated with higher risk of general anaesthetic.

MRI
- Whole-body STIR imaging can be useful to show multifocal extent of disease.

PET
- Most lymphomas are PET positive.
- Increasingly being used to determine 'active disease' during treatment.

⚠ Caution should be taken in imaging these patients. If lying flat, positive pressure ventilation in patients with vascular compression can reduce cardiac venous return, and cause cardiorespiratory arrest.

Differential diagnosis
- Normal thymus: does *not* cause deviation of airway or vessels
- TB: can be very similar in appearance.
- Germ cell tumour: anterior mediastinal mass more commonly mixed attenuation, with areas of fat, fluid or calcification.

Management and prognosis
- Chemotherapy.
- Radiation.
- Bone marrow transplant.
- Hodgkins disease has a good outcome—90% cure.

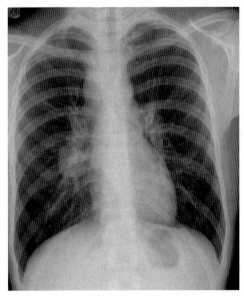

Fig. 2.18 CXR of a teenager with right paratracheal and hilar lymphadenopathy due to lymphoma.

Inhaled foreign body

A foreign body within the airway causes a ball valve effect: trapping air more distally. The most common age is 8 months–3 years. Aspiration may not be witnessed. Patients may present acutely with wheezing, or cough. Others have a chronic presentation, with infection, or wheeze not responding to medical treatment.

▶High index of suspicion required to make diagnosis as there may be no history of aspiration.

Imaging findings

Radiographs

- Increased lung volume on the side of aspiration, this is more obvious on expiratory films.
- The foreign body is not often visualized (often organic material, e.g. peanuts).
- Mediastinal shift to contralateral side.
- Consolidation/atelectasis more common in chronic cases.

Differential diagnosis

- Viral infection/ bronchiolitis, can cause patchy volume loss and asymmetrical lung volumes.
- Extrinsic compression of airway:
  - bronchogenic cyst.
  - lymphadenopathy.
- Swyer–James syndrome/bronchiolitis obliterans–assymetrical lungs.

Management and prognosis

- Endobronchial removal of foreign body.
- Delay in diagnosis can cause chronic complications, e.g. bronchiectasis.

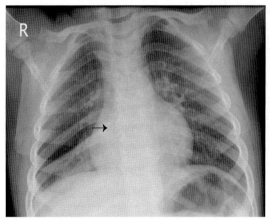

Fig. 2.19 The right upper lobe is hyperinflated due to an inhaled felt tip pen lid in the right main bronchus (black arrow).

Kawasaki's disease

Kawasaki's disease (mucocutaneous lymph node syndrome) is a systemic vasculitis which often affects the coronary arteries, resulting in aneurysm formation. It is the commonest cause for acquired coronary artery disease in children. Japan has the highest rate per population (M>F). Aetiology is unknown but an infective cause with an abnormal immune response is suggested.

Clinical presentation

There are three phases;

- Acute febrile phase (<11 days): pyrexia, hand and feet erythema, swollen tongue and oral mucosa, arthralgia, acute cholecystitis, myocarditis and pericarditis.
- Subacute phase (11–21 days): fever resolves, general irritability, conjunctival infection, desquamation of feet and toes, aneurysm formation.
- Chronic phase: clinical symptoms resolve, cardiac and aneurysmal complications including arrhythmias, functional abnormalities and myocardial infarction.

Imaging findings

Radiographs

- Can be normal.
- Cardiomegaly and signs of heart failure.

Echocardiography

- Coronary artery involvement is in the proximal part at branching points.
- Myocardial dysfunction.

MRI

- Cardiac wall thinning.
- Infarcted myocardium.
- Abnormal wall motion.
- Coronary artery aneurysms.
- Larger vessels can also be involved.
- Coronary artery involvement is in the proximal part or at branching points.

Angiography

- Multiple fusiform and saccular coronary aneurysms.
- Multiple aneurysms throughout the vascular tree.

Ultrasound

- Lymphadenopathy.
- Dilated gallbladder or 'hydrops'.

Differential diagnosis

- Vasculitis, polyarteritis.
- SLE.
- Takayasu's.

Management and prognosis

High-dose anti-inflammatory drugs, intravenous gamma globulin. Imaging follow-up of any aneurysm. Occasionally surgical intervention for severe aneurysm formation.

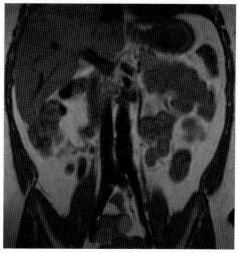

Fig. 2.20 Coronal MR image shows irregularity and slight dilation of the descending aorta in a patient with Kawasaki's disease.

Congenital cardiac disease

Congenital cardiac disease is a complex spectrum of abnormalities. Any child with a suspected congenital heart abnormality should be referred to an appropriate centre where a multidisciplinary approach is undertaken to confirm the nature of the underlying disorder and the appropriate management strategy, be it medical or surgical.

Clinical presentation may be in the neonatal period or later in life. In the neonate, the presence or absence of cyanosis is an important discriminating factor but cyanosis may take weeks to develop. In the older child, the presentation may be with heart failure, shortness of breath, repeated chest infections or a failure to thrive. Historically, certain classical radiographic findings of many of the congenital cardiac disorders have been described. In some circumstances, these findings represent a relative failure of management that does not reflect current surgical practice. In the vast majority of cases, the diagnosis of congenital cardiac disease is made with echocardiography, cardiac angiography, and increasingly cardiac MRI.

Neonatal congenital heart disease

During fetal life, there is a high pulmonary vascular resistance with pulmonary arterial and aortic pressures being equal. There is shunting of blood from the right to left atrium through the foramen ovale and from the pulmonary artery to descending aorta via the ductus arteriosus. Following birth and the child's first breaths, the pulmonary vascular resistance falls, causing an increase in pulmonary blood flow. The presentation of the neonate with a congenital heart defect will depend on the cardiac response to this fall in the pulmonary vascular resistance. Closure of the ductus arteriosus within the first couple of weeks of life will determine the time of presentation of duct dependent lesions.

Clinical presentation

Cyanosis +/− respiratory distress, cardiac failure +/− cyanosis and cardiovascular collapse.

Left to right shunts

Cardiac anomalies which result in shunting of blood from the systemic circulation (left side of the heart) to the pulmonary circulation (right heart). This results in volume overloading of the receiving cardiac chamber and in more chronic cases, those chambers distal to the connection. This includes ventricular and atrial septal defects (VSD and ASD), which are the commonest defects.

Cardiac MRI

Cardiac catheterization is an invasive procedure associated with significant radiation exposure with a morbidity and mortality risk. MRI is increasingly used to provide diagnostic as well as functional evaluation of cardiac lesions.

Techniques

Cardiac and respiratory gating

Images are acquired within a short time period which is synchronized to the cardiac cycle using high-quality electrocardiogram (ECG) monitoring. In some patients, they can be acquired using breath hold sequences. In less cooperative or sicker patients, there may also be respiratory motion synchronization using a bellows device. Both techniques add increased imaging times.

Cine MRI

Cardiac gated gradient echo sequences can produce multiple images over the cardiac cycle. These can be displayed as a cine loop to demonstrate the cardiac motion. This technique can identify high-flow blood as signal voids.

Blood-flow analysis

ECG gated velocity and coded cine MRI can be used to measure blood flow and assess velocity and quantity.

Imaging sequences

- 'Black blood images':
  - Cardiac gated spin echo or double inversion recovery.
  - Excellent for depicting anatomy.
  - Measurement of sizes of defects.
  - Size of anatomical structures.
- 'Bright blood':
  - T2* gradient recalled echo (GRE) steady state sequences.
  - Useful for flow abnormalities.
  - Steady state free precession.
  - Useful in identifying turbulent flow through a stenosis and regurgitant flow.
  - Post-processing will allow functional evaluation of flow including ejection fraction.
- MR angiography.
  - Post-gadolinium sequences with multiple projection of images will show complex anatomical relationships.

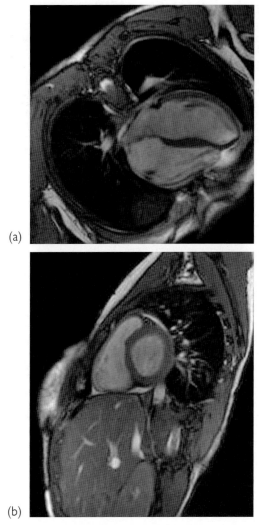

(a)

(b)

Fig. 2.21 Axial (a) and oblique sagittal (b) MR images showing cardiac anatomy. Using the axial plane as a template additional images can be obtained through the ventricles and outflow tracts.

Atrial septal defect (ASD)

Defects of the atrial septum can occur in isolation or with other congenital heart diseases. The size of the defect may vary and is characterized by its location.

Types of ASD

- Patent foramen ovale: a physiological communication which usually closes after birth due to increasing left atrial pressure. Persistence of the foramen occurs with right to left shunts due to elevated right atrial pressure. Causes include tricuspid atresia, Ebstein's anomaly and hypoplastic right ventricle.
- Ostium primum defect: located in the anterior inferior aspect of the atrial septum. Often associated with defects in the mitral valve.
- Secundum defect: bordered by the fossa ovalis.
- Sinus venosus defect: in the upper atrial septum and contiguous with the SVC. Associated with anomalous connection of the right pulmonary veins to the SVC.

Clinical presentation

Often asymptomatic with a systolic murmur, feeding difficulties and failure to thrive, paradoxical emboli. Pulmonary hypertension is now rare, as the defect is usually diagnosed and treated.

Imaging findings

Echocardiography

▶Is the imaging modality of choice.
- Can assess degree of flow across the defect.

Radiographs

- Small defects can be normal.
- Large defects:
  - Cardiomegaly.
  - Possible increased size of pulmonary artery.
  - Increased pulmonary vasculature.
  - In long-term untreated cases, pulmonary hypertension will cause decrease in the size of peripheral pulmonary vessels.

MRI

- Size and position of defect.
- Can evaluate shunt severity.
- Quantify flow.
- Associated cardiac lesions.

Differential diagnosis

- VSD.
- AVSD.
- PDA.
- Scimitar syndrome.

Management and prognosis

Often spontaneous closure of secundum defects. Other defects may require transcatheter or primary surgical closure.

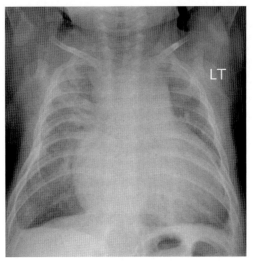

Fig. 2.22 AP radiograph showing an enlarged heart in a young patient. The right atrium is prominent and there is pulmonary plethora.

Ventricular septal defect

Commonest congenital heart abnormality. The size of VSDs is variable. The size of the VSD is compared with the size of the aortic valve opening, with large VSDs being of a similar or greater size than the aortic opening.

Types of VSD

- Membranous or peri-membranous just below the outflow tract beneath the aortic valve (80%).
- Inlet (10%) beneath the tricuspid valve:
  - this is associated with atrioventricular septal defect (AVSD).
- Muscular (5–10%).
- Outlet (5%).

Clinical presentation

Small VSDs are asymptomatic but the child has a murmur. Larger defects cause tachycardia, tachypnea, and failure to thrive. Not usually symptomatic at birth due to high neonatal pulmonary vascular resistance that limits left to right shunting. Larger defects usually present in the first few months of life.

Imaging findings

Echocardiography

▶The imaging modality of choice.
- Characterizes site, type and haemodynamics of the defects.

Radiographs

- Limited role in confirming the diagnosis.
- Small VSDs often have a normal radiograph.
- Large VSD:
  - Cardiomegaly.
  - Increased size of pulmonary artery.
  - Plethoric lungs.
  - Small aorta.
  - Cardiac failure.

MRI

- Can delineate anatomy and quantify function.
- Gated spin echo and cine imaging.
- Shunt volume estimation.

Differential diagnosis

- AVSD defects.
- Patent ductus arteriosus (PDA).

Management and prognosis

Most small VSDs will close spontaneously. Larger defects are treated medically and may require surgical closure. Closure either via percutaneous approach or open heart surgery.

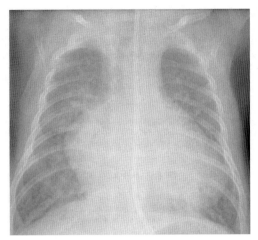

Fig. 2.23 AP CXR of a child with a VSD. There is cardiomegaly and pulmonary plethora.

Patent arterial duct (ductus arteriosus)

In utero, the ductus arteriosus connects the pulmonary artery and descending aorta which allows shunting of blood from the pulmonary to the systemic circulation. The ductus usually closes within the first few days of life. A patent ductus arteriosus can be an isolated finding and is a cause of increased pulmonary blood flow. It can be familial. Presentation depends on duct size.

Associations

- Lung disease, eg. hyaline membrane disease.
- Congenital heart disease, hypoplastic left heart syndrome (HLHS), transposition of great vessels, pulmonary atresia.

Prematurity

Premature infants, particularly those of low birthweight and with respiratory disease, have delayed closure. It may be an asymptomatic finding or the infant may develop cardiac failure if the shunt is large. Chest radiographs may be normal or may show pulmonary plethora. Echocardiography will demonstrate the shunt and may show left atrial, left ventricle and PDA enlargement.

Term infants

A patent ductus arteriosus can be an isolated finding. Presentation depends on duct size. Small ducts may be detected as an asymptomatic murmur. With large shunts, the child may have poor weight gain and cardiac failure. Left untreated, there may be development of pulmonary hypertension with shunt reversal.

Imaging

Echocardiography

▶Initial imaging modality of choice.
- Will demonstrate the shunt and may show left atrial, left ventricle and PDA enlargement.

Radiographs

- Chest radiograph may be normal with small shunts.
- Large shunts:
  - Cardiomegaly.
  - Left atrial and ventricular enlargement.
  - Pulmonary plethora.

MRI

- Sagittal oblique plane through aortic arch depicts ductus.

Differential diagnosis

- Other causes of left to right shunt (VSD, ASD, AVSD).
- Persistent fetal circulation.

Management and prognosis

Medical therapy or transcatheter closure.

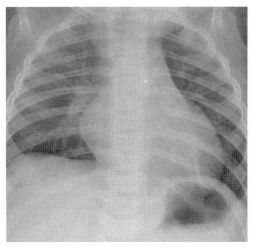

Fig. 2.24 AP radiograph showing PDA. Occlusion device *in situ*.

Tetralogy of Fallot

One of the commoner causes of cyanotic congenital heart disease that presents beyond the neonatal period.

It is an association of:

- right ventricular outflow obstruction (either subpulmonic or infundibular).
- over-riding aorta.
- VSD (usually perimembranous).
- right ventricular hypertrophy.

This creates an outflow obstruction to the right ventricle with an initially normal size heart and reduced pulmonary vascularity. It is associated with a right-sided aortic arch, aberrant subclavian artery, anomalies of the coronary arteries and trisomy 21.

Clinical presentation

Varying degrees of cyanosis. In older children cyanotic episodes are relieved by squatting. The child may be clubbed, have decreased exercise tolerance, arrhythmias, strokes due to paradoxical emboli and endocarditis.

Imaging findings

Radiographs

- Normal-sized heart at birth.
- Develops a boot-shaped heart due to concavity of the pulmonary bay and an elevated apex due to right ventricular hypertrophy.
- Right aortic arch (25%).
- Pulmonary vascularity is reduced or can be disorganized.

Echocardiography

- Will demonstrate all the features.
- Doppler is useful for assessing the size and direction of the VSD and pressure gradients across the valves.

MRI

- Cardiac gated imaging will demonstrate the anatomy of the heart and pulmonary vessels.
- It is possible to calculate the ventricular volumes and degree of outflow stenosis.

Differential diagnosis

- Pulmonary atresia with VSD and aorto–pulmonary collaterals.
- Pulmonary atresia with intact ventricular septum and cardiomegaly with atrial enlargement at birth.
- Tricuspid atresia.

Management and prognosis

- Palliative shunt (Blalock–Taussig shunt).
- Complete repair.
- Pulmonary valve or conduit replacement in adult life after early complete repair.

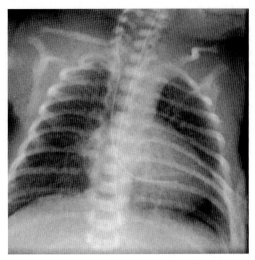

Fig. 2.25 AP radiograph showing a classic 'boot-shaped' heart due to ventricular enlargement with concave pulmonary artery segment with pulmonary oligaemia.

Vascular rings

In early fetal development each of the six branchial arches is supplied by its own aortic arch. Most of these obliterate. Failure of this can lead to vascular anomalies which encircle and compress the airway and oesophagus causing stridor, respiratory distress or feeding difficulties. The location and pattern of tracheal and oesophageal indentation is useful in determining the cause of compression.

Double aortic arch

Both the left and right aortic arch is present (R>L). They unite posteriorly to form the descending aorta which is usually left-sided. The right arch is usually larger than the left. The right subclavian and common carotid artery arise from the right arch. The left subclavian and occasionally the left common carotid arise from the left arch.

Radiographs
- Right-sided indentation of the trachea by the right aortic arch.

Barium swallow
- Right-sided indentation on the AP view with possibly a smaller lower left indentation.
- There is posterior indentation on the lateral view.

MRI and CT angiography
- Will confirm the presence of the double aortic arch.

Right aortic arch, aberrant left subclavian and ligamentum arteriosus (ductus)

The right aortic arch encircles the trachea. The aberrant subclavian passes posterior to the trachea with the ligamentum (or ductus) passing to the more anterior left pulmonary artery.

Aberrant right subclavian artery

Common incidental finding. Posterior indentation of the oesophagus on a barium swallow. Most children are treated conservatively.

Pulmonary sling

If the left pulmonary artery originates from the right pulmonary artery, it will pass posteriorly between the trachea and oesophagus and can cause compression of the right main bronchus which may in turn lead to hyperinflation of the right lung. A barium swallow will show the abnormal left pulmonary artery lying posterior to the trachea but indenting the oesophagus anteriorly.

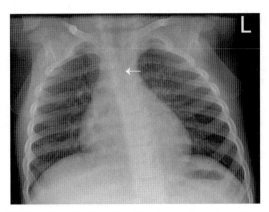

Fig. 2.26 Chest X-ray of an infant with stridor with a double aortic arch. The larger right-sided arch is seen to indent the trachea.

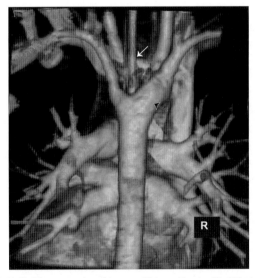

Fig. 2.27 3D CT reconstruction of the same child, posterior view. The NG tube (white arrow) is seen to pass between the double aortic arch. The right aortic arch (black arrow) is larger than the left.

Aortic coarctation

Narrowing of the aorta obstructs normal arterial blood flow and increases left ventricular pressure. The coarctation may be pre-ductal (infantile), juxta or post-ductal or abdominal. It is associated with a bicuspid aortic valve, VSD and PDA. This is an acyanotic disorder, with a normal-size heart and pulmonary vasculature.

Clinical presentation

Often asymptomatic, in severe cases it can lead to congestive heart failure, hypertension and left ventricular hypertrophy. There is a differential in blood pressure between the arms and legs.

Imaging findings

Radiographs

- Rib notching (over 5 years of age), due to collateral circulation.
- Post-stenotic dilatation of the descending aorta.
- Rounded cardiac apex due to left ventricular hypertrophy.

Echocardiography

- Primary diagnostic investigation in infancy.
- Post-surgical surveillance.

MRI

- Oblique sagittal plane (black blood images) will show the level and size of the coarctation.
- Perpendicular images will assess cross-sectional diameter.
- Cine images will show a jet of blood across the coarctation.
- Numerous collateral vessels across the chest wall and ribs.
- Gradient assessment across the coarctation.

Differential diagnosis

- Arteritis.
- Pseudocoarctation.
- Interrupted aortic arch.

Management and prognosis

Surgical resection with an end-to-end or graft anastomosis.

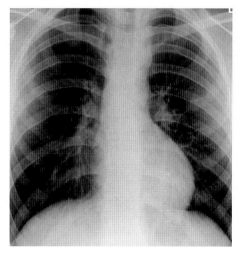

Fig. 2.28 AP radiograph shows rib notching and post-stenotic dilatation in the descending aorta.

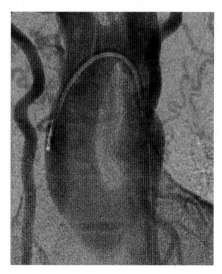

Fig. 2.29 Angiogram showing coartation of the aorta. Numerous collateral vessels have formed.

Scimitar syndrome

This is hypoplasia of the right lung with an abnormal connection between the right pulmonary vein and IVC. There is often an anomalous arterial connection between the right lung base and systemic circulation. As a consequence venous flow from the right lung is returned to the right atrium, creating a left to right shunt and causing volume overload. This is an acyanotic condition with increased pulmonary vascularity.

Clinical presentation

Depends on the size of the left to right shunt. In severe cases presentation is in the newborn with congestive heart failure and pulmonary hypertension. In milder cases it is in the older child, and is associated with recurrent infections of the right lung base.

Imaging findings

Radiographs
- Curved vessel at the right medial cardiophrenic angle which increases in size towards the diaphragm (like a 'curved sword'—scimitar).
- Hypoplasia of the right lung.
- Prominent right atrium.
- Increased pulmonary vascularity.

Echocardiography
- No right pulmonary veins entering the left atrium.
- Abnormal connection to inferior vena cava (IVC).

Angiography (conventional/CT/MRI)
- The 'Scimitar vein' connects to IVC.
- Abnormal systemic arterial supply to the right base.

Differential diagnosis
- Pulmonary sequestration.
- Anomalous pulmonary venous connections.
- Pulmonary hypoplasia.

Management and prognosis

Embolization of systemic arterial supply. Surgical repair of severe shunts to avoid pulmonary hypertension.

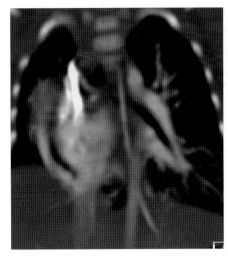

Fig. 2.30 Coronal CT angiogram demonstrates right heart dilatation and abnormal venous drainage supply of the right lung to the inferior vena cava.

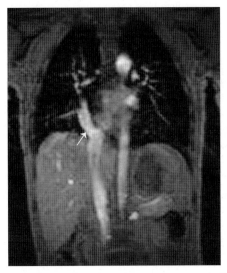

Fig. 2.31 Coronal MR images show abnormal venous connection to the IVC.

Uncommon congenital cardiac conditions

The following conditions, while very serious and potentially life-threatening, are relatively rare. Typically the diagnosis is made on clinical findings and echocardiography. The classical radiographic findings may not be present as these are often associated with untreated disease.

D-Transposition of the great arteries

This is less common than tetralogy of Fallot, but the most common cause of cyanosis in the neonate. The great vessels arise off the inappropriate ventricle. This is incompatible with life unless there is a connection between the pulmonary and systemic circulation: through a patent foramen ovale, a ventricular septal defect or patent ductus arteriosus.

Clinical presentation

Severe cyanosis not improving with oxygen, cardiomegaly and increased pulmonary vascularity. A large VSD will cause congestive heart failure in the neonatal period.

CXR findings

There may be cardiomegaly with narrowing of the superior mediastinum ('egg-on-side'-shaped heart).

Pulmonary atresia

This can occur with or without a VSD, the presence of which is used to classify the lesion. Both types are characterised by the underdevelopment of the right ventricular outflow tract and pulmonary valve. There is extreme outflow obstruction with the entire cardiac output going into the dilated overriding ascending aorta. It presents with progressive cyanosis after birth, following closure of the ductus arteriosus, causing cardiomegaly.

CXR findings

'Boot-shaped heart', oligaemic lungs. A right-sided aortic arch is common.

Ebstein's anomaly

This is downward displacement of the septal and posterior leaflets of the tricuspid valve. It can be asymptomatic at birth with a normal-size heart (the heart can also be enlarged at birth), but it will cause cyanosis and severe cardiomegaly with normal to decreased pulmonary vasculature. It is associated with chronic right heart failure and arrhythmias.

CXR findings

Massive right-sided cardiomegaly, causes the so-called 'box-shaped' heart. The cardiac enlargement with a small vascular pedicle and superior mediastinum can mimic the appearances of a large pericardial effusion.

Tricuspid atresia

Congenital absence or agenesis of the tricuspid valve. It is associated with a VSD and a right aortic arch. Neonates often present with cyanosis in the first 24hrs of life, but may present later in life with congestive heart failure.

With a small VSD the heart is normal in size, when the VSD is large the heart is typically enlarged.

Truncus arteriosus

This is a common arterial trunk arising from the heart, giving rise to the aorta, pulmonary arteries and coronary arteries. Associated with a right-sided aortic arch, absent thymus and parathyroid glands (DiGeorge syndrome). It presents with increasing cyanosis and progressive congestive heart failure as the pulmonary vascular resistance falls due to shunt reversal and development of pulmonary hypertension.

CXR findings

Cardiomegaly, pulmonary plethora, narrow mediastinum due to absent thymus.

Total anomalous pulmonary venous return (TAPVR)

This is failure of the connection between the pulmonary veins and the left atrium. There are three types:

- Type I: supracardiac TAPVR common pulmonary vein joins the left innominate vein.
- Type II: cardiac TAPVR common pulmonary vein joins the coronary sinus.
- Type III: infracardiac TAPVR common pulmonary vein joins the portal vein, ductus venosus or inferior vena cava.

Types I and II present with congestive cardiac failure, while Type III presents with severe cyanosis at birth.

CXR findings

Type I: 'snowman heart'.
Type II: cardiomegaly and plethoric lungs.
Type III: small heart and interstitial oedema.

Hypoplastic left heart syndrome

Hypoplasia/atresia of the ascending aorta, aortic valve, left ventricle and mitral valve. Most severe congenital heart lesion presenting in the neonatal period. There is a rapid deterioration after birth with cyanosis and congestive heart failure after closure of PDA.

CXR findings

Cardiomegaly and interstitial oedema.

Anomalous origin of the left coronary artery

The left coronary artery arises from an abnormal position, most commonly from the pulmonary artery. It causes poor ventricular function and tortuous collateral coronary circulation. Presents in infancy with symptoms related to the degree of cardiac ischaemia such as irritability, wheezing or failure to thrive.

CXR findings

Cardiomegaly with or without interstitial oedema.

Gastrointestinal (GI)
Clinical presentations and role of imaging

Helen Williams

Abdominal distension

Bowel dilatation
- Obstruction.
- Ileus.
- Other causes.

Peritoneal fluid
- Ascites.
- Blood, e.g. post-trauma.

Organomegaly
- Liver.
- Spleen.
- Kidney.
- Adrenal.

Abdominal mass

Obesity

See related sections on bowel dilatation (📖 p. 128, 130, 132, 133), ascites (📖 p. 124, 125) and abdominal mass (📖 p. 120–123).

Role of imaging in abdominal distension

Investigation will depend on organs(s) or pathological process involved, clinical context, history and examination findings. These are general, non-inclusive guidelines.

Radiographs
- Suspected bowel obstruction or ileus.
- Suspected bowel perforation.

Ultrasound
- Initial evaluation of masses and organomegaly.
- Confirm or detect and quantify ascites.
- Suspected intussusception.
- Detection of localized fluid collections/abscesses.

Fluoroscopy
- Upper or lower GI obstruction: selected cases.
- Suspected H-type tracheo-oesophageal fistula (ToF) causing gaseous bowel distension.

CT
- Acute trauma where visceral, vascular or osseous injury is suspected.
- Tumours: staging and follow-up.
- Evaluation of masses.
- Evaluation of localized fluid collections/abscesses.

MRI
- Tumours: staging and follow-up.
- Evaluation of masses.

Abdominal pain: acute

Infancy

Surgical

- Intussusception (📖 p. 190).
- Strangulated hernia.
- Bowel volvulus (📖 p. 162).
- Appendicitis (📖 p. 172).
- Testicular torsion (📖 p. 244).
- Meckel's diverticulitis.
- Hirschsprung's disease (📖 p. 150).

Medical

- Urinary tract infection (UTI) (📖 p. 194).
- Pneumonia (📖 p. 160).
- Food intolerance/allergy.
- Constipation (📖 p. 104).
- NAI.
- Lead poisoning.
- Porphyria.
- Vasculitis, e.g. Henoch–Schönlein purpura (HSP), Kawasaki disease.
- Discitis (rare) (📖 p. 378).

Childhood/adolescence

Infective

- Mesenteric adenitis.
- Pneumonia (📖 p. 60).
- UTI (📖 p. 194).
- Acute hepatitis.
- Gastrointestinal infections.
- Discitis (rare) (📖 p. 378).

Surgical

- Appendicitis (📖 p. 172).
- Trauma.
- Testicular torsion (📖 p. 244).
- Pancreatitis.
- Meckel's diverticulitis.
- Cholecystitis/gallstones (📖 p. 273).
- Renal calculi/renal colic.

Medical

- Peptic ulceration.
- IBD (📖 p. 176, 180).
- Acute nephritis.
- Constipation (📖 p. 104).
- Food intolerance/allergy.
- Vasculitis, e.g. HSP, Kawasaki disease.
- Sickle cell crisis.
- DKA.
- Porphyria.

Gynaecological
- Menstruation.
- Ovulation (mittelschmirtz).
- Pelvic inflammatory disease (PID).
- Ectopic pregnancy.
- Haematocolpos.
- Ovarian cyst or tumour.

Psychological

Role of imaging in acute abdominal pain

Investigation will depend on organs(s) or pathological process involved, clinical context, history and examination findings. These are general, non-inclusive guidelines.

Suspected surgical conditions will require prompt evaluation by an experienced surgeon.

❶ Imaging for suspected NAI should be discussed early with a consultant radiologist.

Radiographs
- CXR: suspected pneumonia, gut perforation (erect CXR).
- AXR: children with symptoms and signs suggestive of obstruction, ileus, toxic dilatation of the colon or gut perforation, renal calculi.

Ultrasound
- Suspected intussusception.
- Suspected cholecystitis/gallstones, renal calculi.
- UTI: not responding to treatment, detection of complications.
- Gynaecologic conditions: mass, ectopic pregnancy, haematocolpos.
- May demonstrate inflamed appendix or detect appendicitis 'mimics'.
- May demonstrate bowel wall thickening or localized fluid collections/abscesses, e.g. IBD.

Fluoroscopy
Upper GI contrast study
- Suspected midgut malrotation and volvulus.

Small bowel contrast studies
- Detection of small bowel involvement with Crohn's disease.

CT
- Acute abdominal trauma.
- May detect other causes of acute abdominal pain, e.g. appendicitis, but not indicated for primary diagnosis.

MRI
- Suspected discitis.

Radio-isotope studies
Meckel's scan
- Identification of ectopic gastric mucosa in Meckel's diverticulum or duplication cyst.

Abdominal pain: chronic/recurrent

- **Chronic abdominal pain** = long-lasting intermittent or constant abdominal pain that is functional or organic (disease-based).
- **Functional abdominal pain** = pain without demonstrable evidence of a pathologic condition. The most common cause of chronic abdominal pain in children. Generally a diagnosis of exclusion when there are no alarm symptoms or signs, normal physical examination and negative stool sample tests. Usually no requirement for additional diagnostic tests including imaging.

Organic causes of chronic abdominal pain

Gastrointestinal
- Gastric ulceration.
- Oesophagitis/gastritis.
- Mesenteric adenitis.
- Gastrointestinal infections.
- Recurrent pancreatitis.
- Cholecystitis/gallstones (🕮 p. 273).
- IBD (🕮 p. 176–80).
- Food intolerance/allergy.
- Constipation (🕮 p. 104).
- Midgut malrotation with intermittent or chronic volvulus.

Urinary tract
- UTI (🕮 p. 194).
- Renal calculi/renal colic.
- PUJ obstruction (🕮 p. 228).

Metabolic
- DKA.
- Hypoglycaemia.
- Hypercholesterolaemia.
- Porphyria.

Miscellaneous causes
- Lead poisoning.
- Referred pain, e.g. from the chest or spine.
- Hereditary angioedema/C1 esterase inhibitor deficiency.

Functional abdominal pain
- Functional dyspepsia.
- Irritable bowel syndrome.
- Abdominal migraine.
- Functional abdominal pain syndrome.

Role of imaging in chronic abdominal pain

Radiographs
- Limited role in detection of renal tract calcification.

Ultrasound
- Suspected cholecystitis/gallstones.
- Suspected renal tract obstruction or calculi.
- UTI: not responding to treatment, detection of complications or underlying structural abnormality.

Fluoroscopy
Upper GI contrast study
- Suspected midgut malrotation and volvulus.

Small bowel contrast studies
- Detection of small bowel involvement with Crohn's disease.

Radio-isotope studies
Meckel's scan
- Identification of ectopic gastric mucosa in Meckel's diverticulum or duplication cyst.

Blood in the stool

- **Haematochezia** = fresh blood in the stool.
- **Melaena** = black, tarry consistency stool containing altered blood.

Neonatal period

- Swallowed maternal blood, e.g. during birth or from a cracked nipple.
- Associated with GI infection (often + mucus).
- Anal fissure.
- Rectal trauma:
  - Constipation (📖 p. 104).
  - Rectal thermometer.
- Cow's milk protein intolerance.
- NEC (📖 p. 174).
- Gut ischaemia, e.g. volvulus or mesenteric thrombosis.
- Bleeding diatheses.
- Haemorrhagic disease of the newborn.
- Gastric mucosal ulceration:
  - Stress.
  - Meckel's diverticulum (📖 p. 154).
  - Ectopic gastric mucosa in intestinal duplication cyst (📖 p. 148).
- Factitious: blood added to stool (Munchausen syndrome by proxy).

After the neonatal period

- Swallowed blood from nose or throat, e.g. nose bleed, tonsillitis.
- Anal fissure.
- Haemorrhoids.
- Rectal trauma:
  - Constipation (📖 p. 104).
  - Rectal thermometer.
  - Sexual abuse.
- Associated with GI infection (often + mucus):
  - *Shigella.*
  - *Salmonella.*
  - *Campylobacter.*
- Intussusception (📖 p. 190).
- HSP.
- Haemolytic uraemic syndrome (HUS).
- Food intolerance/allergy e.g. cow's milk protein.
- IBD (📖 p. 176, 180).
- Bleeding diatheses.
- Oesophagitis.
- Gastric mucosal ulceration:
  - Stress.
  - Meckel's diverticulum.
  - Ectopic gastric mucosa in intestinal duplication cyst.
  - Zollinger–Ellison syndrome.
- Variceal bleeding 2° to portal hypertension.
- Gut ischaemia: volvulus or mesenteric thrombosis.
- Intestinal polyps (may be familial) or telangiectasis.
- Vascular malformations affecting the gut.
- Factitious: blood added to stool (Munchausen syndrome by proxy).

Role of imaging: blood in the stool

Radiographs
- Neonates suspected of having NEC.
- Symptoms and signs suggestive of obstruction, ileus, toxic dilatation of the colon or gut perforation.
- Limited role in suspected intussusception, to demonstrate bowel obstruction or free intraperitoneal air.

Ultrasound
- Suspected intussusception.
- To detect the imaging features of portal hypertension.
- Detection of localized fluid collections/abscesses e.g. in NEC, IBD.
- May demonstrate bowel duplication cyst.
- May demonstrate bowel-wall thickening in IBD, HSP etc.

Fluoroscopy
Upper GI contrast study
- Suspected midgut malrotation and volvulus.

Small bowel contrast studies
- Detection of small bowel involvement with Crohn's disease.
- May demonstrate small bowel polyps.

Catheter angiography
- May identify bleeding site in acute blood loss.

CT
- Limited role, e.g. detection of localized abscess/collections in patients with IBD.

Radio-isotope studies
Labelled red cell studies
- May identify bleeding site in acute blood loss.

Meckel's scan
- Identification of ectopic gastric mucosa in Meckel's diverticulum or intestinal duplication cyst.

Constipation

This term has a different meaning to different people. It may be taken to mean *unusually hard stools*, the *infrequent passage of stools*, or *delay in the passage of stools*. There is a wide variation of normality or physiological variation in all of these, so constipation can be difficult to define. Constipation may be associated with soiling.

Normal physiological variation
- Normal infrequent stools.
- Normal hard stools.

Dietary
- Low fibre diet.
- Starvation or dehydration.

Drugs

Bowel and related disorders
- Obstruction or ileus.
- Hirschprung's disease (🕮 p. 150).
- Anorectal malformations (🕮 p. 140).
- Stricture, e.g. IBD, post-NEC.
- Anal fissure.
- Coeliac disease.
- Cystic fibrosis (CF).
- Prune belly syndrome.

Psychological
- Habit, withholding stools or inappropriate toilet training.

Neurological disorders
- Cerebral palsy.
- Learning disability.
- Hypotonia.
- Spinal cord lesions, e.g. 'tethered cord', spina bifida.

Metabolic causes (all rare)
- Hypercalcaemia.
- Hypothyroidism.
- Rickets (🕮 p. 348).
- Lead poisoning.

Role of imaging in constipation

Radiographs

There is no role for routine abdominal radiography in the investigation of constipation. In selected cases it may be helpful, e.g. in order to demonstrate efficacy of treatment. Radiographs are also used in transit studies.

Fluoroscopy

Contrast studies may be indicated in carefully selected cases to demonstrate size and extent of rectal and colonic dilatation prior to surgery.

MRI

MRI of the spine is the investigation of choice when a congenital spinal abnormality is suspected. Patients usually have intractable constipation and associated neurological abnormality on examination, e.g. affecting the lower limbs. MRI may demonstrate size and extent of distal bowel dilatation prior to surgery.

Radio-isotope studies

Defecating proctography is used in selected cases to investigate constipation and rectal transit in adults. It has no established role in children.

Diarrhoea

Loose stools, not an increased frequency of bowel motion. The two may coexist.

Newborn period

- Breast feeding: stools often explosive, may be bright green.
- Phototherapy for jaundice.
- NEC (📖 p. 174).
- Excess sugar in feeds.
- Drugs: directly or in breast milk.

After the newborn period

Acute diarrhoea

- GI infection:
  - Viral.
  - Bacterial.
  - Protozoal.
- Parenteral response to acute non-GI infection.
- Starvation stools.
- Acute appendicitis or appendix abscess (📖 p. 172).
- Intussusception (📖 p. 190).
- Drugs, e.g. antibiotics, laxatives.
- Ingestion of fruit or fruit juice.
- HUS.
- Addisonian crisis.
- Hirschsprung's disease-related enterocolitis (📖 p. 150).

Chronic diarrhoea

- Chronic GI infection.
- Toddler diarrhoea.
- Fecal retention or organic constipation with overflow diarrhoea.
- IBD (📖 p. 176, 180).
- Food intolerance or allergy:
  - Monosaccharide (e.g. fructose, galactose).
  - Disaccharide (e.g. lactose).
  - Cow's milk protein.
  - Gluten (coeliac disease).
- CF.
- Other causes of malabsorption, e.g. Schwachman–Diamond syndrome.
- Acrodermatitis enteropathica (autosomal recessive [AR] disorder → zinc deficiency).
- Immunodeficiency.
- Phenotypic diarrhoea.
- Short bowel syndrome.
- Hormone-secreting tumours, vasoactive intestinal peptide (VIP), e.g. ganglioneuroma.
- Psychogenic.
- Laxative abuse.

Role of imaging in diarrhoea

Radiographs
- Suspected NEC.
- Suspected toxic dilatation of the bowel.
- Suspected bowel perforation (detection of free intraperitoneal gas).

Ultrasound
- Suspected intussusception.
- Detection of localized fluid collections/abscesses, e.g. in NEC, IBD.
- May demonstrate bowel-wall thickening, e.g. IBD, HSP.
- May demonstrate features of acute appendicitis or appendix abscess.
- May identify hormone-secreting tumours.

Fluoroscopy
Small bowel barium/contrast studies
- Crohn's disease: assessment of small bowel involvement.
- Short gut syndrome: demonstration of bowel length and motility.

Contrast enema
- Hirschprung's disease: demonstration of transition zone/calibre change.

CT
- Detection of localized abscesses, e.g. appendix abscess, IBD.
- Detection and staging of hormone-secreting tumours.

MRI
- Evaluation of perianal Crohn's disease.
- Detection and staging of hormone-secreting tumours.
- Recent use in selected cases for assessment of small bowel involvement in IBD.

Dysphagia

Dysphagia is difficulty swallowing. This may present with discomfort during swallowing, hesitation in swallowing, choking, drooling or return of fluid or food through the nose or mouth.

Congenital malformations

- OA (☐ p. 168)- complications following repair.
- H-type tracheo-oesophageal fistula (TOF) (☐ p. 168).
- Micrognathia.
- Macroglossia.
- Cleft palate.

Oesophageal disorders

- Stricture or stenosis.
- Reflux oesophagitis (☐ p. 186).
- Scalding or caustic burns.
- Infection, e.g. candidiasis, CMV in immunocompromised patients.
- Connective tissue disorders.

Pharyngeal or oesophageal obstruction

- Enlarged tonsils (☐ p. 470).
- Retropharyngeal abscess (☐ p. 468).
- Foreign body including food bolus.
- Mediastinal mass, e.g. tumour, duplication cyst, lymph nodes.
- Vascular ring.
- Goitre (☐ p. 424).
- Cardiac enlargement.

Inflammatory /infective lesions

- Herpetic gingivo-stomatitis.
- Epiglottitis.
- Peritonsillar abscess.

Neuromuscular causes

- Normal preterm infants.
- Hypotonia.
- Cerebral disorders, e.g. causing developmental delay, stroke, tumour.
- Pharyngeal inco-ordination.
- Pharyngeal paralysis:
  - Bulbar palsy.
  - Guillain-Barré syndrome.
  - Drugs.
  - Möebius syndrome.
  - Botulism.
  - Myasthenia gravis.
  - Myotonic dystrophy.
  - Pontine glioma (☐ p. 510).
- Congenital hypothyroidism.

Psychological

Role of imaging in dysphagia

Radiographs

Limited role in detection of radio-opaque foreign bodies.

Fluoroscopy

Upper GI contrast studies in acute and chronic dysphagia
- Detection of anatomical abnormalities, e.g. stricture, extrinsic impression from vascular ring.
- Demonstrate abnormal motility, e.g. reflux oesophagitis, connective tissue disorders, post-OA repair.

Tube oesophagram
- Selected patients suspected of having an H-type TOF.

Videofluorosopy
- Pharyngeal swallowing disorders ± suspected aspiration.

CT and MRI

Limited role.
- Demonstration and characterization of thoracic masses.
- Demonstration of mediastinal vascular anatomy and vascular ring.

Haematemesis

Oesophagus

- Reflux oesophagitis.
- Oesophageal ulceration including gastro-oesophageal reflux (GOR).
- Hiatus hernia.
- Variceal bleeding: chronic liver disease with portal hypertension.
- Mallory–Weiss tear.

Stomach

- Ulceration.
- Erosions.

Duodenum

- Ulceration.
- Erosions.

Miscellaneous causes

- Swallowed blood:
  - During delivery.
  - Cracked nipple: breastfeeding.
  - Nose bleed.
  - Tonsillitis.
- Coagulation disorders including haemorrhagic disease of the newborn.
- Swallowed foreign body.
- Intestinal polyps.
- Connective tissue disorders.
- Drugs.
- Upper intestinal vascular malformation.
- Hereditary telangiectasia (Osler–Weber–Rendu syndrome): telangiectases not usually prominent until >20 years.

Role of imaging in haematemesis

Imaging has a very limited role in the investigation of haematemesis. Radiographs may be used to detect radio-opaque foreign bodies. Oesophageal varices may be detected on ultrasound, upper GI contrast studies, CT and MR Imaging but the investigation of choice is upper GI endoscopy.

Salivary gland swelling: acute

The most common cause in a child is infection, especially viral.

Infection

- Viral:
  - CMV.
  - Epstein–Barr virus (infectious mononucleosis).
  - Mumps.
  - Toxoplasmosis.
  - Other viruses.
- Bacterial. Usually infants, immunocompromised or patients with chronic disorders. Intraparotid abscess may develop:
  - *Staph. Aureus.*
  - *Strep. Viridans.*
  - Secondary to URTI with seeding to intraparotid nodes.
  - Mycobacterial infection: TB or non-tuberculous infection (more often subacute or chronic symptoms).

Duct obstruction

- Sialolithiasis: stones are more common in the submandibular duct (90%) due to alkaline, viscous secretions and upward direction of flow in the duct.
- Stricture.

Role of imaging in salivary gland swelling: acute or chronic

Radiographs

Limited role: detection of radio-opaque salivary calculi.

Ultrasound

Modality of choice for investigation of acute and chronic salivary gland swelling. Can identify masses, diffuse disorders, sialectasis and stones within the gland or duct.

Fluoroscopy

Main indication for sialography is suspected duct obstruction by stone or stricture. Detection of sialectasis.

MRI

Imaging method of choice for suspected neoplasia and for staging tumours. May help characterize lymphatic and vascular malformations.

Salivary gland swelling: chronic

Infection
- Mumps.
- Mycobacterial infection: TB or non-tuberculous infection.
- Cat scratch disease.
- HIV: lymphoproliferative changes or cystic lesions.
- Actinomycosis.

Duct obstruction
- Sialolithiasis.
- Stricture.
- Ranula: usually related to the sublingual glands.

Chronic parotitis
- Autoimmune disorders:
  - Sjögren's syndrome.
  - SLE.
  - Raynaud's disease.
- Chronic recurrent parotitis (juvenile recurrent parotitis).

Non-infective granulomatous disorders
- Sarcoidosis.

Masses
- Lymphatic and vascular malformations (📖 p. 458).
- Mucous retention cyst.
- Branchial apparatus cyst (📖 p. 438).
- Lymphoepithelial cysts (associated with HIV infection).
- Tumours:
  - Haemangioma (📖 p. 480).
  - Pleomorphic adenoma: most common benign salivary gland neoplasm in childhood.
  - Mucoepidermoid carcinoma: most common malignant neoplasm in childhood.
  - Acinic cell carcinoma.
  - Adenocarcinoma.
  - Warthin's tumour.
  - Sialoblastoma.
  - Secondary involvement, e.g. rhabdomyosarcoma, lymphoma.

Vomiting

Newborn/infant

- Normal posseting.
- GOR (📖 p. 186).
- Overfeeding.
- Infection:
  - GI.
  - UTI (📖 p. 194).
  - Meningitis.
  - Septicaemia.
- Midgut malrotation with volvulus (📖 p. 162) ❶ Suspect in any child with bile-stained vomiting.
- Other causes of neonatal intestinal obstruction: see related sections (📖 p. 132, 133).
- Pyloric stenosis (📖 p. 188).
- Raised intracranial pressure, e.g. haemorrhage, oedema, tumour.
- Metabolic disorders.
- Drugs and poisons, e.g. antibiotics.
- Electrolyte or acid-base disturbance, e.g. congenital adrenal hyperplasia (CAH), DKA.

Infant/older child

- GOR (📖 p. 186).
- Oesophageal obstruction, e.g. stricture, achalasia.
- Bezoar (📖 p. 184).
- Overfeeding.
- Infection:
  - GI.
  - UTI (📖 p. 194).
  - Meningitis.
  - Septicaemia.
- Acute abdominal causes (surgical):
  - Intestinal obstruction (📖 p. 128, 132, 133).
  - Intussusception (📖 p. 190).
  - Appendicitis (📖 p. 172).
  - Mesenteric adenitis.
  - Midgut malrotation with volvulus (📖 p. 162) ❶ Suspect in any child with bile-stained vomiting.
  - Testicular torsion (📖 p. 244).
- Electrolyte or acid-base disturbance, e.g. DKA.
- Food intolerance/allergy.
- IBD (📖 p. 176, 180).
- Raised intracranial pressure, e.g. haemorrhage, oedema, tumour.
- Metabolic disorders.
- Drugs and poisons, e.g. antibiotics.
- Travel/motion sickness.
- Migraine.
- Cyclical vomiting.
- Psychological: eating disorders e.g. bulimia nervosa.

Role of imaging in vomiting

Radiographs
- Suspected bowel obstruction or ileus.
- Suspected bowel perforation.

Ultrasound
- Suspected intussusception.
- Pyloric stenosis with equivocal test feed.
- May detect inflamed appendix.

Fluoroscopy
Upper GI contrast study
- Suspected midgut malrotation with volvulus requires urgent surgical assessment + upper GI contrast study.
- Suspected oesophageal obstruction.
- Suspected bezoar.

Small bowel barium/contrast studies
- Crohn's disease: assessment of small bowel involvement.

Contrast enema
- Neonatal lower GI obstruction.
- Other causes of colonic obstruction, e.g. stricture.

CT
- Suspected acute intracranial haemorrhage.
- Detection of tumours: acutely when MRI not available.
- May detect acute abdominal causes e.g. appendicitis but not indicated for primary diagnosis.

MRI
- Detection and staging of CNS tumours: modality of choice.

Weight loss

Infection

- Any acute infection:
  - Gastrointestinal.
  - Chest.
  - Urinary tract.
  - CNS.
  - Musculoskeletal.
  - Septicaemia.
- Chronic infection:
  - Especially chest (e.g. TB), gastrointestinal.
  - HIV/AIDS.

Persistent vomiting

Persistent diarrhoea

Chronic diseases

- Chest:
  - Chronic lung disease of prematurity (📖 p. 23).
  - CF (📖 p. 66).
  - Severe asthma (📖 p. 22).
- Renal disease and renal failure.
- Gastrointestinal:
  - IBD (📖 p. 176, 180).
  - Food intolerance/allergy.
  - Malabsorption.
- Chronic liver disease.
- Degenerative muscle disorders: especially in late stage of the disease.

Endocrine disorders

- Diabetes mellitus.
- Diabetes insipidus.
- Thyrotoxicosis.
- Addison's disease.

Malignancy

- Any primary tumour: particularly neuroblastoma, diencephalic syndrome 2° CNS tumour.
- Disseminated malignancy.

Drugs

- Stimulants for hyperactivity.
- Thyroxine.

Emotional causes

- Child abuse or neglect.
- Depression.
- Anorexia nervosa.

Role of imaging in weight loss

Radiographs
- Acute or chronic lung infection.
- Limited role in monitoring of chronic lung diseases.

Ultrasound
- Assessment of abdominal mass/suspected tumour.
- Monitoring of renal disease.
- Evaluation of thyroid enlargement and masses.

Fluoroscopy
Small bowel barium/contrast studies
- Crohn's disease: assessment of small bowel involvement.

CT
- Detection and staging of tumours.

MRI
- Evaluation and staging of tumours: modality of choice for the CNS.
- Recent use in selected cases for assessment of small bowel involvement in IBD.

Gastrointestinal (GI)
Differential diagnosis

Helen Williams

Abdominal calcification: neonate

Diffuse peritoneal
- Meconium peritonitis 2° to intrauterine perforation.
- Peritonitis 2° to rupture of hydrometrocolpos.

Bowel wall
- Bowel atresia (📖 p. 152).
- Meconium ileus (📖 p. 156).
- Intrauterine volvulus.

Intraluminal
- Intestinal obstruction: small bowel atresia, Hirschprung's disease (📖 p. 150), anorectal malformations (📖 p. 140) (usually indicates fistula to urinary tract).
- Multiple gastrointestinal atresias with AR inheritance.

Hepatic
- Congenital toxoplasmosis, rubella, CMV, herpes (TORCH) infection.
- Tumours: haemangioma, haemangioendothelioma, hepatoblastoma, metastatic neuroblastoma, teratoma (📖 p. 284–298).
- Portal vein thromboemboli.
- Ischaemic infarcts.

Urinary tract
- Medullary nephrocalcinosis:
  - Frusemide.
  - Preterm infants.
  - Renal papillary necrosis.
  - Renal tubular acidosis.
- Cortical nephrocalcinosis:
  - Acute cortical necrosis.

Adrenal
- Following adrenal haemorrhage.
- Neuroblastoma (📖 p. 260).

Abdominal calcification: child

Bowel wall
- Rarely seen in duplication cysts (📖 p. 148).

Intraluminal
- Swallowed foreign bodies.

Hepatic/biliary
- Hepatoblastoma (📖 p. 286).
- Hepatocellular carcinoma.
- Healed granulomatous disease, e.g. TB.
- Hydatid disease.
- Hepatic abscess.
- Gallstones.

Urinary tract
- Renal or bladder calculi (📖 p. 196).
- Renal infection:
  - TB.
  - Hydatid.
  - Xanthogranulomatous pyelonephritis.
- Medullary nephrocalcinosis (the first three account for 70% of cases):
  - Hyperparathyroidism.
  - Renal tubular acidosis.
  - Medullary sponge kidney.
  - Renal papillary necrosis.
  - Hypercalcaemia/hypercalciuria.
  - Ex-preterm infants (including frusemide and corticosteroid therapy).
  - Primary hyperoxaluria.
- Cortical nephrocalcinosis:
  - Acute cortical necrosis.
  - Chronic glomerulonephritis.
  - Chronic transplant rejection.

Adrenal
- Cystic disease usually 2° to adrenal haemorrhage.
- Tumours: teratoma, neuroblastoma and ganglioneuroma.
- Wolman's disease.

Splenic
- Sickle cell anaemia.
- Post-infarction.
- Granulomatous diseases, e.g. TB.
- Rarely in the wall of cysts.

Pancreatic
- CF (📖 p. 66).
- Chronic pancreatitis.
- Pancreatic pseudocyst.

Abdominal mass: neonate

Renal

- Hydronephrosis: PUJ/VUJ (vesico-ureteric junction) obstruction
  (📖 p. 228), PUV (📖 p. 218), ureterocele, prune belly syndrome.
- Multicystic dysplastic kidney (MCDK) (📖 p. 224).
- Autosomal recessive polycystic kidney disease (📖 p. 222).
- Mesoblastic nephroma (📖 p. 232).
- Nephroblastomatosis (📖 p. 236).
- Renal vein thrombosis.
- Renal ectopia (📖 p. 210).
- Wilm's tumour (📖 p. 234).

Genitourinary

- Hydrocolpos: in association with vaginal obstruction, urogenital sinus or
  cloacal abnormality (📖 p. 254).
- Ovarian cyst.
- Ovarian torsion.

Gastrointestinal

- Duplication cyst (📖 p. 148).
- Mesenteric or omental cyst (📖 p. 160).
- Lymphatic malformation.
- Meconium pseudocyst (📖 p. 158).

Adrenal/retroperitoneal

- Adrenal haemorrhage.
- Neuroblastoma (📖 p. 260).
- Teratoma.

Hepatic/biliary

- Diffuse hepatic enlargement:
  - Congenital (TORCH) infection (📖 p. 272).
  - Metastatic neuroblastoma.
  - Cardiac failure.
- Tumours:
  - Haemangioma.
  - Haemangioendothelioma.
  - Hepatoblastoma (📖 p. 286).
- Hepatic cyst.
- Choledochal cyst (📖 p. 278).

Splenic

- Splenic cyst.

Abdominal mass: child

Renal
- Hydronephrosis.
- Cystic renal disease, e.g. autosomal recessive polycystic kidney disease (ARPKD) (📖 p. 222).
- Wilm's tumour (📖 p. 234).
- Infiltration, e.g. lymphoma.

Genitourinary
- Hydrocolpos (📖 p. 254).
- Ovarian cyst.
- Ovarian tumour, e.g. teratoma (📖 p. 252).
- Pregnancy.

Gastrointestinal
- Appendix mass or abscess (📖 p. 172).
- Duplication cyst (📖 p. 148).
- Mesenteric or omental cyst (📖 p. 160).
- Lymphatic malformation.

Adrenal/retroperitoneal
- Neuroblastoma (📖 p. 260).

Hepatic/biliary
- Hepatomegaly. Multiple causes including:
  • Storage disorder.
  • Other metabolic disorders, e.g. tyrosinaemia.
  • Infection.
  • Cardiac failure.
- Tumours:
  • Hepatoblastoma, hepatocellular carcinoma (📖 p. 286).
  • Metastatic disease.
  • Mesenchymal hamartoma (📖 p. 284).
- Hepatic cyst or abscess.
- Choledochal cyst (📖 p. 278).

Splenic
- Splenic cyst.
- Splenomegaly. Multiple causes including:
  • Infection.
  • Storage disorder.
  • Haematological causes, e.g. chronic haemolysis, leukaemia.
  • Malignancy, e.g. lymphoma.
  • Portal hypertension.

Ascites: neonate

Bulging of flank lines and hazy appearance of the entire abdomen. Gas filled loops of bowel displaced centrally—'floating' on supine AXR.

Any cause of hypoalbuminaemia (e.g. reduced hepatic synthesis, protein loss from the GI or renal tract, or nutritional) can cause ascites.

Hydrops fetalis
- Immune hydrops, e.g. Rhesus incompatibility.
- Non-immune hydrops: mostly cardiac causes.

Cardiac/vascular
- Cardiac failure.
- IVC thrombosis.

Lymphatic obstruction
- Chylous ascites: can be caused by malrotation and volvulus.
- Lymphangiectasia.
- Trauma.

Hepatic/biliary
- Neonatal hepatitis (📖 p. 268).
- Portal vein obstruction (e.g. thrombosis) or compression.
- Hepatic vein obstruction, e.g. thrombosis.
- Liver failure with hypoalbuminaemia.
- Rupture of common bile duct (CBD): spontaneous or 2° to obstruction.
- Rupture of choledochal cyst.

Renal
- Urine ascites 2° to rupture of upper urinary tract usually in association with lower urinary tract obstruction:
  - PUV (📖 p. 218).
  - VUJ obstruction.
  - PUJ obstruction (📖 p. 228).
  - Extrinsic bladder mass.
  - Neuropathic bladder.
- Traumatic bladder rupture (e.g. catheterization).

Genitourinary
- Ruptured hydrocolpos or ovarian cyst.

Gastrointestinal
- Bowel perforation with meconium peritonitis (📖 p. 158).
- NEC (📖 p. 174).
- Rupture of mesenteric or omental cyst (📖 p. 160).

Ascites: child

Cardiac/vascular

- Cardiac failure.
- Constrictive pericarditis.
- IVC thrombosis.

Lymphatic obstruction

- Lymphoma.
- Post-irradiation.
- Chylous ascites.
- Trauma.
- Parasitic infection, e.g. filariasis.

Hepatic

- Cirrhosis.
- Hepatic vein obstruction, e.g. thrombosis.
- Liver failure with hypoalbuminaemia.

Renal

- Nephrotic syndrome with hypoalbuminaemia.
- Peritoneal dialysis.

Gastrointestinal

- Poor nutrition.
- Protein-losing enteropathy which may be secondary to cardiac or other systemic disease.

Peritoneal

- TB.
- Bacterial infection.

Malignancy

- Metastatic disease, e.g. lymphoma.

Bowel stricture or narrowing

Small bowel
- Crohn's disease (□ p. 176).
- Adhesions: constant angulation of bowel with normal mucosa.
- Infection, e.g. TB.
- Chemical irritation, e.g. enteric-coated potassium chloride tablets.
- Post-NEC (□ p. 174).
- Post-operative anastamotic stricture.
- Post-radiation therapy.
- Bowel wall haematoma, e.g. HSP, trauma.
- Extrinsic compression from enteric duplication cyst.
- Neoplastic, e.g. lymphoma, tumours 2° to polyposis syndromes, metastatic disease (rare).

Large bowel
- IBD: Crohn's or ulcerative colitis (UC) (□ p. 176, 180).
- Post-NEC (□ p. 174).
- Peri-colic abscess.
- Infection:
  - TB.
  - Parasites: amoebiasis, schistosomiasis.
- Food intolerance/allergy: cow's milk protein.
- Ischaemic, e.g. vasculitis, post-HUS.
- Post-operative anastamotic stricture.
- Post-radiation therapy.
- Extrinsic compression, e.g. enteric duplication cyst.
- Neoplastic, e.g. lymphoma, tumours 2° to polyposis syndromes.
- Fibrosing colonopathy: associated with high dose pancreatic enzyme supplementation in CF.

Colonic wall thickening and oedema

Any cause of colitis

- NEC (📖 p. 174).
- IBD:
    - Crohn's disease (📖 p. 176).
    - UC (📖 p. 180).
- Infections:
    - Viral, e.g. CMV, HSV, rotavirus.
    - Bacterial, e.g. *Salmonella, Shigella, Campylobacter, Yersinia, E. Coli*.
    - Parasitic, e.g. amoebiasis, schistosomiasis, strongyloidiasis.
- Pseudomembranous colitis: *Clostridium difficile*.
- Hirschprung's associated enterocolitis (📖 p. 150).
- Neutropenic colitis (typhlitis).
- Chemotherapy and radiation therapy.
- Food intolerance/allergy: cow's milk protein.
- Behçet's syndrome.
- Ischaemic colitis: very rare in children, e.g. vasculitis, hypovolaemic shock.

Miscellaneous causes

- Hereditary angioedema/C1 esterase inhibitor deficiency.
- HUS.
- Iatrogenic: detergent, caustic and herb enemas.

Colonic dilatation

Colitis

May lead to **toxic dilatation** (transverse colon diameter >5.5cm in an adult, with mucosal abnormalities and loss of haustral pattern) especially 2° to IBD, infectious colitis, pseudomembranous colitis, Hirschprung's associated colitis, chemotherapy and radiotherapy.

Mechanical obstruction

- Hirschprung's disease (📖 p. 150) (dilated proximal bowel).
- Large bowel stricture.
- Hernia.
- Peritoneal adhesions.
- Extrinsic compression, e.g. enteric duplication cyst, peri-colic abscess.
- Neoplasia: very rare in children, e.g. lymphoma, tumours 2° polyposis syndromes.

Electrolyte or acid-base disturbance

Pseudo-obstruction

Gasless abdomen

High obstruction
- Pure OA (📖 p. 168).
- Duodenal atresia, stenosis or web (📖 p. 144).
- Midgut malrotation and volvulus (📖 p. 162).
- Congenital peritoneal (Ladd's) bands.
- Annular pancreas.
- Hypertrophic pyloric stenosis (📖 p. 188).
- Extrinsic compression of bowel, e.g. enteric duplication cyst, choledochal cyst.

Vomiting

Excess NG aspiration

Fluid-filled bowel
- Obstruction.
- Paralytic/adynamic ileus.
- Gastroenteritis.
- Mesenteric infarction.
- Bowel wash out.

Ascites

Congenital diaphragmatic hernia
- Bowel in the chest.

Gastric dilatation

Swallowed air
- Excessive crying.
- Emotional distress.

Acute gastric dilatation
- Post-surgery.
- Abdominal trauma.
- Severe pain or abdominal inflammation.
- Immobilization.
- Drugs.
- Vagal nerve division/damage.
- Electrolyte or acid-base disturbance.

Bezoar

Gastric outlet obstruction
- Pyloric stenosis (📖 p. 188).
- Antral web.
- Inflammatory disorder, e.g. Crohn's disease.
- Peptic stricture.
- Gastric volvulus.
- Extrinsic compression, e.g. gastric duplication cyst.

Duodenal obstruction
- Duodenal atresia (📖 p. 144).
- Duodenal web or stenosis (📖 p. 146).
- Midgut volvulus (📖 p. 162).
- Annular pancreas.
- Congenital peritoneal (Ladd's) bands.
- Acute pancreatitis.
- Extrinsic compression, e.g. duodenal duplication cyst.

Mucosal ulceration

Mouth and pharynx (not detected using imaging)

- Aphthous ulcers.
- Infection, e.g. herpes gingivostomatitis, cocksackie virus (hand, foot and mouth disease, herpangina), bacterial infections.
- Drugs.
- Steven's–Johnson syndrome.
- Behçet's syndrome.
- Crohn's disease.
- Trauma.
- Chemotherapy and radiation therapy.
- Neutropenia: multiple causes.
- HIV.
- Iron and vitamin deficiencies: folate, zinc, vitamin B12.

Oesophagus

- Causes of oesophageal ulceration except different infective agents: candida, CMV, HSV (usually immunocompromised patients).
- GOR.
- Barrett's oesophagus.
- Caustic ingestion.
- Epidermolysis bullosa dystrophica.
- Graft versus host disease (GVHD).
- Frequent vomiting: e.g. bulimia nervosa.

Stomach and duodenum

- Peptic ulceration.
- Crohn's disease (📖 p. 176).
- Drugs, e.g. corticosteroids, NSAIDs.
- Stress, e.g. severe acute or prolonged illness, burns.
- Zollinger–Ellison syndrome.
- Corrosive ingestion.
- Stasis 2° to pyloric or duodenal obstruction.

Small bowel

- Crohn's disease (📖 p. 176).
- Infections, e.g. *Yersinia, salmonella*, TB.
- Drugs, e.g. non-steroidal anti-inflammatory drugs (NSAIDs).
- Food intolerance/allergy, e.g. coeliac disease.
- Chemotherapy and radiation therapy.
- Behçet's syndrome.
- Polyarteritis nodosa (PAN).

Large bowel

- Colitis, e.g. IBD, infective, ischaemic.
- Behçet's syndrome.
- Radiation therapy.
- Churg–Strauss syndrome.

Neonatal high intestinal obstruction

Presentation is relatively early with obstructive symptoms (e.g. vomiting). Higher level of obstruction → earlier presentation and relatively ↓ abdominal distension. Causes of 'high' obstruction incorporate bowel as far as the jejunum.

Gastric

- Pyloric atresia: very rare.
- Antral or pyloric web.

Duodenal obstruction

- Duodenal atresia (📖 p. 144).
- Duodenal stenosis or web (📖 p. 144).
- Midgut malrotation and volvulus (📖 p. 162).
- Congenital peritoneal (Ladd's) bands.
- Annular pancreas.
- Extrinsic compression of bowel, e.g. enteric duplication cyst, choledochal cyst.

Jejunal atresia

- Generally proximal atresia (📖 p. 152).

Neonatal low intestinal obstruction

Usually present relatively later with abdominal distension and delayed passage of meconium. Vomiting and ↑ gastric aspirates relatively late. Most will be investigated with enema to define level of obstruction and evaluate colon calibre.

▶ It is generally not possible to differentiate small from large bowel in neonates.

Small bowel causes

- Jejunal or ileal atresia (📖 p. 152).
- Meconium ileus (📖 p. 156).
- Inguinal hernia.

Large bowel causes

- Neonatal functional colonic obstruction (📖 p. 166):
  - Meconium plug syndrome.
  - Small left colon syndrome.
- Inspissated milk curd (usually premature neonates).
- Hirschprung's disease (📖 p. 150).
- Anorectal malformations (📖 p. 140).
- Colonic atresia (rare).

Neonatal microcolon

A small calibre colon on lower GI contrast studies. No absolute measurements for diagnosis.

Underused colon 2° to lack of intraluminal content

- Distal ileal atresia (📖 p. 152).
- Meconium ileus (📖 p. 156).

Total colonic aganglionosis

Oesophageal stricture

- Peptic stricture 2° to gastro-oesophageal reflux.
- Caustic ingestion.
- Epidermolysis bullosa dystrophica.
- Infective oesophagitis (usually immunocompromised patients):
  - CMV.
  - *Candida albicans.*
  - HSV.
- Post-operative: oesophageal atresia repair.
- Crohn's disease (📖 p. 176).
- Behçet's syndrome.
- Chronic granulomatous disease.
- GVHD.
- Radiation therapy and chemotherapy.

Pneumatosis intestinalis

Gas in the bowel wall.

Primary
- Idiopathic.

Secondary
- NEC (📖 p. 174).
- Steroids and other immunosuppressive therapy.
- Connective tissue disorders:
  - Dermatomyositis.
  - Scleroderma.
  - JIA (📖 p. 356).
- Leukaemia.
- Colitis and enteritis:
  - IBD (📖 p. 176, 180).
  - Bowel ischaemia.
  - GI infections particularly rotavirus, CMV colitis, cryptosporidiosis in immunocompromised patients.

Pneumoperitoneum

Free air or gas in the peritoneal cavity.

Perforation of a gas containing abdominal viscus

- Toxic dilatation of the stomach.
- Peptic ulcer: rare in children, associated with steroids and acute stress.
- Bowel obstruction.
- Bowel inflammation:
  - NEC (📖 p. 174).
  - IBD (📖 p. 176, 180) including toxic megacolon.
  - Infections particularly with immunosuppression.
  - Appendicitis (📖 p. 172) although rare to get free air.
- Traumatic.
- Rupture of mural 'cysts' in pneumatosis coli.

Iatrogenic

- Post-laparotomy, laparoscopy or insertion of peritoneal catheter/drain.

Intrathoracic causes

- Pneumomediastinum: gas can track into the peritoneum via the retroperitoneal space.
- Pneumothorax: through a congenital pleuroperitoneal fistula.

Gynaecologic causes

Rare in children unless sexually active or following abuse.

Small bowel dilatation

Air swallowing
- Crying and emotional distress.
- Habitual.

Mechanical obstruction
- Peritoneal adhesions (large or small bowel).
- Congenital peritoneal (Ladd's) bands.
- Stricture (large or small bowel).
- Hernia.
- Distal intestinal obstruction syndrome (DIOS) in CF.
- Hirschprung's disease (📖 p. 150).
- Inspissated milk curd (usually premature neonates).

Paralytic/adynamic ileus
- Post-surgery.
- Abdominal trauma.
- Drugs.
- Electrolyte or acid-base disturbance.
- Immobility.

Vascular insufficiency
- Midgut volvulus (📖 p. 162).

Malabsorption
- Multiple causes including;
- Food intolerance causing malabsorption:
  - Monosaccharide (e.g. fructose, galactose).
  - Disaccharide (e.g. lactose).
  - Cow's milk protein.
  - Gluten (coeliac disease).
- Gastrointestinal infections.

Rare causes
- Idiopathic intestinal pseudo-obstruction.
- Total intestinal aganglionosis.
- Scleroderma.
- Lymphoma.

Gastrointestinal (GI)
Disorders

Helen Williams

Anorectal malformations (ARM)

Spectrum of distal bowel abnormalities. Incidence 1/5000 live births, 60% ♂. Clinically no anal opening. Classification is controversial with several alternative systems. ARM can be divided into **high**, **intermediate** or **low** according to relationship to the pelvic floor (puborectalis muscle).

Alternative classification subdivides into four categories:

- **Ectopic anus** (most common): terminal bowel opens at an abnormal location including scrotum, perineum, vulva, vestibule, urethra, vagina, or cloaca. Results from failure of the hindgut to descend properly to join the anus and empties ectopically through a fistula.
- **Imperforate anus**: terminal bowel ends blindly without a fistula. Two types: *anal atresia* and *anorectal atresia* depending on the length of the atretic portion.
- **Rectal atresia**: anus is present and open but a variable segment of rectum above it is atretic and there is no fistula.
- **Anal or rectal stenosis**: incomplete atresia.

Associated anomalies found in >50%. Many are part of vertebral, anorectal, tracheal, oesophageal, renal abnormalities (VATER) or vertebral, anorectal, tracheal, oesophageal, renal, limb abnormalities (VACTERL) association. Also ↑ incidence of spinal dysraphism and cord abnormalities. 12–22% associated with cardiovascular abnormalities, mostly ToF and VSD. Renal dysplasia and vesico-ureteric reflux (VUR) are associated. Affected ♀ have a high incidence of genital abnormalities such as bicornuate uterus, uterus didelphys or vaginal septum. Cryptorchidism seen in ~20% affected ♂.

Currarino's triad is a rare association of anomalies including an anorectal malformation (ARM), lumbosacral abnormalities and a pre-sacral mass (teratoma, anterior meningocele or enteric cyst).

▶ Radiology alone is insufficient in differentiating high and intermediate lesions from low lesions but has an important role in conjunction with clinical examination.

Imaging findings

Radiographic signs

- Distal bowel obstruction: multiple dilated bowel loops.
- ± Intraluminal meconium calcification.
- ± Gas in bladder in ♂, vagina in ♀.
- Lateral prone cross table with buttocks raised ('invertogram') taken at ~24 hours may help define level of obstruction in relation to the pubococcygeal line (M-line). Can be unreliable:
  - Crying, straining or ↑ distension of pouch: high lesions appear low.
  - Meconium-packed pouch: low lesions appear high.

Ultrasound

- Can show distance from rectal pouch to the skin surface.
- <10mm low lesion, 10–15mm intermediate or high lesion.
- Similar reliability and pitfalls to invertogram.
- May demonstrate associated genital or renal abnormalities.

Fluoroscopy

Findings dependent on type of malformation and associated genitourinary abnormalities.

- Micturating cystourethogram (MCUG) may demonstrate neurogenic bladder, VUR, recto–vesical or recto–urethral fistula.
- Cloacogram: if single perineal orifice.
- Fistulogram = distal colonogram: performed electively prior to definitive repair:
  - Water-soluble contrast injected into defunctioned distal bowel stoma under gentle pressure (inflate catheter balloon).
  - Lateral view demonstrates any fistulous connection with urethra, bladder or vagina requiring dissection and surgical division.

MRI

- Demonstrates anatomy and integrity of pelvic musculature and anal sphincter.
- Demonstrates associated spinal dysraphism.

Differential diagnosis

Other causes of neonatal distal bowel obstruction (ileal atresia, meconium ileus, functional colonic obstruction, Hirschprung's disease), cloacal exstrophy.

Management and prognosis

High and intermediate lesions are treated with colostomy and delayed definitive repair including deep perineal exploration. Low lesions are repaired by anoplasty and avoid colostomy. Faecal and urinary continence may be affected, and sexual function. Overall prognosis partly dependent on associated congenital abnormalities.

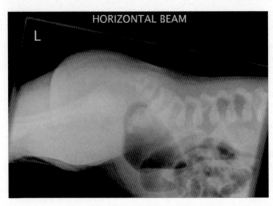

Fig. 3.1 Invertogram taken at 24 hours of age in a male infant with a high lesion.

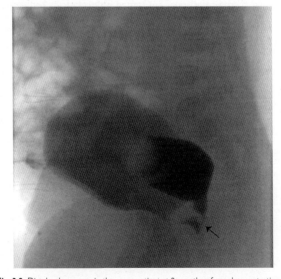

Fig. 3.2 Distal colonogram in the same patient at 2 months of age demonstrating fistula between the distal colon and posterior urethra (arrow), with retrograde filling of the urinary bladder.

Duodenal atresia and duodenal stenosis

Most common cause of upper GI obstruction in a neonate. Both thought to be caused by failure of vacuolization/re-canalization of the duodenum during gut development. Alternative theory is inadequate endodermal proliferation. Atresia/stenosis usually located in second or third part of duodenum. Often antenatally detected: dilated stomach and proximal duodenum on U/S + polyhydramnios in 40%.

Clinical presentation

Within several hours of birth with vomiting, bile-stained in 85% (obstruction distal to ampulla of Vater). Similar presentation to midgut malrotation and volvulus.

Associations: 30% of patients with duodenal atresia have Down's syndrome, 28% have midgut malrotation. Other abnormalities found in 50%: other intestinal atresias, CHD, abnormalities of situs, ARM, renal, gallbladder and biliary abnormalities.

All intrinsic duodenal abnormalities are associated with ↑ incidence of annular pancreas (33%) and pre-duodenal portal vein.

Imaging findings

Radiographic signs

- Characteristic 'double-bubble' appearance: dilated gas-filled stomach and proximal duodenum.
- May not be apparent if NG tube *in situ*: inject air to confirm prior to radiograph.
- If there is distal gas on AXR, proceed to upper GI contrast study to confirm stenosis and exclude midgut malrotation + volvulus.

Differential diagnosis

Midgut malrotation + volvulus, duodenal web, enteric duplication cyst causing extrinsic duodenal compression.

Management and prognosis

Surgical repair: commonly duodeno-duodenostomy. Correction of dehydration and any electrolyte disturbance prior to surgery. Survival >90% with surgical correction.

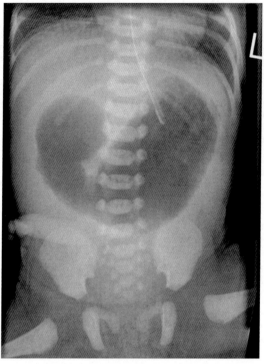

Fig. 3.3 Characteristic 'double-bubble' appearance in a neonate with duodenal atresia.

Duodenal web

Intrinsic duodenal obstruction by a web-like diaphragm located in second to third part of duodenum. The diaphragm usually has a central aperture ranging in size from pinhole to larger, allowing passage of bowel contents and gas, but in doing so the diaphragm becomes stretched like a windsock, projecting distally within the duodenal lumen.

Clinical presentation: high-grade or complete obstruction presents early within hours or days of birth (+ may be detected antenatally). Lesser degrees of obstruction may present later in infancy, childhood or even adulthood. Vomiting is bile-stained in 85%. Later presentation with variable symptoms: vomiting, food intolerance, dehydration, electrolyte and acid-base disturbance, GOR, pancreatitis, abdominal pain.

Associations: 30% have Down's syndrome. 28% have midgut malrotation. ↑ Incidence of other intestinal atresias, CHD, pyloric stenosis, VATER association, biliary abnormalities.

All intrinsic duodenal abnormalities are associated with ↑ incidence of annular pancreas (33%) and pre-duodenal portal vein.

Imaging findings

Radiographic signs

- High-grade obstruction: 'double-bubble' appearance.
- AXR may be normal if mild narrowing.

Fluoroscopy

- Dilated stomach and proximal duodenum.
- Intrinsic duodenal web may be seen:
  - Slight indentation in duodenal contour at attachment.
  - Circumferential membrane or diaphragm.
  - Redundant membrane ballooned like a windsock.

Differential diagnosis

Midgut malrotation + volvulus, duodenal atresia or stenosis, enteric duplication cyst causing extrinsic duodenal compression.

Management and prognosis

Surgical repair: duodeno-duodenostomy for complete obstruction, resection of web. Correction of dehydration and any electrolyte disturbance prior to surgery. Excellent prognosis following correction.

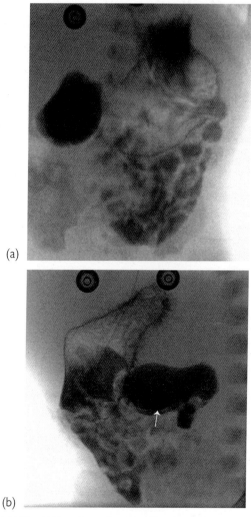

(a)

(b)

Fig. 3.4 (a) AP and (b) lateral images from upper GI contrast study in a neonate with a duodenal web. There is proximal duodenal dilatation and a thin membrane (arrow) with windsock configuration within the dilated duodenum on the lateral view creating a double-lumen.

Enteric duplication cysts

Congenital cystic mass related to the bowel with smooth muscle wall, and epithelial lining of alimentary tract mucosa. May secrete alimentary tract substances. 50–60% contain gastric mucosa or pancreatic tissue. Usually integrated within gut wall, rarely communicate with the true gut lumen. Can be located anywhere from tongue to anus. Frequency: ileum> oesophagus > colon > jejunum > stomach > duodenum > rectum. 75% abdominal, 20% thoracic, 5% thoraco-abdominal. Synchronous lesions occur in 10–20%. Tubular duplications may extend above and below the diaphragm.

Often incidental finding on antenatal or postnatal ultrasound (US). Most present in childhood. May become symptomatic due to compressive effects on adjacent structures, e.g. airway. Can enlarge with haemorrhage or cyst infection.

Complications: ulceration and bleeding (especially if contain ectopic gastric mucosa), volvulus, small bowel obstruction, rupture. Imaging modality depends on location.

Imaging findings

Fluoroscopy

● Extrinsic impression upon contrast-filled bowel.
● Rarely contrast may enter cyst if it communicates with gut lumen.

Ultrasound

● Unilocular cyst with well-defined double-layered wall:
  • Echogenic internal layer: mucosa.
  • Hypoechoic outer layer: muscle wall.
● Layered echogenic debris within cyst.
● Calcification within cyst wall rare.

CT

● Well-defined cystic lesion with relatively thick enhancing wall.
● Debris: fluid levels may be seen.

MR Imaging

● Findings as for CT but useful for defining intraspinal extension and vertebral abnormalities in neurenteric cysts.

Differential diagnosis

Mesenteric cyst, lymphatic malformation, ovarian cyst or teratoma, urachal cyst, choledochal cyst, hydrometrocolpos. In oral cavity: ranula, thyroglossal cyst or lingual thyroid, haemangioma, dermoid cyst.

Management and prognosis

Surgical resection. Generally good prognosis if uncomplicated.

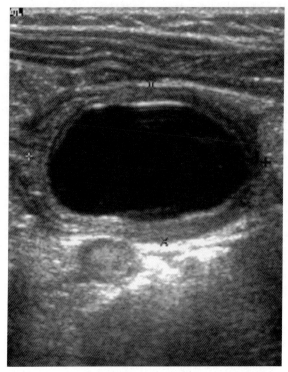

Fig. 3.5 Ultrasound of a small bowel duplication cyst showing the double-layered wall.

Hirschprung's disease (HD)

Absence of ganglion cells in part of, or the entire colonic wall resulting in a state of permanent contraction and bowel obstruction. Disease is continuous extending from the anus proximally. ♂>♀ 4:1. Uncommon in premature infants. 8–10% of cases are familial. Associations: Down's syndrome (in 15–20% of patients with Hirschprung's disease), congenital heart disease (CHD), genitourinary (GU) abnormalities, congenital deafness, central hypoventilation syndrome, ileal atresia. Classified according to transition between affected aganglionic and normal ganglionic bowel: 70–80% **short segment**: rectosigmoid involved; 15–25% **long segment**: transition above the rectosigmoid; **total colonic**: transition usually in distal ileum; **ultra-short segment**: transition at anorectal verge (very rare); **total intestinal aganglionosis** (very rare).

Clinical presentation

90% diagnosed in newborn period usually with failure to pass meconium by 24–48hrs, abdominal distension and bowel dilatation ± bilious vomiting. Late presentation with constipation since birth. At any age can present with Hirschprung's associated enterocolitis even after treatment.

▶ Enema can suggest Hirschprung's disease, but definitive diagnosis made by rectal biopsy showing absence of ganglion cells on acetylcholinesterase staining.

Imaging findings

Radiographic signs
- Multiple loops of distended bowel.
- Paucity of rectal gas.

Fluoroscopy
❶ Enema contraindicated in symptomatic acute colitis.
- Water-soluble contrast enema: neonates.
- Barium enema: infants and older children.
- Early lateral and AP views of rectosigmoid essential.
  - Rectum smaller than sigmoid (R/S ratio <1).
  - Transition zone from abnormally small affected colon to normally innervated dilated proximal colon.
  - Total colonic aganglionosis → microcolon.
  - May be normal in very short segment Hirschprung's Disease (HD) or delayed cases.
  - Spasm of affected colon → serrated/'sawtooth' mucosal pattern.
  - Associated colitis → colon thickened and ulcerated.

Differential diagnosis

With microcolon: meconium ileus, ileal atresia, small calibre colon associated with prematurity, colonic atresia.
No microcolon: neonatal functional colonic obstruction (meconium plug syndrome/small left colon syndrome), midgut volvulus, allergic colitis (milk allergy).

Management and prognosis

Surgical resection of affected colon. Frequently defunctioning colostomy performed with delayed definitive procedure. If untreated can lead to toxic megacolon, sepsis and death. 90% satisfactory outcome after treatment, although increased incidence of constipation and incontinence following surgery.

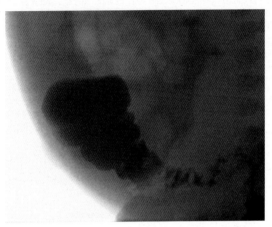

Fig. 3.6 Neonatal enema showing spasm and 'sawtooth' appearance of the rectum and sigmoid with dilated bowel proximally.

Jejunal and ileal atresia

Congenital absence or occlusion of the small bowel lumen. Stenotic segments may occur and there may be multiple atresias. The level of the most proximal atresia determines the level of bowel obstruction: jejunum → proximal obstruction; mid-distal ileum → distal obstruction. Aetiology uncertain. May be 2° to *in-utero* vascular ischaemic insult. There are rare hereditary forms associated with multiple atresias and prematurity. Abnormalities may be detected antenatally: dilated, echogenic bowel loops on U/S, ± signs of meconium peritonitis.

Clinical presentation

Within first few days of life. Early presentation with high atresia: bile-stained vomiting. Distal atresia: abdominal distension, failure to pass meconium and bile-stained vomiting.

Associations: other abnormalities found overall in 10%. Malrotation, volvulus, omphalocele, gastroschisis, meconium ileus; rarely total colonic aganglionosis, ARM, biliary atresia. Higher incidence of associated anomalies in jejunal atresia compared with ileal atresia. Potential complications: short gut, gut dysmotility, functional obstruction.

Imaging findings

Radiographic signs

- Dilated loops of bowel: number of dilated loops determines level of obstruction.
- Few loops = proximal (jejunal) obstruction.
- Multiple loops = distal (ileal or colonic) obstruction.
- ± Signs of perforation.
- ± Evidence of meconium peritonitis.

Fluoroscopy

- In cases of distal bowel obstruction: water-soluble contrast enema often helpful to determine likely cause prior to surgery.
- Microcolon:
  - Distal ileal atresia ± reflux of contrast into blind-ending distal ileum.
  - Meconium ileus.
  - Total colonic aganglionosis.
- Normal or almost normal calibre colon:
  - Jejunal and proximal ileal atresia.
  - Late *in-utero* midgut volvulus.
  - Ileal duplication cyst causing extrinsic compression.

▶ If enema normal in cases of presumed distal obstruction may need to exclude midgut volvulus with upper GI contrast study.

Differential diagnosis

Other causes of distal bowel obstruction: meconium ileus, neonatal functional colonic obstruction, Hirschprung's disease.

Management and prognosis

Surgical resection of affected bowel and very dilated segments. Correction of dehydration and any electrolyte disturbance prior to surgery. Prognosis depends on amount of functional residual bowel and presence of associated abnormalities.

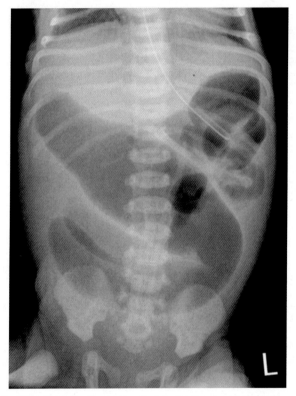

Fig. 3.7 AXR of a neonate presenting with abdominal distension and bilious vomiting on day 2 of life. There are multiple loops of dilated bowel. Uncomplicated ileal atresia was found at laparotomy.

Meckel's diverticulum

Persistent remnant of the vitellointestinal duct, usually found within 2 feet of the ileocaecal valve. Wall consists of same layers as adjacent small bowel. May contain ectopic gastric or pancreatic tissue. Variable size, typically 5–6cm (2 inches). Population incidence 2 %, ♂=♀. A small percentage become symptomatic. Symptoms may occur at any age but most <2yrs. Complications: ulceration of gastric mucosal tissue → pain, bleeding or perforation (rare), intussusception (acts as lead point), volvulus or torsion.

Clinical presentation

GI blood loss (may be occult/chronic, or acute frank blood loss per rectum (p.r.), intermittent abdominal pain, small bowel obstruction, abdominal mass.

Imaging findings

Radiographic signs

- AXR usually normal.
- May show right lower quadrant (RLQ) mass, displacement of bowel loops or obstruction.
- Diverticula occasionally contain enteroliths (mimicking appendicitis).

Ultrasound

- Thick-walled tubular structure.
- Heterogeneous mass in the right iliac fossa (RIF) mimicking appendicitis.
- May be hyperaemic 2° to inflammation.
- Rarely cystic appearance due to secretions from ectopic mucosa.

Fluoroscopy

- Lumen can fill with contrast.
- Indirect evidence of mass and inflammatory changes in adjacent bowel.

CT

- Mimics appendicitis.
- Thick walled blind ending tubular structure near caecum.
- Inflammatory changes in surrounding mesentery.
- Abscess or free air following perforation.

Radioisotope studies

▶ ^{99m}Tc pertechnetate scan is most specific test for detection of ectopic gastric mucosa within Meckel's diverticulum.

- Pertechnetate accumulates in mucus secreting cells (not parietal cells).
- Uptake parallels that of gastric mucosa in the stomach, increased conspicuity with time.
- Commonly seen in the RIF.
- No movement of radioisotope with peristalsis unless active bleeding.

▶ False positive pertechnetate scan: ectopic gastric mucosa in duplication cyst, renal excretion mimicking focal ectopic uptake, appendicitis or IBD may accumulate tracer 2° to hyperaemia.

▶ False negative pertechnetate scan: lack of sufficient gastric mucosa to localize isotope, uptake obscured by isotope in bladder from renal excretion (minimize by lateral image or emptying bladder).

Differential diagnosis

Appendicitis and other inflammatory processes such as IBD, enteric duplication cyst containing ectopic gastric mucosa, bleeding from enteric vascular malformation.

Management

Surgical resection, including those found incidentally on imaging or at laparotomy (appendicectomy also usually performed).

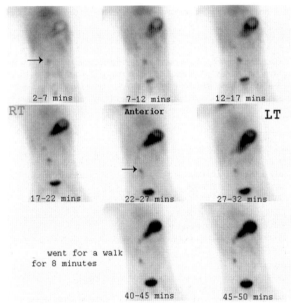

Fig. 3.8 ^{99m}Tc pertechnetate scan demonstrating uptake in ectopic gastric mucosa of a Meckel's diverticulum in the right iliac fossa (arrows). The activity parallels that in the normal gastric mucosa.

Meconium ileus

Distal small bowel obstruction in neonates due to impaction of abnormally thick, tenacious meconium in the distal ileum. Almost always associated with CF. Primary presentation in ~15% of patients with CF, associated with poorer lung disease outcomes and ↓ survival. Diagnosis can be suggested antenatally by dilated echogenic bowel on U/S, or pseudocyst.

Clinical presentation

Usually <24hrs of age with bilious vomiting, abdominal distension and failure to pass meconium.

Complications: volvulus, intestinal atresia, perforation with meconium peritonitis or pseudocyst formation.

▶ Water-soluble contrast enema often therapeutic in uncomplicated cases, need to reach dilated loops of bowel proximal to the obstruction. May need repeating if incomplete response. ❶ Risk of perforation (up to 3%). Indications for surgery: clinical deterioration, failure of therapeutic enema, perforation.

✒ Gastrograffin (meglumine diatrizoate) is hyperosmolar so draws water into the gut even when dilute. Can result in large fluid shifts and ↑ morbidity. Most radiologists favour other water-soluble agents for enema.

▶ All infants with meconium ileus require testing for CF.

Imaging findings

Radiographic signs

Uncomplicated meconium ileus
- Multiple dilated gas-filled bowel loops of bowel ≈ low obstruction.
- May be mottled lucencies in the RLQ due to impacted meconium 'soap bubble' appearance.
- Paucity of air–fluid levels due to viscid meconium is suggestive.

Complicated meconium ileus
- Soft tissue mass or gasless abdomen.
- Speckled or curvilinear calcification on peritoneal surface or within pseudocyst.

Ultrasound
- Multiple dilated, echogenic, thick-walled bowel loops.
- Ascites following volvulus or perforation.
- Peritoneal calcification or pseudocyst mass following perforation.

Fluoroscopy
- Microcolon (underused as succus entericus has not reached colon).
- Meconium pellets (tubular filling defects) in small calibre terminal ileum.
- Dilated bowel proximally.

Differential diagnosis

With microcolon: ileal atresia and total colonic aganglionosis.
Without microcolon: neonatal functional colonic obstruction.

Management and prognosis

Prognosis poor without relief of obstruction. Failure rate of enema 30–40% → laparotomy + enterotomy and removal of obstructing meconium.

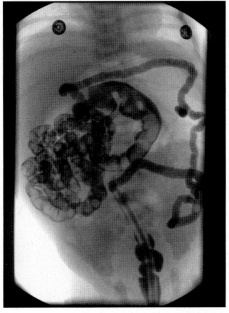

Fig. 3.9 Meconium ileus. Neonatal enema showing a microcolon and inspissated meconium plugs in the distal ileum.

Meconium peritonitis

Sterile chemical peritonitis following *in-utero* bowel perforation and peritoneal contamination with meconium. On entering the peritoneum, a foreign body inflammatory reaction is elicited within 24hrs. Most common sequel of healed meconium peritonitis (86% of cases) is the presence of scattered calcified peritoneal plaques on AXR, either focal or diffuse. Meconium reaching the scrotum via a patent processus vaginalis can cause a sterile inflammation of the paratesticular tissues. Subsequent fibrosis and calcification may mimic a testicular or paratesticular tumour. If the bowel perforation does not heal and meconium continues to spill into the peritoneal cavity, a meconium *pseudocyst* forms. Depending on its size this can cause mass effect on the bowel (→ obstruction) and other structures. May be detected or suspected antenatally.

Clinical presentation

Signs may be detected on antenatal or post-natal imaging: peritoneal calcification, ascites, abdominal mass (pseudocyst), bowel obstruction.

Associated abnormalities: meconium ileus, bowel atresia, bowel obstruction, *in utero*-volvulus, intrauterine vascular insufficiency of unknown cause.

Imaging findings

Radiographic signs
- Linear, curvilinear or punctate peritoneal calcification.
- Soft tissue mass (pseudocyst).
- Ascites.
- Dilated bowel loops.

Ultrasound
- Punctate echogenic foci ± acoustic shadowing.
- Dilated bowel loops.
- ± Ascites.
- ± Heterogeneous soft tissue mass (pseudocyst), may have calcified wall.

Fluoroscopy
- Upper GI contrast study: may be normal or show malrotation.
- Enema may show normal calibre or microcolon.

Differential diagnosis

CF with meconium ileus; viral infection (CMV, parvovirus B19) causing atresia or perforation; intrauterine vascular insufficiency associated with mechanical obstruction 2° to atresia, volvulus, intussusception, mesenteric hernia or congenital peritoneal (Ladd's) bands.

Management

Surgical management of pseudocyst and associated conditions.

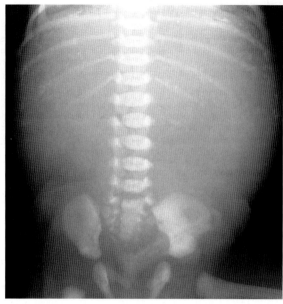

Fig. 3.10 AXR of a neonate showing a distended, gasless abdomen with punctate peritoneal calcification. The underlying diagnosis was meconium ileus and CF.

Mesenteric and omental cysts

Also known as mesenteric lymphatic malformations. Rare congenital malformations of the lymphatic system usually found in the small bowel mesentery (60%), less commonly in the colonic mesentery or omentum. Most present <5yrs of age. Size ranges from <1cm to 40cm. Jejunal cysts contain chylous fluid; ileal and colonic cysts contain serous fluid.

Clinical presentation

Abdominal distension (most common) ± pain, abdominal pain, vomiting.

Complications: small bowel obstruction, torsion, infection, haemorrhage or rupture. May mimic other acute abdominal pathology, e.g. appendicitis. Rarely obstruct the biliary system or renal tract.

Imaging findings

Radiographic signs

- AXR often normal.
- May show soft tissue mass, displacement of bowel loops or obstruction.

Ultrasound

- Predominantly anechoic, well-defined cyst.
- ± Thin septations: may be multiple.
- ± Smaller internal cysts.
- ± Debris or fluid–fluid levels.

CT

- Well-defined cyst: variable attenuation depending on content, e.g. chyle containing fat, haemorrhage, infected cysts etc.
- ± Thin septations: not as well demonstrated as on US.
- ± Smaller internal cysts.
- ± Debris, fluid–fluid levels, fat–fluid levels.
- Wall enhancement if inflamed.
- Rarely calcification in the wall.

MR Imaging

- Hypointense on T1-WI, hyperintense on T2-WI.
- Haemorrhage or fat can → T1 and T2 hyperintensity.
- Septations and internal cysts better seen.

▶ Large cysts displace bowel, dependent on location. Omental cysts are anteriorly located and displace the bowel posteriorly.

Differential diagnosis

Duplication cyst, ovarian cyst, pancreatic pseudocyst, localized fluid collection or abscess.

Management

Open or laparoscopic enucleation or marsupialization of cyst. Bowel resection may be required.

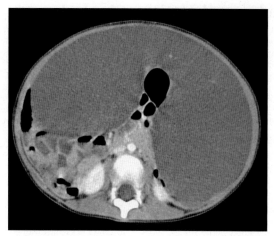

Fig. 3.11 Two-year-old child with abdominal distension. Enhanced CT scan showing large, anteriorly located omental cyst, with posterior displacement of bowel.

Midgut malrotation and volvulus

Malrotation is a general term used to describe the anatomical situation when the normal process of embryonic gut rotation, positioning and fixation is arrested or altered at any stage. Malrotated gut has a short mesenteric base and propensity to twist/volve about its mesentery causing interruption of its blood supply which may → infarction of extensive amounts of gut. Volvulus can be intermittent but renders the entire small bowel at risk of ischaemia and necrosis. Incidence ~ 1/500 live births, ♂ slightly >♀. Symptoms can occur at any age. Most present in the first week of life, up to 80% in the first month of life. Malrotated gut is also prone to obstruction by congenital bands of fibrous tissue (Ladd's bands) traversing the bowel externally, usually extending from the caecum or ascending colon to the right upper quadrant (RUQ) and duodenum.

Clinical presentation

Bile-stained vomiting in most patients 2° to obstruction distal to the ampulla of Vater, due to associated volvulus or obstruction by Ladd's bands. Volvulus may present as acute abdomen (abdominal distension, bloody stools, peritonitis and shock 2° to bowel ischaemia) with poorer prognosis.

Atypical presentations: intermittent abdominal pain or vomiting, constipation, diarrhoea, malabsorption, failure to thrive (FTT). Children outside the neonatal period and even adults may have insidious presentation with chronic symptoms lasting from weeks to years. Occasionally incidental finding during GI contrast study or laparotomy for another reason.

Associations: expected finding in patients with exomphalos, gastroschisis and congenital diaphragmatic hernia with low incidence of volvulus. Other congenital malformations including small bowel atresias, cloacal extrophy, heterotaxy syndromes, Down's syndrome.

▶▶ A diagnosis of malrotation and volvulus must be considered in a child of any age with bile-stained vomiting.

Imaging findings

Radiographic signs

- AXR usually normal.
- Relative distension of the stomach and proximal duodenum.
- Proximal small bowel in the RUQ.
- Dilatation of multiple bowel loops may indicate volvulus + bowel ischaemia.

Ultrasound

- Abnormal relationship of superior mesenteric artery (SMA) superior mesenteric vein (SMV):
  • SMV may be anterior or to the left of the SMA.
  • Often obscured by gas so cannot be assessed.
- 'Whirlpool sign': swirling of bowel about the mesenteric vessels.

❶ US is not accurate enough to be the primary test for malrotation or volvulus in the acute situation.

Fluoroscopy
- Upper GI contrast study is imaging modality of choice.
- Diagnosis based on abnormal position of duodeno-jejunal flexure (DJF).

▶ The normal DJF is located to the left of the left spinal pedicle, at the level of the duodenal bulb or higher, on AP view. On lateral view duodenum typically courses posteriorly then inferiorly.
- Malrotation is not a single distinct entity with identical anatomical features in all patients.
- DJF abnormality may be low, midline, to right of the spine, unable to determine position, proximal bowel in right side of abdomen.
- On lateral view duodenum may not take initial posterior course.
- Signs of volvulus:
  - Spiral/'corkscrew' configuration of proximal bowel.
  - Proximal duodenal obstruction: usually second part.
- Pitfalls:
  - Rarely DJF position may appear normal with malrotation ± volvulus.
  - 'Normal variants': duodenum inversum, redundant duodenum or mobile DJF.

▶ Contrast enema may show abnormally positioned caecum or colon: not reliable for 1° diagnosis.

CT
- Abnormal relationship of SMA/SMV.
- ± Swirling of bowel about the mesenteric vessels.
- ± Bowel distension, pneumatosis, free intraperitoneal gas or fluid.

Differential diagnosis

Bilious vomiting: duodenal stenosis or atresia, proximal jejunal atresia, severe GOR, ileus 2° to electrolyte imbalance, GI infection.

Management and prognosis

Ladd's procedure: de-rotation of bowel volvulus, resection of ischaemic non-viable bowel if present and division of obstructing peritoneal bands. Division of ligament of Treitz, duodenum straightened and bowel placed in a position of 'non-rotation' (small bowel on the right side and large bowel predominantly on the left). Prognosis dependent on amount of residual viable gut. Increased morbidity and mortality with bowel necrosis and hypovolaemic shock.

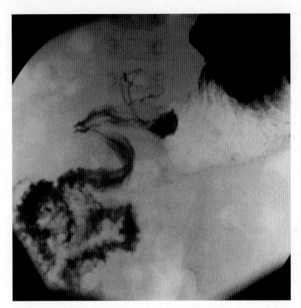

Fig. 3.12 Upper GI contrast study showing malrotation with volvulus. The duodenum and proximal jejunum is in the RUQ with a spiral/corkscrew configuration of the duodenum/proximal small bowel.

Neonatal functional colonic obstruction

Common cause of distal bowel obstruction in neonates 2° to transient colonic inertia with failure of normal peristalsis in normally innervated colon. Includes *meconium plug syndrome* and *small left colon syndrome*, but completely distinct from meconium ileus. No histological or surgical abnormality. Incidence: ♂=♀. Aetiology uncertain, but may be 2° to immaturity of ganglion cells or hormone receptors.

Associations: maternal diabetes, prematurity, sepsis, traumatic delivery, antenatal administration of magnesium sulphate (for pre-eclampsia) and psychotropic drugs.

Clinical presentation

Within 1-2 days of birth with abdominal distension, failure to pass meconium and occasionally bilious vomiting in otherwise well neonate.

▶ Imaging modality of choice is water-soluble contrast enema, procedure often hastens recovery.

Imaging findings

Radiographic signs

- Multiple dilated gas-filled bowel loops of bowel ≈ low obstruction.

▶ Non-specific signs. It is not possible to differentiate dilated large from small bowel in neonates on AXR, regardless of position.

Differential diagnosis

Hirschsprung's disease, meconium ileus, ileal atresia, immature colon associated with prematurity, colonic atresia (rare).

Fluoroscopy

- Rectum > sigmoid (rectosigmoid ratio >1).
- Reduced calibre descending and sigmoid colon.
- Abrupt change to normal or increased calibre at splenic flexure.
- ± Multiple filling defects (meconium plugs) particularly in left colon.
- Passage of meconium plugs during or soon after study.

Differential diagnosis

Long segment Hirschsprung's disease.

Management and prognosis

Excellent prognosis with conservative management. Repeat contrast enemas may be required. Potential risk of fluid shifts, electrolyte imbalance and perforation with contrast studies.

▶ Suction rectal biopsy performed to exclude long segment Hirschsprung's disease, especially if prolonged symptoms.

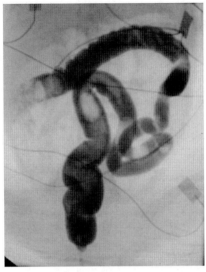

Fig. 3.13 Pre-term neonate with bowel obstruction. Contrast enema showing plugs of meconium in a normal calibre colon.

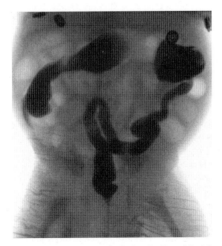

Fig. 3.14 Neonatal contrast enema showing reduced calibre of the left colon with abrupt transition to normal calibre at the splenic flexure. The patient was an infant of a diabetic mother.

Oesophageal atresia (OA) and tracheo-oesophageal fistula (TOF)

Spectrum of abnormalities. Aetiology uncertain, primitive foregut is a common channel in the embryo and forms both trachea and oesophagus. Postulated abnormal division in first month of embryonic life. Incidence 2.4/10 000 births, usually sporadic.

Five main types according to atretic portion and location of fistula:
- Type A: OA with proximal atretic pouch and distal TOF (82%).
- Type B: Pure OA without TOF (9%).
- Type C: Isolated TOF (H-type) without OA (6%).
- Type D: OA with proximal and distal TOF (2%).
- Type E: OA with proximal TOF and distal atretic pouch (1%) – see Figs 3.15–3.17.

Clinical presentation

Antenatal US diagnosis: polyhydramnios, small or non-visualized stomach, dilated upper pouch. Postnatally: excess oral secretions, choking, cyanosis (especially with feed), abdominal distension (with H-type and distal TOF only). H-type usually presents later: recurrent chest infections. Location of fistula usually C7–T2.

Associations: other atresias, cardiac, renal, limb and spinal abnormalities. Often part of VATER and VACTERL associations. Need renal and cardiac US, spinal radiograph (CXR and AXR usually suffice). Many have tracheo-malacia ('TOF cough'), possibly due to antenatal compressive effect of dilated pouch on trachea.

▶ Diagnosis made clinically + CXR/AXR. H-type TOF diagnosis from contrast oesophagram (supine oblique, lateral or prone).

Imaging findings

Radiographic signs
- Gas in dilated upper oesophageal pouch +/–tip of enteral tube.
- + Gas in distal bowel with TOF.
- Gasless distal bowel if no TOF.
- ± Vertebral abnormalities, cardiac abnormalities, evidence of distal bowel atresia.

❶ Note side of aortic arch: thoracotomy for repair done on opposite side. 5% have right-sided aortic arch (AA).

Fluoroscopy
Pre-operative imaging
- Contrast oesophagram to detect H-type TOF.
- Contrast studies in pure OA to determine length of gap.

Post-operative imaging
- Early contrast study: identify leaks and recurrent fistula before feeding.
- Later contrast studies:
  - Identify anastomotic strictures (related to technique, ischemia and GOR) and recurrent fistula.
  - Dysmotility 2° to surgical manipulation and vagal disruption in most.
  - High incidence of GOR.

Differential diagnosis

OA: traumatic oesophageal perforation with enteral tube, laryngotracheal cleft with high fistulous connection. H-type TOF: GOR with aspiration, aspirated FB, CF, immunodeficiency, congenital lung lesion.

Management and prognosis

Surgical repair in first few days of life, except pure OA which has delayed repair following gastrostomy insertion for feeding. Long-gap OA may require delayed repair, gastric 'pull-up' or oesophageal substitution (e.g. jejunal interposition) depending on length of gap. Long term post-surgical issues: recurrent fistula in up to 10%; recurrent post-op anastamotic/ oesophageal strictures require dilatation. Post-operative survival 75–95% but dependent on other associated abnormalities, especially cardiac.

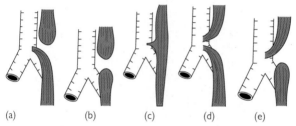

(a)   (b)   (c)   (d)   (e)

Fig. 3.15 Types of OA and TOF.

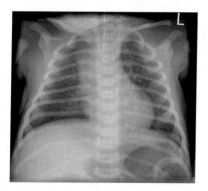

Fig. 3.16 OA with replogle tube in upper oesophageal pouch. Gas in the stomach and proximal bowel indicates the presence of a TOF.

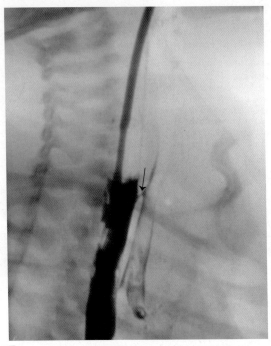

Fig. 3.17 Contrast oesophagram showing isolated H-type TOF (arrow) in an infant with recurrent chest infections.

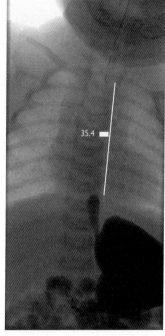

Fig. 3.18 Fluoroscopic study to assess length of the gap between the proximal and distal oesophagus in pure OA, prior to repair. Contrast has been introduced via the gastrostomy and refluxes into the distal oesophagus. Note the replogle tube in proximal oesophageal pouch.

Appendicitis

Acute inflammation of the appendix 2° to obstruction of the appendicular lumen → distention → ischaemia + superimposed bacterial overgrowth → perforation. ↑ Morbidity with perforation. Most frequent indication for abdominal surgery in children. Average age: late teens to early twenties but can affect any age group. ♂slightly>♀.

Most common presentation: RLQ pain (pain may begin in peri-umbilical region and migrate to RLQ) associated with nausea, vomiting and anorexia, ↑ white cell count (WCC), and inflammatory markers. Often non-specific signs in younger children, can lead to delayed diagnosis and ↑ rate of perforation.

▶ Primarily a clinical diagnosis. Imaging aids diagnosis in atypical cases or with non-specific symptoms and signs. Can lead to earlier diagnosis and also useful in differentiating between other causes of RIF pain, e.g. ovarian pathology, mesenteric adenitis.

Imaging findings

Radiographic signs
● Calcified appendicolith is specific and diagnostic.

Other signs may be associated:
● RLQ mass.
● Bowel dilatation due to ileus or rarely small bowel (SB) obstruction.
● Free intraperitoneal air rare.

Ultrasound
● Distended, non-compressible, fluid filled tubular structure >6mm diameter.
● Appendicolith + acoustic shadowing.
● Point/rebound tenderness using ultrasound probe.
● ± ↑ flow on colour Doppler.
● Free intraperitoneal fluid.
● Dilated fluid-filled bowel loops.
● 'Appendix mass' consisting of inflammatory tissue + matted bowel loops following perforation and sealing off by mesentery.
● Abscess may form after perforation.

CT
● Calcified appendicolith may be seen.
● Distended fluid-filled appendix with wall thickening and enhancement.
● Peri-appendicular soft tissue stranding.
● Thickening and enhancement of the caecum and terminal ileum.

Other CT findings especially with perforation
● Enlargement of regional lymph nodes.
● Small bowel dilatation + fluid.
● Localized fluid collections.
● Free intraperitoneal fluid.

Differential diagnosis

Mesenteric adenitis, haemorrhagic ovarian cyst, ovarian torsion, Meckel's diverticulum, IBD, omental infarction.

Management and prognosis

Appendicectomy: open or laparoscopic. Conservative management + delayed appendicectomy if appendix mass formation. Continued clinical deterioration is indication for earlier surgery. Prognosis good with early diagnosis and surgery. ↑ Morbidity with delayed diagnosis and perforation, including post-operative complications such as pelvic abscess.

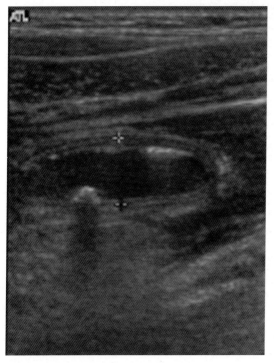

Fig. 3.19 Ultrasound of appendicitis. The inflamed appendix is a non-compressible, blind-ending tubular structure. This example contains small amounts of air which is echogenic with acoustic shadowing.

Necrotizing enterocolitis (NEC)

Idiopathic bowel disease usually affecting premature neonates (up to 90%), particularly <1000g. Aetiology: likely related to combination of infection and ischaemia, possibly as yet unidentified endotoxin or organism. Acute inflammation + mucosal ulceration → transmural necrosis. Location typically terminal ileum and right colon but any part of small or large bowel including stomach can be affected.

Risk factors: hypoxia, perinatal stress, birth asphyxia, congenital heart disease (esp. cyanotic), umbilical artery catheterization, maternal cocaine use, placental insufficiency. ↑ Incidence in enterally fed infants.

Clinical presentation

Abdominal distension, loose/bloody stools, feed intolerance, ↑ NG gastric aspirates (often bilious), generalized sepsis, bradycardia and apnoea, temperature instability, mild respiratory distress.

▶ Primarily a clinical diagnosis, AXR may be normal but done to support or confirm diagnosis and detect complications, especially perforation which is an indication for surgery.

Imaging findings

Radiographic signs

- Focal or generalized bowel dilatation (ileus).
- Separation of bowel loops.
- Fixed configuration of bowel loop(s) on serial AXR.
- Pneumatosis intestinalis: 'bubbly' (submucosal) or curvilinear (subserosal) lucencies (50–75% of patients).
- Gas in the portal venous system—branching lucencies over the liver.
- Pneumoperitoneum: perforation 2° to full thickness bowel necrosis: may require lateral decubitus or cross table lateral AXR to confirm.
- ± Ascites: central displacement of bowel loops ('floating').

Ultrasound

- Thickened bowel wall.
- Increased (inflamed) or decreased (necrotic) bowel wall vascularity.
- Ascites.
- Focal collection(s) of fluid.

Fluoroscopy

▶ contrast studies contraindicated in acute presentation. Used to detect strictures (occur in 10–20% of survivors).

Differential diagnosis

Bowel obstruction, non-specific gaseous distension of bowel.

Management and prognosis

Isolate and barrier nurse infant, stop all enteral feeds and commence iv fluids/parenteral nutrition (PN), iv antibiotics. Fulminant disease may require resuscitation with albumin/fluid bolus. Monitor with serial AXR. Involve surgeons in moderate–severe disease. Indications for surgery: perforation, progressive clinical deterioration despite resuscitation and conservative management. Prognosis: overall mortality 20–30%. (<1500g 10–44%, >2500g 0–20%).

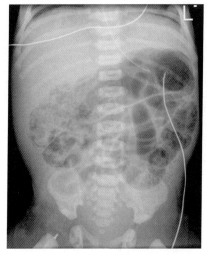

Fig. 3.20 Multiple loops of distended bowel and extensive pneumatosis in a term neonate with congenital cardiac disease and NEC.

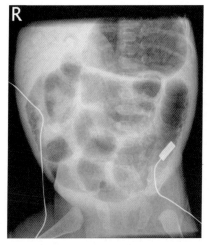

Fig. 3.21 Pre-term neonate with NEC. In addition to gastric and bowel dilatation with widespread pneumatosis, there is extensive portal gas.

Crohn's disease

Chronic, idiopathic, recurrent, granulomatous (non-caseating) inflammatory bowel disease characterized by segmental transmural inflammation and 'skip' lesions. AKA *regional enteritis*. May affect any part of the alimentary tract from mouth to anus, terminal ileum affected in 95% of cases. 25% of cases occur in childhood but peak incidence from 18–25 years, with smaller peak of incidence at 60–80 years. ♂=♀. Aetiology unknown but genetic, immunological, infective, environmental and psychologic factors implicated.

Clinical presentation

Variable. Most common symptoms and signs are recurrent diarrhoea, colicky abdominal pain, rectal bleeding, weight loss, malaise, anorexia, anaemia. Disease characterized by exacerbations and remissions with prolonged, unpredictable course. Other signs and symptoms: malabsorption 2° to interruption of enterohepatic bile salts in TI, erythema nodosum, pyoderma gangrenosum. Perianal/perirectal disease found in up to 80%.

Complications: fissures, sinus tracts, fistulas and abscesses, toxic megacolon, bowel strictures and obstruction, perforation, gallstones, sclerosing cholangitis, pancreatitis, ankylosing spondylitis, arthritis, oxalate urinary calculi, growth retardation.

Imaging findings

Ultrasound

- May demonstrate bowel wall thickening and abscesses.

Fluoroscopy

Early changes on barium studies

- Lymphoid hyperplasia: tiny, round uniform nodules/filling defects (lymphoid follicles) in the bowel wall.
- Shallow 'aphthous' ulcers.
- Cobblestone mucosal pattern: combined transverse and longitudinal ulceration.
- Thickened mucosal folds and featureless mucosa ('Moulage sign').
- Deep, fissuring ('rose-thorn') ulcers.
- Bowel wall thickening.

Late changes on barium studies

- Luminal narrowing and strictures: especially in the TI.
- Skip lesions.
- Sacculations (antimesenteric border) 2° to ↑ intraluminal pressure.
- Loss of haustration.
- Post-inflammatory pseudopolyps.
- Perianal/perirectal disease: ulcers, fissures, sinuses, stenosis.

CT

Similar findings to barium studies on enhanced scans, more sensitive for extramural/mesenteric disease and abscesses.

- Acute phase demonstrates mural stratification, 3-layered bowel wall:

- Inner ring: soft tissue density mucosa.
- Middle ring: low-density submucosal oedema and fat.
- Outer ring: soft tissue density muscularis propria and serosa.
- Target or double halo sign: intense enhancement of inner and outer ring with ↓ attenuation middle ring.
- Chronic phase: luminal narrowing and loss of mural stratification.
  - Homogeneous thickened bowel wall.
  - Enlarged mesenteric lymph nodes.
  - Mesenteric changes: fat opacification, abscesses, hypervascularity.
  - 'Vascular jejunization' of the ileum/the 'comb sign' = multiple tubular tortuous opacities on the mesenteric side of the ileum aligned like the teeth of a comb (= ↑flow in the vasa recta and fibro-fatty proliferation in the mesentery).
  - Fistulas and sinus tracts.

MRI
- Imaging modality of choice for perianal/perirectal disease.
- Also demonstrates extent and severity of bowel and mesenteric inflammatory changes.

Radioisotope studies
- ^{99m}Tc labelled white cell scans correlate well with disease activity.

Differential diagnosis
Ulcerative colitis, infectious colitis, appendicitis, mesenteric adenitis, lymphoma.

Management and prognosis
Depends on extent and severity of disease. Medical management: bowel rest, aminosalycilates, steroids, antibiotics, immunosuppressant drugs and antibody therapy. Surgical management: resection of affected bowel, strictureplasty, fistulotomy.

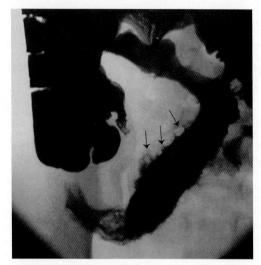

Fig. 3.22 Small bowel barium study demonstrating distal small bowel ulceration (arrows).

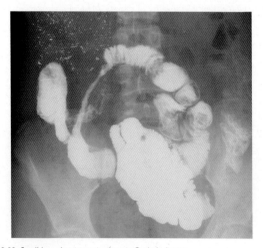

Fig. 3.23 Small bowel stricture in chronic Crohn's disease.

Ulcerative colitis (UC)

Chronic, idiopathic, recurrent inflammatory bowel disease primarily affecting the colorectal mucosa and submucosa. Affects the rectum and extends proximally to affect part of, or the entire colon. Inflammation primarily involves the mucosa and extends to involve the submucosa and muscularis, with crypt micro-abscesses. Uncommon in children, peak incidence 20–40 years. Smaller peak of incidence at 55–65 years. ♂<♀. Aetiology unknown but genetic, familial, immunological, infective, environmental, hormonal, vascular traumatic and psychologic factors implicated.

Clinical presentation

Most common symptoms and signs recurrent bloody mucus diarrhoea, rectal bleeding, tenesmus, fever, weight loss, crampy abdominal pain. Disease characterized by exacerbations and remissions. Other signs and symptoms: iritis, erythema nodosum, pyoderma gangrenosum, liver disease (primary sclerosing cholangitis, chronic active hepatitis, fatty liver, pericholangitis, cirrhosis), digital clubbing, arthritis and rheumatoid arthritis.

Complications: toxic megacolon, strictures, perforation, growth retardation in childhood, increased risk of colorectal carcinoma in long-term sufferers, annual increase of 10% after first decade of UC, 50% after 25 years.

Imaging findings

Radiographic signs

- Diffuse colonic dilatation.
- Colonic mural thickening ± mucosal oedema ('thumb-printing').
- Loss of colonic haustration.

Fluoroscopy

Acute changes on single or double contrast enema

- Colorectal spasm with incomplete filling.
- Fine granular mucosal pattern: oedema and hyperaemia.
- Mucosal ulceration: stippling and 'collar button' ulcers.
- Inflammatory polyps and post-inflammatory pseudopolyps.

Chronic changes on single or double contrast enema

- Colonic shortening.
- Narrowed and rigid 'lead-pipe' colon.
- Loss of colonic haustration.
- Benign strictures.
- Proctitis: reduced calibre and thickening or absence of rectal valves.
- Widened pre-sacral space (>1.5cm).
- ± 'Backwash ileitis' = involvement of the terminal ileum by inflammatory and ulcerative changes, may be featureless and dilated.

CT

- Colorectal luminal narrowing.
- Diffuse, symmetrical, continuous, concentric colonic wall thickening.
- Smooth contour of outer wall.

- Enhancing inner ring of mucosa and outer muscularis of bowel wall with non-enhancing oedematous middle layer of submucosa ('target' or 'halo' sign).
- Mural stratification: ability to distinguish layers of bowel wall.
- Widened pre-sacral space.

Radioisotope studies
- ^{99m}Tc-labelled white cell scan evaluates disease activity.

Differential diagnosis
Crohn's disease, pseudomembranous colitis, infectious colitis, typhlitis.

Management and prognosis
Depends on extent and severity of disease. Medical management: aminosalicylates, steroids, immunosuppressant drugs and leukotriene B4 inhibitors. Surgical management: proctocolectomy + ileostomy or ileal pouch formation.

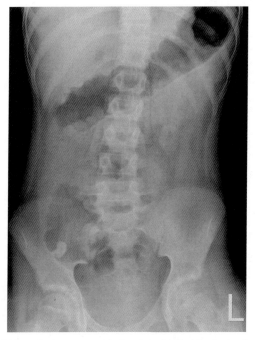

Fig. 3.24 Pan-colitis in a teenager with ulcerative colitis. The left colon is collapsed and empty. There is dilatation of the ascending and transverse colon which is thickened with 'thumbprinting'.

Achalasia

Abnormal motility and failure of relaxation of the distal oesophagus usually due to absence of the myenteric plexuses in the lower oesophagus. Can also occur 2° to vagus nerve damage. Rarely inherited as AR condition. Primarily a disorder of adults from third to fifth decades. Only 5% of all cases occur <14yrs of age, usually older children but any age can be affected. Rare associated syndrome of achalasia, alacrimia (↓ tear production) and ACTH resistant adrenocortical insufficiency = triple A syndrome/Allgrove's syndrome—AR inheritance.

Clinical presentation

Dysphagia, worse with solids, food regurgitated on pillow, aspiration, nocturnal cough or stridor.

▶ Early diagnosis may be made with oesophageal manometry.

Imaging findings

Radiographic signs

- CXR may show parenchymal changes 2° to aspiration.
- Air filled dilated oesophagus ± air–fluid level.
- Absent stomach gas bubble in 1/3.

Ultrasound

- Transoesophageal US: thickening of the circular and longitudinal muscle layers in lower oesophagus.
- Transabdominal US: dilated oesophagus containing fluid and debris.

Fluoroscopy

- Early achalasia:
  • Disordered motility.
- Later signs:
  • Disordered motility.
  • Dilated oesophagus with distal obstruction.
  • Tapering of contrast column and 'beaked' appearance.
  • Intra-oesophageal debris and air–fluid level.

Differential diagnosis

Pseudoachalasia: malignant infiltration of distal oesophagus causing obstruction simulating achalasia, occurs in adults.

Management and prognosis

Surgical: Heller's myotomy (open or endoscopic), division of circular muscle at the level of the gastro-oesophageal junction, following suction of any accumulated oesophageal debris endoscopically. Balloon dilatation carries ↑ risk of perforation. Pulmonary complications in up to 1/3, long term ↑ risk of oesophageal carcinoma affecting middle 1/3 of oesophagus.

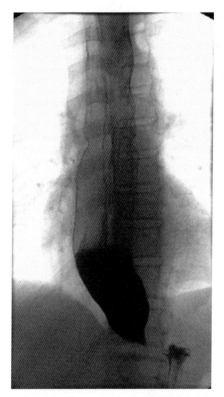

Fig. 3.25 Image from upper GI contrast study showing dilated oesophagus with an air–fluid level. There is characteristic tapering of the distal oesophagus with obstruction at the gastro-oesophageal junction.

Bezoar

Concretions of swallowed hair, fruit or vegetable fibres or similar substances found in the gastrointestinal tract, and conforming to the shape of the containing viscus. Usually found in the stomach or proximal small bowel but may extend or move into more distal bowel. Age at presentation: infancy to adolescence. ↑ Incidence with impaired gastric emptying, ↓ acid production. *Lactobezoar* = undigested milk curds; associated with incorrectly reconstituted milk formula. *Trichobezoar* = hair ball; ↑ incidence in childhood, ♀ patients, developmental delay or psychological/psychiatric illness, may be accompanying alopecia. *Phytobezoar* = fruit or vegetable matter; ↑ incidence post partial gastrectomy or gastrojejunostomy and with ↓ gastric motility.

Clinical presentation

Vomiting, abdominal distension, abdominal mass, anorexia, weight loss, halitosis.

Complications: obstruction, ulceration ± haematemesis, perforation.

Imaging findings

Radiographic signs

- Non-specific 'mottled' soft tissue density in stomach similar to undigested food.
- May be signs of intestinal obstruction.

Fluoroscopy

- Irregular filling defect in stomach or bowel outlined by contrast.
- Partial or complete obstruction.

Differential diagnosis

❶ Appearance mimics retained food: check when the patient last ate.

Management

Laparotomy + enterotomy to remove bezoar. Laparoscopic procedure or endoscopic removal. Conservative management may be tried but ↑ risk of complications with persisting bezoar.

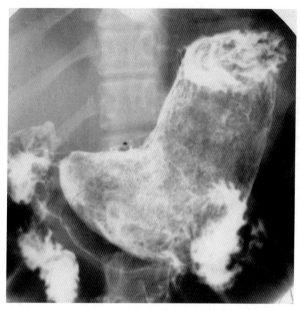

Fig. 3.26 Image from an upper GI contrast study in a patient with a large trichobezoar, which is outlined by barium.

Gastro-oesophageal reflux

Retrograde passage of gastric contents into the oesophagus. Can be considered a normal physiological phenomenon, occurring intermittently especially after meals. Most common presentation: effortless regurgitation, non-bilious vomiting (sometimes forceful), irritability, failure to thrive due to insufficient caloric intake. Less common presentations: wheeze, cough (due to reflux into the airway) and hoarseness. Can occur at any age but ↑ incidence <2yrs. Symptoms improve as toddlers become more upright. Complications: Oesophagitis (± stricture formation), pulmonary aspiration.

▶ The diagnosis is suspected from symptoms and usually prompts treatment without further investigation.

Indications for further investigation (upper GI endoscopy, pH studies or radiology): suspected alternative or predisposing condition (e.g. duodenal obstruction or midgut malrotation), failure to respond to medical management, to detect complications, atypical history, pre-operative assessment.

Imaging findings

Radiographic signs
- Usually normal.
- Hiatus hernia may be seen.

Ultrasound
- Retrograde passage of gastric contents into lower oesophagus may be seen but upper extent cannot be determined.

Fluoroscopy
- Often normal, without detection of reflux as this occurs intermittently.
- Reflux of contrast into oesophagus allowing assessment of proximal extent.
- Abnormal swallowing ± aspiration.
- Dysmotility: disordered peristalsis, delayed clearance of contrast, intra-oesophageal reflux (to and fro movement).
- Oesophageal stricture.
- Schatzki ring: narrow ring-like constriction in lower oesophagus.
- Hiatus hernia.

Radioisotope studies
- ^{99m}Tc sulphur colloid added to feed.
- Activity detected above level of gastro-oesophageal junction.
- Activity may be detected in lungs if aspiration occurring.

Differential diagnosis
Other causes of oesophagitis, pyloric stenosis, duodenal stenosis or web, antral/pyloric web, achalasia.

Management and prognosis

Medical management includes feed thickeners, antacids, drugs that ↓ gastric acid production. Approx 1% require surgical treatment with fundoplication.

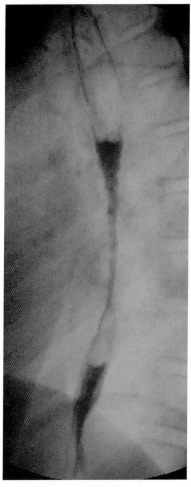

Fig. 3.27 Long narrow stricture of the distal oesophagus 2° to reflux in a child.

Pyloric stenosis

Thickening and hypertrophy of pyloric muscle occurring in early infancy, causing progressive gastric outlet obstruction. Incidence ~2/1000 live births. Unknown aetiology but may have genetic/familial basis as there is frequently positive family history. Other associations: erythromycin exposure, e.g. in breast milk, eosinophilic gastroenteritis, ↑ incidence in CF.

Clinical presentation

Usually with progressive non-bilious vomiting, characteristically projectile and weight loss. ♂>♀ (4–5:1), age 2–12 weeks. Later presentation in pre-term infants. Electrolyte disturbance: hypochloraemic alkalosis and dehydration may be present, exaggerated gastric peristaltic waves may be seen on abdominal inspection.

▶ Primarily a clinical diagnosis. Hypertrophied pylorus ('olive') is palpated in the upper abdomen during test feed. US used in equivocal cases or with atypical history. AXR and upper GI contrast studies should not be used routinely for diagnosis.

Imaging findings

Radiographic signs

- Distended stomach with paucity of bowel gas distally.
- Stomach may not be distended if recently vomited.

Ultrasound

- Elongated pyloric channel (>16mm).
- Thickened pyloric muscle (>3.5mm single wall thickness).
- Increased pyloric diameter (>12mm).
- Gastric hyperperistalsis.
- Failure of pyloric channel to open during dynamic examination.
- Echogenic mucosal layer may also look hypertrophied.

Fluoroscopy

- Distended stomach with hyperperistalsis.
- Narrow elongated pyloric channel ('string sign'/tram-track of contrast).
- Hypertrophied pyloric muscle indents duodenal bulb ('mushroom sign').
- ± GOR (often prominent).

Differential diagnosis

Transient pylorospasm (lacks muscle thickening but pyloric channel elongated), GOR, other causes of high intestinal obstruction, e.g. duodenal stenosis or web, annular pancreas, malrotation with midgut volvulus, choledochal cyst.

Management and prognosis

Correction of electrolyte imbalance and fluid resuscitation. Surgical pyloromyotomy: open or laparoscopic. Non-surgical treatment not widely used in the UK. Prognosis excellent following intervention.

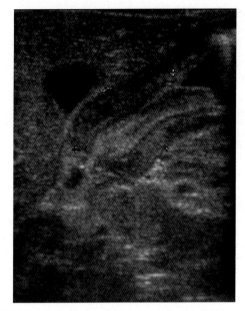

Fig. 3.28 Ultrasound showing elongated pyloric channel with thickened pyloric muscle layer.

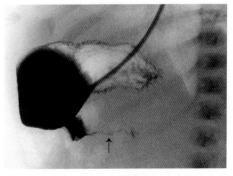

Fig. 3.29 Lateral image from upper GI contrast study showing narrow, elongated pyloric channel outlined by 'string' of contrast (arrow).

Intussusception

Occurs when a segment of bowel invaginates or telescopes into a contiguous segment distally. The proximal segment of bowel is called the *intussusceptum* and the distal segment of bowel the *intussuscipiens*. 90% of cases are idiopathic ileocolic intussusception = most common cause of small bowel obstruction in infant-toddler age group. Peak incidence 2 months–3 years, ↑ incidence in winter and spring with viral illnesses.

Atypical age at presentation should alert to the possibility of a pathological lead point, e.g. Meckel's diverticulum, duplication cyst, lymphoma. Other associations: Henoch–Schönlein purpura: haematoma in bowel wall acts as lead point, post-operatively jejunal or ileal (small bowel to small bowel) intussusception may occur – usually self limiting.

Clinical presentation

Usually abrupt onset intermittent abdominal pain, often associated with 'drawing-up' the knees, lethargy and pallor. Vomiting and diarrhoea may occur ± blood in the stools. *Redcurrant jelly* stools = mixture of stool, mucus and blood clot (late sign). Frequently preceding upper respiratory tract infection or gastroenteritis. Patients often dehydrated at presentation. Some have palpable sausage shaped abdominal mass commonly in RUQ, rarely intussusception visible at the anus.

Complications: bowel wall congestion from venous obstruction → bowel ischemia and necrosis → perforation, peritonitis, shock, even death.

Imaging findings

Radiographic signs

- Soft tissue mass with concentric lucencies (target sign)
- Colonic crescent of gas outlining the intussusception (meniscus sign).
- Non-specific signs include:
  - Paucity of gas in RLQ.
  - Soft tissue mass in RUQ obscuring liver edge.
  - Non-visualization of air-filled caecum.
  - Small bowel obstruction.

▶ Role of AXR in suspected intussusception is debatable. Specific signs of intussusception are rarely seen.

Ultrasound: diagnostic imaging modality of choice

- Mass with alternating rings of hyper- and hypoechogenicity ('target sign') in transverse section.
- Layered or 'pseudo-kidney' appearance in longitudinal section.

Fluoroscopy

❶ Absolute contraindications to radiological reduction: dehydration or hypovolaemic shock, perforation or peritonitis. Relative contraindications: atypical presenting age, long history.

▶ Recommended maximum 3 attempts using gas/air pressure up to 120mmHg, 3 minutes per attempt.

- Pneumatic enema: rounded mass that moves retrogradely with increased pressure. Reduction of intussusception → resolution of mass and air enters small bowel.
- Contrast enema: similar findings to air but positive contrast.

CT

- Mass with alternating rings of high and low attenuation.
▶ Not advocated as a diagnostic tool for suspected intussusception.

Differential diagnosis

Appendicitis, gastroenteritis, ovarian pathology, Meckel's diverticulum.

Management and prognosis

Patients require surgical assessment, iv access, fluid resuscitation and pain relief prior to attempted non-surgical (image-guided) reduction with gas/air or hydrostatic enema, under fluoroscopic control. Some centres perform hydrostatic or pneumatic reduction with US guidance. Those who have failed non-surgical reduction or are unsuitable for image-guided reduction require surgery. Prognosis excellent for un-complicated intussusception with prompt diagnosis and non-surgical treatment.

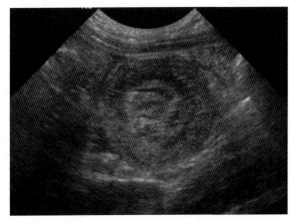

Fig. 3.30 Transverse ultrasound of intussusception showing 'target' sign of bowel layers.

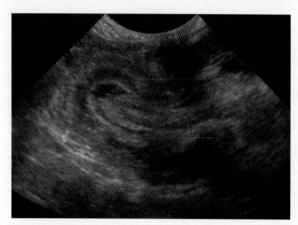

Fig. 3.31 Longitudinal ultrasound of intussusception.

Genitourinary (GU)
Clinical presentations and role of imaging

Karl Johnson

Urinary tract infection

This is the commonest condition affecting the GU tract in children. Infection can involve the upper renal tract (pyelonephritis) or the lower renal tracts (cystitis and urethritis). It can present with a wide variety of signs and symptoms.

- Signs:
  - Haematuria.
  - Altered urine colour.
  - Offensive smell.
  - Pyrexia of unknown cause.
- Symptoms:
  - Asymptomatic bacteruria can occur in pre-school girls but is very uncommon in boys.
  - Dysuria (pain/discomfort on micturition, commoner in the older child).
  - Stranguary (slow painful drop by drop passage of urine).
  - Anorexia.
  - Lethargy.
  - Poor feeding.
  - Nausea.
  - Abdominal pain.
  - Altered frequency.
  - Enuresis.
  - Loss of bladder control.
  - Septicaemia in severe cases.

Diagnosis

- Clean catch of urine recommended.
- Dip stick of urine positive for nitrates and leucocyte esterase.
- Microscopy and culture of mid stream sample.

Role of imaging

The role of imaging in the acute stage and in the follow up of children with a UTI is controversial.

▶ Prompt diagnosis and appropriate antibiotic prophylaxis is the most important part of management.

The aim of imaging is to detect a possible precipitating cause, congenital abnormalities, any abnormal renal morphology, signs of chronic renal disease and in children who do not respond quickly to therapy. The significance of the presence of renal scarring and vesico-ureteric reflux is debated.

Ultrasound

▶ The primary imaging investigation. If the child is systemically well with a normal ultrasound no other imaging warranted for a single UTI.

- Can exclude an underlying or predisposing cause for the UTI:
  - Congenital renal abnormalities (📖 p. 210)
  - Renal tumours.
  - Renal abscess.
  - Hydronephrosis/obstruction.
  - Bladder abnormalities (📖 p. 216).
  - Renal calculi.

- Relatively sensitive in detecting renal scars which may imply previous episodes of infection.
- In the acute phase an acute pyelonephritis will show a swollen echogenic kidney.

Nuclear medicine
- DMSA
  - ▶The most sensitive investigation to detect renal parenchymal scarring.
  - Unable to differentiate acute infection from a renal scar and therefore delay in the DMSA some 2–3 months following the acute infective episode is often practiced in many institutions.
  - Will provide an estimation of split renal function. A difference in activity of 10% between the kidneys is within normal limits.
- MAG 3
  - Obstruction.
  - Split renal function.
  - Vesico-ureteric reflux.

Radiographs
- Not indicated in acute disease.
- Can detect renal calcification in some metabolic and infective conditions.

Fluoroscopy
- A micturating cystourethrogram (MCUG) is used to detect the presence of reflux in children with previous UTIs.
- The relationship between vesico-ureteric reflux, renal infection and renal scarring is not totally understood and the use of an MCUG in the investigation of UTI will vary between institutions.
- Posterior urethral valves.

MR Imaging
- Renal tumour.
- Renal abscess.
- Xanthogranulomatous pyelonephritis (XPGN).
- Hydronephrosis/obstruction.
- Bladder lesions.

CT
- XPGN.
- Renal tumour.
- Renal abscess.
- Calcification.

Haematuria

Haematuria may be macroscopic or microscopic. The presence of macroscopic haematuria is a clinical finding whereas microscopic haematuria is often an incidental finding on urine analysis.

Causes
- Bacterial infection.
- Atypical infections (infectious mononucleosis, acute haemorrhagic cystitis-adenovirus, leptospirosis).
- Tuberculous infection.
- Trauma.
- Renal calculi.
- Henoch–Schönlein purpura.
- Glomerulonephritis (acute and chronic).
- Renal and bladder tumours.
- Haemoglobinopathy.
- Renal vascular malformation.
- Alport's syndrome.
- Haematuria can also occur as a factitious feature of Munchausen's syndrome by proxy.

Role of imaging
Clinical history, examination and laboratory investigation are more important in the initial assessment of haematuria than imaging. Imaging is primarily to exclude a tumour of the renal tract, renal calcification or a vascular malformation.

Radiographs
- Renal tract calcification.
- Some renal stones are radiolucent.

Ultrasound
- Renal tract tumours.
- Renal calculi.
- Bladder lesions (rhabdomyosarcoma).
- Vascular malformation.

MRI
- Vascular abnormalities.
- Renal tract tumours.

Urinary retention

Acute retention is the inability to pass urine with a tense painfully distended bladder. It may be due to pain inhibiting micturition, local compression or obstruction, or a neurological disorder.

In chronic retention the bladder is distended but painless overflow and incontinence occur.

Causes

Pain/discomfort
- Meatal ulcer.
- Cystitis.
- UTI.
- Phimosis.

Obstruction
- Faecal impaction.
- Urethral obstruction/stricture (📖 p. 203).
- Urethral valves (📖 p. 218).
- Impacted stone.
- Trauma.
- Bladder tumour (📖 p. 256).
- Sacrococcygeal tumour.

Neurological
- Spina bifida.
- Spinal cord lesion (📖 p. 518).
- Acute neurological condition.
- Drugs.
- Behavioural.

Role of imaging

Ultrasound
- Enlarged bladder.
- Stones.
- Blood clot.
- Renal vascular malformations.
- Pelvic mass.

MRI
- Spinal cord lesion.

Genitourinary (GU)
Differential diagnosis

Karl Johnson

Renal (flank) mass

Neonate and young infant

- Hydronephrosis.
- Multicystic kidney (📖 p. 224).
- Polycystic kidneys (📖 p. 220–222).
- Renal ectopia.
- Congenital mesoblastic nephroma.
- Renal vein thrombosis.
- Wilms' tumour (📖 p. 234).
- Adrenal lesion (📖 p. 260).

Older child

- Wilms' tumour (📖 p. 234).
- Hydronephrosis.
- Nephroblastomatosis (📖 p. 236).
- Renal tumours (other than Wilms').
- Multilocular cystic nephroma (📖 p. 238).
- Angiomyolipoma (📖 p. 240).
- Polycystic kidneys (📖 p. 220, 222).
- Adrenal mass.

Adrenal/retroperitoneal mass

- Adrenal haemorrhage (typically in the neonate) (📖 p. 264).
- Neuroblastoma (📖 p. 260).
- Ganglioneuroma.

Causes of hydronephrosis

- Congenital.
- Posterior urethral valves and other cause of bladder outflow obstruction (📖 p. 218).
- Pelvi-ureteric junction obstruction (📖 p. 228).
- Ureteric-vesical obstruction.
- Vesico-ureteric reflux (📖 p. 226).
- Neurogenic.
- Prune belly.
- Other cause of renal tract obstruction (stones, blood clot, etc.).

Renal cysts

Renal cysts are usually diagnosed on ultrasound where it is important to demonstrate posterior acoustic enhancement, define the cyst wall and differentiate from hydronephrosis by the lack of communication with the renal pelvis.

Polycystic disease

- Autosomal recessive polycystic disease (📖 p. 222).
- Autosomal dominant polycystic disease (📖 p. 220).

Cortical cysts

- Simple cyst.
- Haemodialysis.
- Cystic nephroma.
- Syndromes:
  - Tuberous sclerosis.
  - Von Hippel-Lindau.
  - Turner's syndrome.
  - Trisomy 13 and 18.

Medullary cysts

- Medullary sponge kidney.
- Papillary necrosis.
- Calyceal cyst.
- Juvenile nephronophthisis.

Intrarenal cysts

- Tuberculous.
- Hydatid.
- Neoplastic.
- Post-traumatic.
- Infection/calculi.

Renal dysplasia

- Multicystic dysplastic kidney (📖 p. 224).
- Focal renal dysplasia.
- Multiple cysts associated with posterior urethral valves (📖 p. 218).

Increase in echogenicity in the neonatal kidney

- Normal.
- Infantile polycystic disease.
- Renal vein thrombosis.
- Cortical nephrocalcinosis.
- Early stages of adult polycystic disease.
- Glomerulocystic disease.
- Congenital/neonatal nephritic syndrome.

Testicular and scrotal lesions

Any lesions in the testes and/or scrotum may cause swelling, tenderness or a hydrocele or a combination of these findings.

Testicular masses

- Germ cell tumours (📖 p. 245):
  - Seminoma.
  - Teratoma.
  - Embryonal carcinoma.
  - Choriocarcinoma.
- Non-germ cell tumours.
- Lymphoma or leukaemia.
- Orchitis (📖 p. 248).

Extra testicular masses

- Varicoele.
- Hydrocele.
- Hernia.
- Testicular torsion (📖 p. 244).
- Appendicular torsion.
- Epididymitis (📖 p. 248).
- Epididymal cyst.
- Scrotal trauma/oedema.

Painful scrotal lesions

- Testicular torsion (📖 p. 244).
- Epididymitis (📖 p. 248).
- Orchitis.
- Incarcerated hernia.
- Appendicular torsion.

Causes of hydrocele

- Congenital.
- Infantile.
- Epididymitis (📖 p. 248).
- Orchitis.
- Testicular or appendicular torsion (📖 p. 244).
- Trauma.

- Neoplasm (📖 p. 245).
- Varicoele.

Bladder masses

- Blood clot.
- Rhabdomyosarcoma (📖 p. 256).
- Ureterocele (📖 p. 216).
- Calculus.
- Infection/debris.
- Foreign body.

Bladder outflow obstruction

- Posterior urethral valves (commonest in boys) (📖 p. 218).
- Ectopic ureterocele (commonest in girls) (📖 p. 216).
- Vesical diverticulum.
- Bladder neck obstruction:
  - Calculus.
  - Foreign body.
  - Ureterocele.
  - Rhabdomyosarcoma.
- Urethral stricture.
- Anterior urethral diverticulum.
- Prune-belly syndrome.
- Meatal stenosis.
- Phimosis.
- A neuropathic bladder with incomplete emptying.

Pelvic masses in girls

- Ovarian cyst.
- Sacrococcygeal teratoma (📖 p. 258).
- Ovarian tumour (📖 p. 252).
- Hydrosalpinx/tubo-ovarian abscess.
- Haemorrhagic cyst.
- Ovarian torsion (📖 p. 250).
- Pregnancy.
- Hydrometrocolpos (📖 p. 254).
- Pelvic/bladder rhabdomyosarcoma (📖 p. 256).
- Bowel duplication.
- Distended bowel, e.g. Hirschprung's (📖 p. 150).
- Distended bladder.

Genitourinary (GU)
Disorders

Karl Johnson

Umbilical catheters

These are catheters placed in either the umbilical artery (UAC) or umbilical vein (UVC) of predominantly premature infants or newborns with the need for vascular access. The umbilical artery line can also be used to monitor arterial pressures and for taking blood samples. It is important to recognize the correct positioning of these lines on plain film to avoid line complications. Thrombus in a peripheral artery can lead to limb ischaemia or septic emboli, or in the portal vein (PV) can lead to portal hypertension or liver abscess.

Normal catheter positions

UVC

Umbilical vein→Left portal vein→ ductus venosus→ middle/left hepatic vein→ IVC.

The tip of the UVC line should lie at approximately T8/9 level, above the level of the diaphragm, into the RA.

UAC

Umbilical artery→ internal iliac artery→ common iliac artery→ aorta

The tip of the UAC line should either lie high (between T6 and T10) or low (below L3) to avoid the major arterial branches of the aorta, e.g. renal arteries at L2.

Complications

- Abnormal position:
  - UVC: in PV, SMV, SVC, internal jugular vein (IJV) or through a patent foramen ovale into a pulmonary artery.
  - UAC: celiac axis, SMA, renal arteries, through the ductus arteriosus into the pulmonary artery.
- Thrombus:
  - Echogenic intravascular material on ultrasound (US).
- Infection.
- Perforation:
  - Liver can lead to ascites.
  - LA wall into the lung.

Imaging findings

Radiographs

- The lines are radio-opaque and should be traced along expected pathway to determine correct positioning.
- Chronic thrombus or perforation may lead to calcification over the liver.

Ultrasound

- The lines appear as two high echogenicity parallel lines.
- Thrombus is an echogenic intraluminal filling defect.

Management and prognosis

Most thrombi are self-limiting but may lead to vascular occlusion and ischaemia. In most cases the advice is either to reposition or remove the catheter.

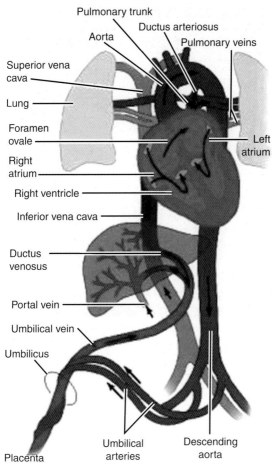

Fig. 4.1 Diagram to show circulation in the fetus.

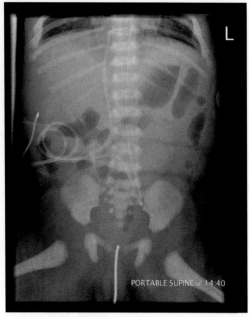

Fig. 4.2 AXR showing correctly positioned UAC and UVC catheters.

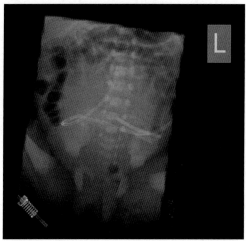

Fig. 4.3 AXR showing incorrectly positioned UVC with the tip lying too low.

Congenital renal abnormalities

In utero, the embryonic kidneys (metanephric blastema) ascend on either side of the spine from level of the bladder to lie at level of the L1 vertebral body by term. The renal pelvis initially lies in an anterior position but rotates 90° medially during the ascent. Alteration in this migration can cause renal tissue to be present anywhere from a pre-sacral position to an intrathoracic location.

Abnormalities may be bilateral, unilateral or cross the midline. They include: pelvic and subdiaphragmatic located kidneys, horseshoe- and pancake-shaped kidneys (fusion of the inferior poles or medial borders of the kidneys respectively), cross-fused ectopia (one kidney crosses the midline and fuses to the lower pole of the contralateral kidney, with this fused mass lying in an abnormal position).

Typically, the renal parenchyma is normal; the isthmus (midline junction) of a horseshoe kidney may contain functional renal tissue or non-functioning fibrosis. In the vast majority of cases, the ureters drain into both sides of the bladder, so with cross-fused ectopia the ureter will traverse the midline.

Simple ectopia is seen in 1 in 900 post-mortem cases. Malpositioned kidneys are more susceptible to trauma, injury, obstruction, infection, VUR and stones. There is an increased incidence of aberrant or multiple renal vessels. Horseshoe kidneys are associated with other congenital anomalies and the VACTERL syndromes (vertebral, anorectal, cardiac, tracheo-oesophageal, renal and limb abnormalities).

Clinical presentation

Can be an incidental finding, may be detected following screening for a UTI. An ectopic kidney may stimulate a pelvic mass.

Imaging

Radiographs

- Ectopic renal tissue may be confused as a midline pelvic mass, displacing bowel gas with renal calcification.

Ultrasound

- Abnormal positioned kidney, hydronephrosis and abnormal orientation of renal pelvis.
- With a horseshoe kidney renal tissue is seen anterior to the aorta.
- Pelvic kidneys may be difficult to visualize.

MRI

- Abnormal location of renal tissue.
- Abnormal vascular supply.
- Hydronephrosis.

Nuclear medicine (DMSA renogram)

- Ectopic renal tissue or absence of activity in renal bed, pelvic kidneys.
- Abnormal renal contours.

Differential diagnosis

- Abdominal mass.
- Severe scoliosis.

Management and prognosis
Treatment of complications: UTI, hydronephrosis, calculi, VUR.

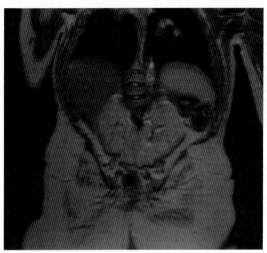

Fig. 4.4 Coronal T2-weighted image of the upper abdomen shows a horseshoe kidney with abnormal orientation of the pelvicalyceal collecting systems.

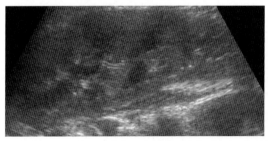

Fig. 4.5 Sagittal ultrasound image of a horseshoe kidney shows there is poor definition of the lower pole of the kidney with continuation of structures across the midline.

Pelvic/renal duplication

Duplicated (or multiple) renal collecting systems arise as a result of two or more ureteric buds that form their own nephrons creating multiple collecting systems. The incidence is up to 50% in the general population and it is commoner on the left.

With two separate pelvicalyceal collecting systems, the two ureters may join above the bladder (partial duplication) or may separately enter the bladder (complete duplication). The ureter draining the superior moiety of the kidney inserts into the bladder inferiorly and medial to the ureter draining the lower moiety (Weigert–Meyer rule). The upper pole tends to obstruct and the lower pole tends to have vesico-ureteric reflux (VUR). It is the lower ureteric orifice which is ectopic and can be associated with an ureterocele.

There is an association with other genital abnormalities, bladder duplications and PUJ obstruction.

Clinical presentation
Often an incidental finding, can be detected on screening following a UTI.

Imaging

Ultrasound
- Band of renal cortex crossing the medullary portion of the kidney.
- Separate renal pelvis.
- Ureterocele.
- Dilatation of the upper pole with normal appearance of the lower pole.

Fluoroscopy
MCUG will show reflux into the lower pole.

MR imaging
- T2WI urography defines the type of collecting system and level of any ureteric fusion.
- Will demonstrate the site of ureteric insertion into the bladder.
- Duplicated kidneys tend to be larger (and/or longer).
- Duplex kidneys may have more than one renal artery and vein (but this can be a finding in normal kidneys).

Nuclear medicine (DMSA renogram)
- Split renal function.
- Scarring.

Differential diagnosis
- Column of Bertin.
- Partial incomplete duplication.
- Upper pole mass (e.g. Wilms').

Management and prognosis
Depending on the complications that arise, ureterocele excision, hydronephrosis treated to improve drainage, infection treated with antibiotics.

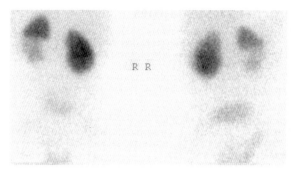

Fig. 4.6 DMSA scan of a duplex system on the left side. The degree of activity in the left upper pole moiety is greater than that in the lower pole.

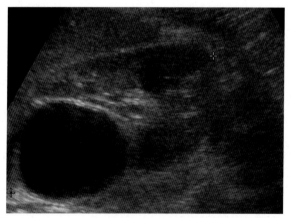

Fig. 4.7 Ultrasound image of a child with duplex kidneys. There is a hydronephrotic left upper pole and normal appearance of the lower pole.

Urachal abnormalities

A variety of developmental anomalies can arise due to persistence of all or part of the connection between the bladder and umbilicus, this includes: a patent urachus, urachal fistula, urachal remnant, urachal cyst, and urachal sinus or urachal diverticulum. M>F.

A urachal fistula is an open channel from the bladder to the umbilicus. A sinus is a persistence of the superficial segment opening onto the skin.

Clinical presentation

Typically diagnosed in the first few months of life but some cysts can be detected later in childhood. Symptoms include persistent urinary tract infections, periumbilical inflammation and periumbilical wetness. A cyst can cause a superior pelvic mass.

Imaging

Ultrasound

- ▶The bladder should be full.
- Fluid along the tract between the dome of the bladder and umbilicus.
- Urachus may be thick but may not contain fluid or it can be continuous with a bladder diverticulum.
- Urachal cyst.

Fluoroscopy (MCUG)

- Patency of the urachus that will fill with contrast.
- Can underestimate the length of the remnant.
- True lateral views are necessary.

MRI

- Urachal cyst may cause a subcutaneous abscess.
- Solid or tubular structures extending through the anterior aspect of the peritoneal cavity to the umbilicus.
- Inflammatory changes around the umbilical (↑signal on T2WI).

Differential diagnosis

- Granulation tissue of the umbilical stump.
- Umbilical hernia.
- Haemangioma of the cord.

Management and prognosis

Resection of the entire tract.

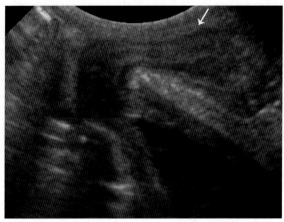

Fig. 4.8 Sagittal ultrasound image of the pelvis showing a patent urachus extending from the bladder to the umbilicus.

Ureterocele

A congenital cystic dilatation of the submucosa of the distal ureter. It may be intravesical (within the bladder) or extravesical. Ectopic ureteroceles are those who orifices are located in an abnormal position within the bladder. Ureteroceles associated with a single kidney and ureter are typically simple and intravesical. With duplex systems the ureteroceles are more likely to be ectopic and extravesical (F >M, L>R, can be bilateral). Increased incidence with duplication/congenital anomalies, hydronephrosis and hydroureter.

Clinical presentation

Can be an incidental finding, is a cause of UTI. Ectopic ureteric insertion (can be a vaginal insertion) is a cause of enuresis and wetting.

Imaging findings

Ultrasound

- Thin walled anechoic cystic structure connected to the distal ureter.
- Associated renal abnormalities and hydronephrosis.

Fluoroscopy (MCUG)

- Best imaged on the initial filling phase.
- Oblique views help visualize.
- When bladder becomes full the intravesical pressure may compress the ureterocele.

MRI

- MR urogram will detect a filling defect in the bladder.
- Sensitive in detecting duplication anomalies.
- Ectopic ureteric insertion.

Differential diagnosis

Bladder tumour (solid lesions).

Management and prognosis

If asymptomatic no intervention is required, may be associated with ectopic ureteric insertion and surgical reimplantation may be necessary. Typically endoscopic incision and deroofing is performed.

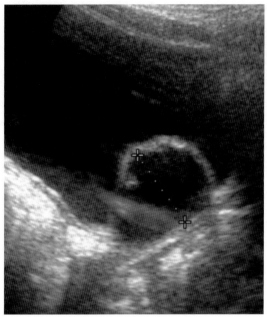

Fig. 4.9 Fluid-filled cystic uretrocele at the bladder base.

Posterior urethral valves

Chronic urethral obstruction due to abnormal thickening and prominence of the muscular folds of the urethra which is only seen in males.

Clinical presentation

Antenatally there may be oligohydramnios and hydronephrosis. If not detected antenatally the onset of symptoms will depend on the severity of the obstruction, there can be hydronephrosis, urinary ascites, urinary tract infection, sepsis, urinary retention, poor urinary stream, abnormal voiding patterns and an enlarged post-voiding bladder.

Imaging findings

Ultrasound

- Antenatally oligohydramnios.
- Hydronephrosis and hydroureters.
- Dilated posterior urethra.
- Dilated or small bladder, but thickened wall and diverticula.

Fluoroscopy (MCUG)

- ▶Must obtain true lateral view of the urethra.
- Abrupt calibre change in the posterior urethra.
- Dilated posterior urethra with a small calibre bulbous penile urethra.
- Enlarged, trabeculated bladder with diverticulum.
- Vesico-ureteric reflux.
- Dilated ureters and hydronephrosis.

MRI

- Antenatally oligohydramnios.
- Urinary ascites.
- Hydronephrosis.
- Bladder wall thickening.

Differential diagnosis

- Anterior urethral valves.
- Voidance dysfunction.
- Mega urethra.
- Post-surgical/traumatic/infected stricture.

Management and prognosis

Surgical resection. There is an increased incidence of voiding problems and UTIs. Can develop chronic renal failure.

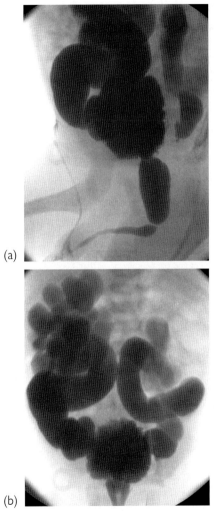

(a)

(b)

Fig. 4.10 (a) Sagittal and (b) coronal fluoroscopic images in a neonatal boy with marked dilatation of the posterior urethra and thickening valve tissue extending across the urethra. The bladder has an irregular trabeculated pattern and there is marked bilateral vesicoureteric reflux into dilated ureters and renal collecting systems.

Autosomal dominant polycystic kidney disease (ADPKD)

An autosomal dominant disorder that causes multiple renal cysts, but it can involve other organs including the liver, pancreas, brain, ovaries and testes. There may also be evidence of cardiovascular disease, abdominal hernias and cerebral berry aneurysms. The number of cysts visible increases with age and initially young children may not have any cysts.

Clinical presentation

It is often an incidental finding or may be detected on familial screening. Symptoms include pain, haematuria and hypertension. It can lead to chronic renal failure (typically in adulthood).

Imaging

Radiographs
- Often normal.
- There may be curvilinear calcification within the cyst wall.
- Can be associated with renal calculi.

Ultrasound
- ▶Enlarged kidneys contain varying number of cysts
- The cysts are simple anechoic structures with posterior acoustic enhancement and are typically larger than 1.0cm in diameter.
- Preservation of cortico-medullary differentiation.
- Surrounding vessels are distorted.
- Haemorrhage may occur within the cyst creating debris or septations.
- Cysts in the liver, pancreas, ovaries or testes are always accompanied by renal cysts.

MRI
- Uncomplicated cysts are ↑signal on T2WI.
- Infection or haemorrhage within the cysts may lead to wall thickening and heterogeneous signal intensity.

Differential diagnosis
- ARPKD (bright kidneys, poor cortico-medullary differentiation, cysts <1.0cm).
- Multiple simple cysts (no family history, no cysts in liver or pancreas, no renal enlargement).
- Tuberous sclerosis (associated clinical features, hyperechogenic angiomyolipoma).
- Post-dialysis.

Management and prognosis

Symptomatic treatment of pain, infection and hypertension, dialysis and transplantation if there is associated renal failure.

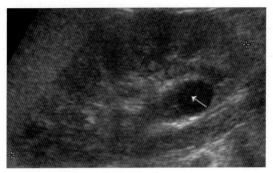

Fig. 4.11 Sagittal ultrasound shows a large anechoic cyst at the lower pole of the left kidney. Two smaller cysts are seen at the upper pole.

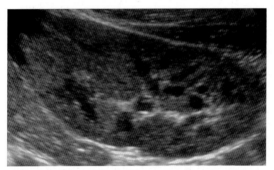

Fig. 4.12 Multiple small cysts are seen throughout the kidney. The cysts are of variable size and occupy all areas (subcortical, central and medullary areas).

Autosomal recessive polycystic kidney disease (ARPKD)

An autosomal recessive disorder, with a wide spectrum of severity that results in multiple, bilateral small renal cysts that involve the collecting ducts and tubules. Associated with pulmonary hypoplasia (which can cause severe respiratory distress) and hepatic fibrosis (which can lead to portal hypertension, requiring transplantation). Is a cause of chronic renal failure requiring dialysis and transplantation.

Clinical presentation

Often the diagnosis is made antenatally. In the neonate there is palpable bilateral renal enlargement and significant renal impairment.

Imaging

Radiographs
- Abdominal distension with large flank masses.
- Pulmonary hypoplasia on the chest X-ray.

Ultrasound
- Antenatally there is fetal oligohydramnios and enlarged kidneys.
- ▶In the neonate there are bilateral enlarged hyperechoic kidneys.
- Renal shape is maintained but there is loss of normal corticomedullary differentiation.
- The cysts are <1cm in diameter and may not be individually identified.
- Focal rosettes of radially orientated dilated collecting tubules.

MRI
- Enlarged kidneys which are ↑ signal T2 WI.
- Small cysts may be detected.

Differential diagnosis
- ADPKD (normal renal echogenicity).
- Asymmetrical large renal cysts.

Management and prognosis

If the kidneys are grossly enlarged they may cause respiratory compromise and surgical removal may be contemplated. Medical management is typically supportive and may include dialysis and transplantation. Liver transplantation may be required if there is progression of the hepatic fibrosis.

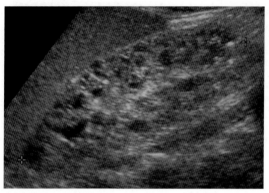

Fig. 4.13 Sagittal ultrasound shows enlarged kidneys in a neonate with multiple small cysts throughout the kidney. There is loss of normal corticomedullary differentiation and increased renal echotexture.

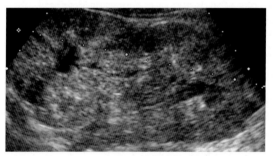

Fig. 4.14 An enlarged echogenic kidney with no discernible corticomedullary differentiation.

Multicystic dysplastic kidney (MCDK)

Multiple cysts of varying sizes replace the normal renal tissue resulting in a non-functioning kidney. It is unilateral, as bilateral disease is incompatible with life. Renal size is variable depending on the number and size of the cysts and any residual renal tissue. Cysts vary in size from a few cms to >10cms. Second commonest cause (after hydronephrosis) of an abdominal mass in a neonate. Over time an MCDK will involute and can disappear. There is high association with abnormalities in the contralateral kidney (PUJ obstruction and VUR) and chromosomal abnormalities.

Clinical presentation

A MCDK presents early in life due to a palpable mass, smaller lesions may be an incidental finding. It can then be complicated by infection, hypertension or a Wilms' tumour.

Imaging

Ultrasound

- ▶Abnormal renal contours with loss of normal corticomedullary differentiation.
- Kidney can be either enlarged or very small.
- Multiple cysts of varying size which do not communicate.
- Intervening renal tissue is echogenic.
- The contralateral kidney should be assessed for evidence of hydronephrosis and enlargement.

Nuclear scintigraphy

- A MAG3 or DMSA study will demonstrate no significant activity in the MCDK.
- A MAG3 will assess any degree of obstruction in the contralateral kidney.

Differential diagnosis

- Hydronephrosis (communication between the dilated calyces, uptake on DMSA).
- Chronic renal disease (small bilateral echogenic kidneys).
- Wilms' tumour (may be cystic).
- Mesoblastic nephroma (uptake on DMSA).

Management and prognosis

Surgical excision if there is recurrent infection, focal enlargement (which may suggest transformation to a Wilms' tumour or hypertension). If asymptomatic serial ultrasounds to monitor involution. Management of any abnormality in the contralateral kidney.

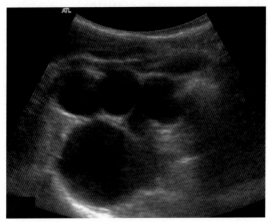

Fig. 4.15 Multiple large anechoic cysts in a dysplastic kidney.

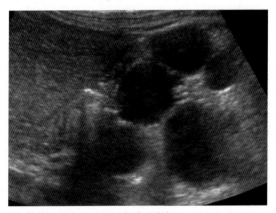

Fig. 4.16 Multiple anechoic cysts in a dysplastic kidney.

Vesico-ureteric reflux (VUR)

Retrograde flow of urine from the bladder into the ureter towards the kidneys. Commonest in children <2yrs, majority of children outgrowing the condition before puberty.

An international reflux study committee grading system exists;

- I Reflux into ureter not reaching the renal pelvis
- II Reflux into the renal pelvis but with normal calyces
- III Calyceal blunting
- IV Calyceal and ureteric dilatation
- V Dilated and tortuous collecting system with intrarenal reflux.

Children with high grade or persistent VUR who have recurrent UTIs are potentially at an increased risk of renal scarring, hypertension and end stage renal disease.

Clinical presentation

Often discovered during the investigation of UTIs or hydronephrosis. In some institutions children with antenatally detected hydronephrosis undergo screening. VUR is associated with other renal abnormalities such as MCDK, ectopic kidneys and neurogenic bladder.

Imaging

Ultrasound

- A normal ultrasound does not exclude significant VUR.
- With high grade VUR there may be ureteric dilatation, hydronephrosis and renal scarring.
- VUR can be detected by instilling ultrasound contrast agents into the bladder followed by imaging of the ureters.

Fluoroscopy

▶MCUG is the most common investigation used to detect VUR. It can be traumatic and its use should be avoided in the older child.

- Early filling images of the bladder (with oblique views) will detect intraluminal filling abnormalities such as ureterocoeles, polyps and masses.
- Contrast in the ureter or renal pelvis confirms VUR.
- Voiding images are important to exclude urethral abnormalities in boys.
- A delayed cross-kidney image will detect high grade reflux.

Nuclear scintigraphy

MAG3 renogram with an indirect cystogram, alternatively isotope can be instilled directly in the bladder.

- These investigations provide less anatomical detail than a MCUG.
- Useful in the follow-up of the older toilet-trained child.

Management and prognosis

Conservative approach in most cases. Medical management predominantly consists of prophylatic antibiotic therapy. Surgical treatment includes ureteric re-implantation and endoscopic vesico-ureteric injections.

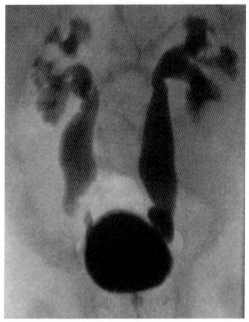

Fig. 4.17 Bilateral vesicoureteric reflux into dilated ureters and dilated renal collecting systems in a girl.

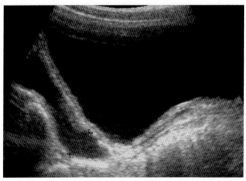

Fig. 4.18 Sagittal ultrasound shows a fluid-filled bladder and dilated ureter extending down to the bladder base.

Pelvi-ureteric junction obstruction (PUJ)

PUJ is the commonest site of upper urinary tract obstruction in children, the degree of obstruction can be variable and result in pelvicalyceal dilatation of varying severity. The dilation involves just the renal collecting system and very proximal ureter. There is an association with an aberrant renal artery running anterior to the ureter, possibly causing the obstruction.

Clinical presentation

Often detected antenatally, but can be associated with UTIs, abdominal pain or haematuria in childhood. It can be an incidental finding on abdominal ultrasound.

Imaging

Radiographs
- ►Not routinely indicated in PUJ obstruction
- A large soft tissue abdominal mass may be seen.

Ultrasound
- ►Hydronephrosis and renal pelvic dilatation with no ureteric dilatation.
- There is communication between the calyces (to differentiate from cystic disease).
- The renal pelvis abruptly tapers at the PUJ.
- There may be renal parenchymal thinning in long-standing cases.
- The presence of echogenic urine suggests possible infection.
- Doppler examination may show an aberrant vessel crossing anterior to the PUJ.
- Serial ultrasounds measuring the AP diameter of the renal pelvis in the transverse plane are useful to monitor disease progression.

Fluoroscopy (IVU)
- Not routinely indicated due to the radiation burden.
- Delayed nephrogram phase as a consequence of the obstruction.
- Dilated renal collecting system but normal ureter.
- A Whitaker test involves monitoring the pressure within the renal pelvis during a fluid infusion to the collecting system (not commonly performed).

MRI
- MR urograms will show renal pelvic dilation and normal calibre ureters.
- Important to demonstrate communication between collecting system and renal pelvis.
- MR angiography will show the relationship of the vessels to the ureter and is useful prior to laparoscopic surgery.

Nuclear scintigraphy (MAG3 renograms)
- Diuretic (frusemide) should be administered at the same time as the isotope to demonstrate hydronephrosis and poor drainage.
- Useful following corrective surgery to assess outcome.
- Will provide a differential measure of renal function.

Differential diagnosis

- Hydronephrosis of other cause, e.g. VUR, MCDK.
- Megacalycosis (idiopathic dilation of calyces, without impaired drainage).

Management and prognosis

Most cases will improve spontaneously and serial ultrasound to monitor progress is the initial approach. In children with systemic symptoms or in whom the dilatation is worsening and there is loss of renal function surgical intervention may be indicated. Pyeloplasty (reconstruction of the PUJ) is the commonest procedure.

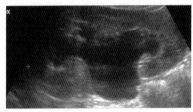

Fig. 4.19 Sagittal ultrasound shows some marked hydronephrosis of the left kidney with dilatation of the renal pelvicalyceal system but no ureteric dilatation distally.

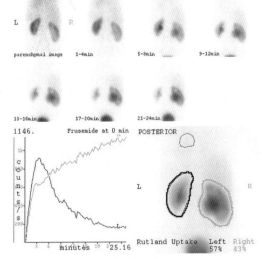

Fig. 4.20 MAG 3 image shows good uptake and excretion of the left kidney. In the right kidney, there is uptake but a minimal amount of excretion. On delayed images, there is shown to be collection of activity within the right collecting system, consistent with PUJ obstruction.

Pyelonephritis

This is acute infection of the renal parenchyma and is distinct and more serious than lower urinary tract or bladder infections. *E. coli* is the commonest infective agent, F>M. The aim should be for a prompt diagnosis to ensure adequate treatment and so avoid any long-term complications, which include perirenal abscesses, renal scarring and urinary obstruction. ▶Severe scarring following repeated infections can cause end-stage renal failure.

Clinical presentation

Pyrexia, general malaise, irritability, abdominal/flank pain, vomiting, an alteration in urinary habit, with loss of bladder control. Positive urine and blood cultures, with a leucocytosis.

Imaging

▶The diagnosis is primarily a clinical one. Imaging may confirm the diagnosis and detect complications. The use and timing of any investigation should be clearly defined in local guidelines.

Ultrasound

- Renal swelling which may be localized or widespread.
- Loss of corticomedullary differentiation.
- Altered echogenicity and irregular renal outline.
- Occasionally rounded mass-like areas may appear within the kidney.
- Reduced perfusion on colour Doppler.
- Detect underlying renal abnormality (hydronephrosis, duplex etc.).

Fluoroscopy

- Vesico-ureteric reflux is associated with pyelonephritis but MCUGs should be avoided in the acute phase.

CT

- Not routinely indicated, due to radiation burden.
- Inflammatory changes in the peri-renal fat following contrast enhancement.
- Wedge-shaped or focal areas of reduced enhancement.
- Contrast enhancement may be streaky.

MRI

- Inflammatory changes in the peri-renal fat.
- T1WI increased signal intensity in renal parenchyma due to oedema.
- Focal areas of reduced signal intensity following gadolinium.

Nuclear scintigraphy (DMSA renograms)

- Focal photopenic areas which may persist for up to 8 weeks after acute infection.
- Similar photopenic areas can be confused with renal scarring.

Differential diagnosis

Renal infarction, scarring or mass.

Management and prognosis

Antimicrobial therapy. Follow-up imaging to assess for vesico-ureteric reflux and congenital anomalies if appropriate. Some authors suggest prophylatic antibiotics should be used in the presence of vesico-ureteric reflux.

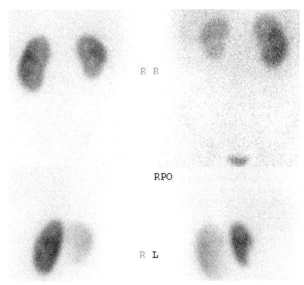

R R

RPO

R L

Fig. 4.21 DMSA scan shows irregularity and loss of normal contour at the lower pole of the right kidney, consistent with renal scarring. Similar appearances would occur with pyelonephritis if the DMSA scan was performed during the acute phase.

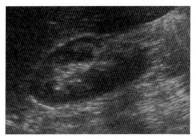

Fig. 4.22 Sagittal ultrasound shows loss of normal renal tissue and parenchymal thinning at the lower pole of the right kidney.

Mesoblastic nephroma

A solitary unilateral hamartomatous renal tumour containing predominantly spindle cells and fibroblasts. Typically benign but can change to become more aggressive, often shows rapid growth. Varies in size from >1cm to >15cm, can involve the entire kidney and cross the midline. Haemorrhage, necrosis, cystic change and hydronephrosis are uncommon. M>F.

Clinical presentation

Causes polyhydramnios antenatally, usually diagnosed in the first 3 months of life as a palpable flank mass. Can cause AV shunting. There is an association with hypercalcaemia and polyuria.

Imaging

Radiographs

- Mass effect and bowel displacement.
- Cardiac enlargement from AV shunting.

Ultrasound

- Renal mass, with displacement of the bowel.
- Variable size and echogenicity (similar to muscle).
- Solid tumour with smooth outline, can have cystic elements.
- No vascular invasion, but can cause venous obstruction.
- Identify a normal adrenal gland to confirm renal origin.
- Polyhydramnios in pregnancy.

CT

- Solid flank mass.
- Calcification atypical.
- Variable enhancement.
- Cystic areas of necrosis and haemorrhage are uncommon.

MRI

- T1WI intermediate to low signal intensity.
- Variable enhancement with gadolinium.
- T2WI increased signal intensity.

Differential diagnosis

- Wilms' tumour (typically older).
- Neuroblastoma (suprarenal location).
- Adrenal haemorrhage (it will evolve over time).
- ARPCKD.
- MCDK.

Management and prognosis

Nephrectomy usually curative, follow-up imaging to exclude local reoccurrence.

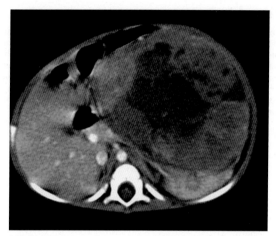

Fig. 4.23 Axial CT post-intravenous contrast image shows a large solid lesion arising from the left kidney. The degree of contrast enhancement within the tumour is reduced compared to the remaining portion of the left kidney.

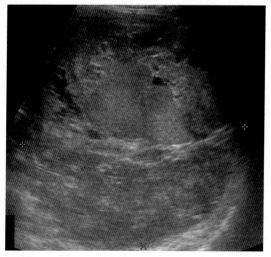

Fig. 4.24 Ultrasound shows a mixed echogenic lesion arising from the upper pole of the left kidney.

Wilms' tumour

A malignant tumour of primitive metanephric cells. It is the commonest abdominal malignancy in children between 1–8yrs age and the third commonest childhood malignancy after leukaemia and CNS tumours. ~ 10% are bilateral. Spread can be local along the renal vein into the IVC and it can also metastasize (commonly to the lungs). There is an association with nephroblastomatosis, Beckwith–Wiedemann syndrome, chromosome 11 abnormality, trisomy 18 and other rare inherited disorders. Children at increased risk should undergo regular ultrasound screening.

Clinical presentation

Commonly an asymptomatic flank mass. There may be haematuria, hypertension, failure to thrive and fever.

Imaging

Radiographs

- Soft tissue mass displacing the bowel.
- Calcification is uncommon (~10%), unlike neuroblastoma.
- Chest radiograph for lung metastases (well-defined 1-5cm rounded opacities).

Ultrasound

- ▶Heterogeneous, mixed echogenic mass involving the kidney with extension into the renal vein and displacement of adjacent organs.
- Focal lesions in the contralateral kidney.
- Echocardiography may be needed to detect cardiac tumour thrombus.

CT

- ▶Large heterogeneous mass replacing the kidney and displacing, but not encasing, adjacent organs.
- Tumour margins are well defined with heterogeneous enhancement.
- Extension into the renal vein and IVC.
- There may be focal lesions in the contralateral kidney (nephroblastomatosis).
- Lung metastases are well defined rounded lesions (1-5cm).

MRI

- ▶Renal-based mass with displacement of adjacent organs (different from neuroblastoma).
- Tumour spread along the renal vein and IVC.
- T1WI-mixed/low signal intensity mass lesion.
- T2WI-high/mixed intensity signal of the mass lesion.
- May contain blood products causing altered signal characteristics.

Differential diagnosis

- Neuroblastoma (calcification, encasement, adrenal origin).
- Multilocular cystic nephroma.
- Nephroblastomatosis.
- Renal cell carcinoma.

Management and prognosis

Pre-operative chemotherapy followed by surgical resection. Radiation and chemotherapy post-operatively.

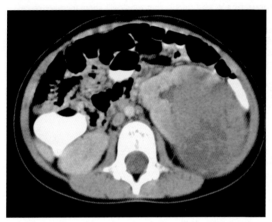

Fig. 4.25 Axial CT shows a large solid lesion arising from the left kidney. Post-intravenous contrast, there is enhancement of the kidneys but reduced enhancement of the Wilms' tumour.

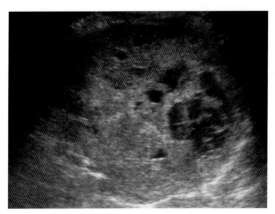

Fig. 4.26 Ultrasound of the left kidney shows a mixed echogenic lesion with some cystic areas within the mass arising from the left kidney.

Nephroblastomatosis

Multiple, diffuse, rests of nephrogenic tissue, typically within the peripheral subcapsular region of the kidney. Usually <3cm in size, each can potentially progress to a Wilms' tumour but most will spontaneously regress. They can occur in the newborn but are rare after 7yrs of age, there is no sex predilection. The majority of cases are sporadic but there is an association with Beckwith–Wiedemann, trisomy 18, aniridia, Drash (gonadal dysgenesis and nephropathy) and WAGR syndromes.

Clinical presentation

Usually an asymptomatic finding, often seen in children with Wilms' tumours (in either kidney), they occur in over 90% of children who have bilateral tumours.

Imaging

Ultrasound
• Hypo or isoechoic ovoid mass in the subcapsular renal parenchyma.
• Homogenous, often multifocal.

CT
• Homogenous low attenuation peripheral nodules.
• Enhances less than renal parenchyma.

MRI
• T1WI, homogenous ovoid mass less or isointense to renal parenchyma.
• T2WI, the lesions are of similar or slightly increased signal intensity to the renal parenchyma.
• Enhancement is less than renal parenchyma.

Differential diagnosis
• Lymphoma/leukaemia (infiltrative masses).
• Pyelonephritis.
• Wilms' tumour.

Management and prognosis

Children with associated syndromes are screened for Wilms' tumours, typically with regular serial ultrasound. If the lesions increase in size may be treated as Wilms' tumour or be biopsied.

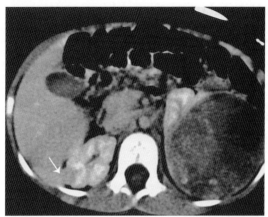

Fig. 4.27 Axial CT images show a large Wilms' tumour in the left kidney. Within the right kidney, there is a focal area of low attenuation (arrowed) of nephroblastomatosis. This enhances less than the surrounding kidney and is in the periphery of the kidney.

Multilocular cystic nephroma

Large benign multiloculated cystic renal tumour, arising from the metanephric blastema (also called cystic nephroma and cystic adenoma). Well-circumscribed mass, fibrous capsule with honeycomb cystic areas of varying sizes ranging from a few centimetres >30cm in size, it can herniate into the renal pelvis.

▶Clinical presentation

Painless, palpable abdominal mass and can cause UTIs and haematuria. M>F under 2yrs, F>M over 50yrs.

Imaging

Ultrasound
- Large well-defined multiloculated cystic mass.
- Anechoic cyst and hypoechoic septa and capsule.
- Many tiny cysts may appear slightly solid.

CT
- ▶Well-defined multiloculated cystic mass.
- Attenuation similar to water.
- Small cyst containing proteinaceous material can appear solid.
- Calcification.
- Enhancement of capsule.

MRI
- T1WI: low signal intensity multiloculated mass.
- T2WI: variable/high signal intensity depending on protein and blood products in the cysts.
- Enhancement of septa.

Differential diagnosis

Simple cyst, MCDK, cystic Wilms' tumour.

Management and prognosis

Complete or partial nephrectomy. Malignant transformation is very rare.

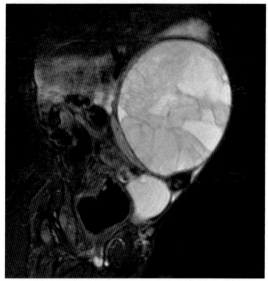

Fig. 4.28 Coronal MR image shows a large cyst with multiple septations within it arising in the upper pole of the left kidney.

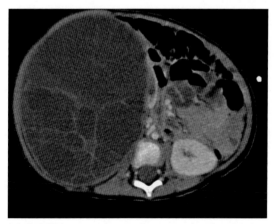

Fig. 4.29 Axial CT showing a multiseptated lesion arising from the right kidney.

Angiomyolipoma

A benign renal tumour composed of abnormal blood vessels, smooth muscle and fat cells. The commonest location is the kidney but they can also occur in the liver, lymph nodes and spleen. They can occur at multiple sites, be bilateral, vary in size, and shape.

Clinical presentation

Most commonly asymptomatic and an incidental finding on abdominal imaging. ▶Common in tuberous sclerosis. If >4cm can cause pain, haematuria, which can be severe and life-threatening. No malignant potential.

Imaging

Ultrasound
- ▶Hyperechoic to renal parenchyma. No acoustic shadowing.
- Well-defined mass.
- Vascular.

CT
- Contain low attenuation intramural fat (5% have no fat).
- Calcification is rare, which suggests a renal cell carcinoma.
- There is marked enhancement following contrast.

MRI
- T1WI: high signal due to fat content.
- T2WI: variable signal intensity depending on tissue content.
- Variable enhancement depending on vascular content.
- Reduced enhancement if they contain a large amount of fat.

Angiography
- Vascular mass with absence of arterial shunting.
- Sunburst appearance of the capillary nephrogram with an onion peel appearance of peripheral vessels in the venous phase.

Differential diagnosis

- Wilms' tumour.
- Renal abscess (ring enhancement).
- Renal lymphoma.
- Renal cell carcinoma (calcification).

Management and prognosis

Lesions <4cm are treated conservatively, those >4cm either partial nephrectomy or partial embolization are recommended.

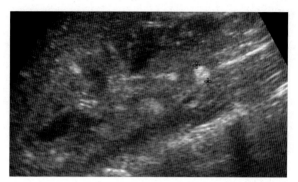

Fig. 4.30 Sagittal ultrasound showing a non-acoustic shadowing echogenic renal mass in a child with tuberous sclerosis, consistent with an angiomyolipoma.

Renal tract trauma

The kidneys are a relatively common site of traumatic injury. Injury is particularly related to blunt deceleration injuries but can occur from penetrative injuries. Motor vehicle/pedestrian accidents are the commonest cause in children. Bladder injury is commoner following pelvic trauma. Severe renal injury is associated with other abdominal injuries, while isolated injuries are typically minor. There is increased risk of injury to the kidney if there is a pre-existing renal abnormality such as an ectopic or horseshoe kidney.

Renal injuries include haematoma (intra-parenchymal, subcapsular, perinephric or within the collecting system), laceration with possible injury to the vascular pedicle, collecting system or proximal ureter.

Imaging

Radiographs

- Insensitive for renal injury.
- Loss of the normal psoas shadow and renal outlines.

Ultrasound

- ▶A normal renal ultrasound does not exclude a traumatic renal injury.
- Echogenic haematoma around the kidney or within the collecting system.
- Renal laceration.
- Damage to vascular supply, Doppler studies can assess vascular flow.
- Echogenic blood within the collecting system or bladder.

CT

- ▶The imaging modality of choice for significant abdominal trauma.
- In cases of trauma imaging should be performed following iv contrast.
- Intra-renal haematoma or contusion appear as ill-defined or rounded lesions with reduced contrast enhancement.
- Non-expanding subcapsular haematoma can cause deformity of the underlying kidney.
- Renal lacerations are areas of low attenuation which extend from the capsule into the parenchyma.
- High attenuation haemorrhage within the renal collecting system, which does not enhance with contrast.
- Extravasation of contrast into the peri-nephric space.
- Haemoperitoneum (blood within the abdomen).
- Devascularized kidneys:
  - Renal infarction, small well-demarcated wedge-shaped areas of low attenuation on post-contrast images.
  - Segmental infarction of the kidney.
  - Renal artery thrombosis/injury: there is preserved subcapsular enhancement due to peripheral vessels but ischaemia of the central kidney (cortical rim sign).
- Delayed images of the bladder may show leakage of contrast due to bladder rupture.
- Delayed renal imaging useful for assessing vascularity of the kidneys and excretion of urine into perirenal spaces creating an urinoma.

Management and prognosis

Non-operative management in the majority of cases. Active bleeding may require embolization or surgery. With urine extravasation catherization or ureteric stenting. Surgery for severe shock and shattered kidneys.

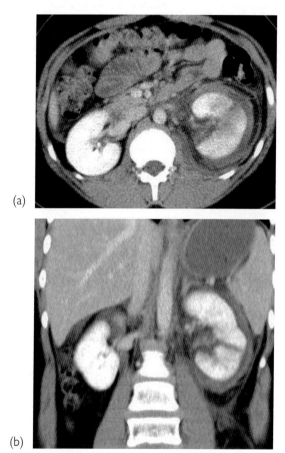

(a)

(b)

Fig. 4.31 (a) Axial and (b) coronal CT images following intravenous contrast shows a large haematoma around the left kidney. There is differential enhancement of the kidney with poor enhancement of the lower pole, consistent with vascular pedicle disruption. There is large laceration within the left kidney.

Testicular torsion

Twisting of the testis and spermatic cord within the scrotum resulting in occlusion of the testicular artery causing infarction of the testis. Majority of cases are spontaneous, but it can occur following trauma. Commoner in infants, adolescents and on the left. Increased incidence in testes where the tunica vaginalis has a high attachment (bell clapper deformity).

Clinical presentation

Acute scrotal pain with a swollen erythematous scrotum, the testicle is elevated and lies in transverse orientation. This is a surgical emergency as testicular infarction and loss of viability will occur.

Imaging

Ultrasound

- ▶Ultrasound may be normal so it cannot totally exclude the diagnosis.
- High frequency (10–15MHz) linear probe is recommended.
- In very acute cases testicular parenchyma may be normal.
- With prolonged torsion the testis and epididymis become enlarged with a mixed echotexture, due to necrosis and haemorrhage.
- The twisted spermatic cord may be visualized.
- There may be a hydrocele.
- Colour Doppler ultrasound will show absent or decreased blood flow to the testis in up to 90% of cases.

Differential diagnosis

- Epidymo-orchitis (epididymal and testicular enlargement, with increased colour Doppler flow).
- Scrotal cellulitis.
- Torsion of the testicular appendage.
- Testicular tumour (localised mass).
- Trauma.
- Hernia.

Management and prognosis

This is an acute surgical emergency requiring detorsion of the testis. Often the controlateral testis is fixed within the scrotum as prophylaxis.

Torsion of the testicular appendage

Spontaneous twisting of the pedunculated vestigial remnant attached to the testis or epididymis, causing ischaemic pain. It is a common cause of scrotal pain in paediatric patients.

It commonly occurs in the pre-teenage years, compared to testicular torsion which is commoner in teenagers.

Clinical presentation

Acute scrotal pain, small tethered mobile lump by the testis, 'blue dot sign' of the ischaemic appendage seen through the scrotal wall.

Imaging
Ultrasound
- Enlarged appendage.
- Hydrocele.
- Periappendiceal hyperaemia on Doppler ultrasound.
- Spherical shape suggests swelling.

Differential diagnosis
- Testicular torsion.
- Epididymo-orchitis.
- Tumour.
- Trauma.

Management and prognosis
Analgesia and anti-inflammatory agents. Antibiotics are not indicated as pain usually resolves.

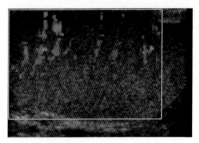

Fig. 4.32 Normal flow within the testis.

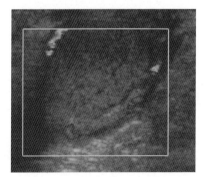

Fig. 4.33 Torted testis showing increased echogenicity. There is some peripheral blood flow but no central blood flow. The margins are swollen and irregular.

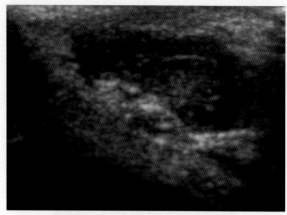

Fig. 4.34 Small irregular post-infarcted testes.

Malignant Testicular Tumours

Testicular tumours account for approximately 2% of paediatric tumours and are uncommon in infants and children. Those tumours which do occur in young children are commonly germ-cell tumours, the commonest being the yolk-sac tumour. Other tumour cell types include Leydig cell, teratoma and seminoma (usually post-pubertal). Secondary malignancies which affect the testes include leukaemia, lymphoma and neuroblastoma. Most tumours are unilateral, up to 10% may be bilateral.

Clinical Presentation

Painless scrotal swelling with a hard mass on palpation. There may be a feeling of heaviness or fullness. In some cases, there may be an acute presentation similar to orchitis. There may be an acute increase in testicular size due to haemorrhage. There may be a hydrocele. Over 70% of tumours produce either beta HCG or alpha-feto protein which can be used as tumour markers. Increased incidence with a family history, cryptorchidism, microlithiasis and trisomy 21.

Imaging

Ultrasound

- Imaging modality of choice.
- Distinguish between intra and extra-testicular masses.
- Tumours seen as focal lesions within the testis are often hypoechoic.
- Cystic changes can occur and there may be fluid to fluid levels due to haemorrhage and necrosis.
- Margins may be smooth or irregular.
- Macrocalcification increases the likelihood of a germ-cell tumour.
- Ultrasound features are non-specific and can overlap with those of infarct, haematoma, abscess or orchitis.

CT and MRI

- Isointense on T1WI.
- Hypointense on T2WI.
- Heterogeneous signal change due to calcification, necrosis and haemorrhage.
- Important to evaluate abdomen and chest for metastatic disease.

Differential Diagnosis

- Orchitis.
- Epididymitis.
- Haemorrhage/trauma.
- Cysts.

Treatment and Prognosis

- Tumour excision and chemotherapy.
- Very good survival rates.

Epididymitis/orchitis

Infection of the epididymis, the testis or both. It can occur in infants, children and adolescents (particularly those who are sexually active). Epididymitis can be bilateral. The commonest causative organisms are *S. Aureus, E. Coli* and viruses.

Clinical presentation

Usually gradual in onset with a painful, swollen erythematous scrotum. There can be systemic or urinary symptoms. Mumps orchitis is associated with fever, myalgia and parotitis.

Imaging

Ultrasound

- ▶Should be performed with high frequency (10–15MHz) linear transducer, examination may be difficult because of patient pain and compliance.
- Increase in size of the affected organs.
- Increased echogenicity.
- Hydrocele and scrotal wall thickening.
- Colour Doppler will show increased vascularity of the involved tissue.
- Chronic infection can lead to abscess formation.

Differential diagnosis

- Testicular torsion (reduced or absent blood flow on colour Doppler).
- Scrotal cellulitis.

Management and prognosis

Conservative management with pain and symptom relief. Antibiotics can be used. Follow-up ultrasound is useful if symptoms do not resolve promptly.

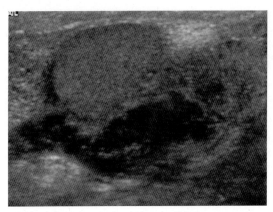

Fig. 4.35 Mixed echogenic texture in an enlarged epididymis.

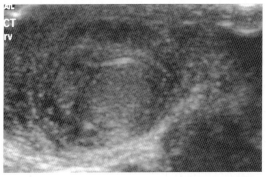

Fig. 4.36 Transverse image showing a markedly thickened and irregular epididymis.

Ovarian torsion

Twisting of the vascular pedicle of the ovary, it may also involve the fallopian tube, resulting in ischaemia and haemorrhagic infarction of the ovary. Approximately 50% of cases occur in pre-menarchal girls but it can occur in the neonate. Cysts, tumours or trauma increases the risk of torsion.

Clinical presentation

Abdominal pain, which may be acute or intermittent, generalized nausea, vomiting and fever. There may be a palpable mass. Right-sided torsions may be confused with appendicitis.

Imaging

Ultrasound

- ▶Unilaterally enlarged ovary (typically twice size of contralateral ovary).
- Variable echogenicity with cystic and solid components.
- Cyst contain debris and septations.
- Smaller peripheral cysts (8–12mm in diameter).
- Ascites.
- Fallopian tube thickened.
- Colour Doppler shows 'whirlpool sign' in the twisted vascular pedicle.
- Can appear normal if the torsion is intermittent.

CT

- Tubal thickening and ovarian mass.
- Ascites which may be of increased attenuation (haemorrhagic).
- Uterus is deviated with a twisted adenexa.
- Lack of contrast enhancement of the ovarian stroma.

MRI

- Tubal thickening.
- Enlargement of the ovary.
- T2WI: hyperintensity of ovarian stoma.

Differential diagnosis

- Appendicitis.
- Pelvic inflammatory disease.
- Ovarian cyst, tumour.
- Endometriosis.
- Pregnancy (particularly ectopic).

Management and prognosis

Surgical de-torsion. Conservation of the ovarian tissue is preferable. Oophoropexy (ovary is sutured to the peritoneum of the posterior abdominal wall).

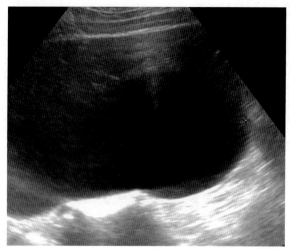

Fig. 4.37 Ultrasound shows a large cyst arising from the ovary, which resulted in ovarian torsion.

Ovarian teratoma

Teratomas may contain any cell type and this can include calcium, bone, hair and fat. Typically, there is a mass arising from the ovary which can vary in size, it has well-defined margins, no surrounding oedema. Larger lesions can occupy the whole pelvis and extend up into the abdomen. It typically occurs during the reproductive years and so presents from adolescence onwards.

Clinical presentation

It may be an incidental finding or may be associated with torsion or rupture. With a torsion the onset of pain is acute. Alternatively teratomas can cause chronic abdominal pain, abnormal uterine bleeding, and urinary or gastrointestinal symptoms.

Imaging

Radiographs
- May see calcification or teeth in the pelvis.
- Mass effect of lesion in the pelvis.

Ultrasound
- Heterogeneous well-circumscribed, echogenic mass with both solid and cystic components.
- Calcification will cause posterior acoustic enhancement.
- There may be fluid–fluid levels due to fat, fluid and haemorrhage within the lesion.

CT
- Useful in determining the presence of fat and calcium within the lesion.
- Variable attenuation depending on the nature of the lesion.

MRI
- Well-defined capsulated lesion may displace adjacent organs.
- Mixed signal intensity lesion.
- Low signal intensity on T1WI due to fat. Calcification of bone will be low signal intensity on both T1WI and T2WI.
- There may be fluid fluid levels due to haemorrhage.

Differential diagnosis

- Other benign ovarian lesions (follicular cyst, cystic adenomas, gonadoblastomas).
- Malignant tumours (germ cell tumours, stromal cell epithelial carcinomas, malignant teratomas).
- Tubular ovarian abscess.
- Ovarian torsion.
- Ectopic pregnancy.

Management and prognosis

May enlarge. Spontaneous haemorrhage or torsion. Prognosis is usually good following resection. A small minority have malignant degeneration. Treatment is with surgical resection (laparoscopic), preserving the ovary.

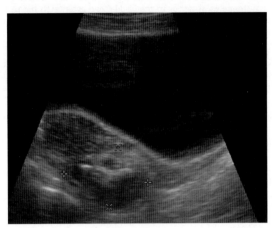

Fig. 4.38 Mixed echogenic lesion in the right ovary.

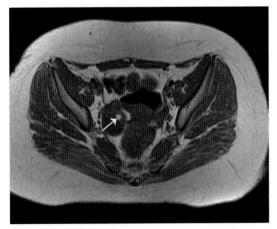

Fig. 4.39 Axial T1WI shows a lesion of mixed signal intensity in the right ovary. The high signal is the result of fat in the lesion.

Hydrometrocolpos

Dilatation of the vagina and/or uterus due to distal vaginal/cervical stenosis, atresia or an imperforate hymen. Hydro (fluid), hemato (blood), metra (uterine), metrocolpos (uterus and vagina).There is cystic/debris-filled mass in the pelvis posterior to the bladder and anterior to the rectum, it can cause secondary hydronephrosis. Prior to the menarche it usually contains cervical mucous and fluid, post menarche it contains blood.

Clinical presentation

Pelvic mass, which in infants can cause secondary urinary tract obstruction and infection, in adolescent girls there is a delayed menarche, and cyclical pelvic pain.

Imaging

Radiographs

- Soft tissue mass in the pelvis.
- Occasional peritoneal calcification.

Ultrasound

- ▶Well defined fluid-filled (+\– debris, blood products) cavity between the bladder and rectum.
- Uterine distension.
- Echogenic debris in the vagina.
- Secondary hydronephrosis.
- Can appear solid.

CT

Fluid-filled cavity, enhancing walls displacing adjacent organs.

MRI

- Mixed signal intensity on both T1WI and T2WI due to blood products.
- Uterine and cervical anomalies.
- Hydronephrosis.

Differential diagnosis

- Pelvic abscess.
- Ovarian tumour or cyst.
- Ovarian/fallopian tube torsion.
- Pelvic rhabdomyosarcoma.
- Sacrococcygeal teratoma.

Management

Drainage of cavity, hymen excised. Vaginal stenosis and focal atresia or uterine abnormalities may require a primary further surgical intervention.

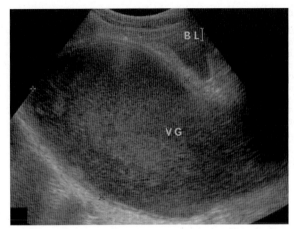

Fig. 4.40 Sagittal images through the pelvis showing a small anterior bladder (BL) anterior to a markedly dilated vagina (VG) with mixed echogenic blood products within it.

Genitourinary rhabdomyosarcoma

Rhabdomyosarcoma is an aggressive malignant tumour that probably arises from primitive muscle cells. It can occur anywhere in the body, pelvis and orbits are common sites, and tend to be large at presentation. There are four histological types: embryonal, botyroid, alveolar and undifferentiated. The tumour can arise from any pelvic organ, particularly bladder, vagina, uterus, prostate, pelvic muscle and paratesticular tissue. Tumour spreads by local extension, lymphatics and blood. Peak incidence is 2–6yrs, M>F. Staging based on tumour size, extension, nodal disease and metastatic spread, survival is based on staging.

Clinical presentation

Large pelvic mass, urinary symptoms (retention, haematuria, frequency), constipation and pain.

Imaging

Radiographs
- Soft tissue mass.
- Calcification.
- Bony destruction.
- Pulmonary metastases on chest X-ray.

Ultrasound
- ▶Solid multilobulated mass of mixed echogenicity.
- Large mass arising in the pelvis or mass within the bladder wall.
- Can be partially cystic.
- Evidence of urinary retention and hydronephrosis.

CT
- Useful in determining site of origin and assessing bone invasion.
- Metastatic spread.
- Heterogeneous invasive mass.
- Pulmonary metastases.

MRI
- ▶Most accurate modality in determining site of origin.
- Variable signal intensity depending on tissue components.
- Local invasion and vascular compression.
- Typically enhances with gadolinium.
- Can assess intra-spinal extension.

Nuclear scintigraphy
- Bone scan: metastatic disease.
- PET scan: metastatic spread and tumour recurrence.

Differential diagnosis
- Sacro coccygeal teratoma.
- Pelvic lymphoma.
- Ovarian tumour.
- Pelvic neuroblastoma.

Management and prognosis

Chemotherapy followed by organ-sparing surgery. Radiation therapy is also used and the gonads are often temporarily moved out of the radiation field.

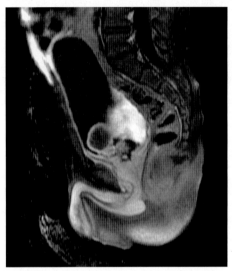

Fig. 4.41 Sagittal T1 WI following the administration of gadolinium shows an enhancing irregular partly cystic partly solid lesion at the bladder base.

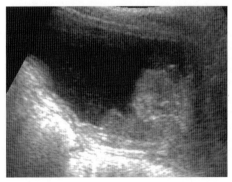

Fig. 4.42 Ultrasound image at the bladder shows a thickened bladder base and an irregular and nodular structure at the bladder base.

Sacrococcygeal teratoma

Proliferation of the pluripotential cells that may be malignant or benign. The tumour may contain any tissue type including hair, teeth, cartilage and fat. Varies in size from few cm to large volume mass. ▶Origin is always at the coccyx, but various types depending on extension can occur.

- Type I external in location.
- Type II dumbbell shaped with external and internal components.
- Type III predominantly internal.
- Type IV entirely internal.

Clinical presentation

Often diagnosed *in utero* or in the newborn if there is an external component. When the mass is entirely internal, diagnosis may be delayed and associated with urinary and bowel symptoms. Those with delayed diagnosis after 1yr have higher malignant potential. Alpha fetoprotein (AFP) useful tumour marker.

Imaging

Radiographs

- Large tissue mass extending outside the infant.
- Calcification, fat and teeth may be present.
- Fat/fluid levels.
- Arise around coccyx.

Ultrasound

- Heterogeneous, mixed echogenic mass.
- Calcification, fat and fluid.
- Mixed vascular pattern.

CT

- A large mass wrapped around the coccyx.
- Fat, calcified and fluid components.
- Often no bony destruction.
- Variable enhancement.

MRI

- Mixed signal intensity on T1 WI and T2 WI depending on cellular components.
- ▶The coccyx is enveloped.
- Variable enhancement with gadolinium.

Differential diagnosis

- Exophytic rhabdomyosarcoma (no bone or hair).
- Myelomeningocoele (contains neural elements).
- Neuroblastoma.

Management and prognosis

Surgical resection. Benign tumours have an excellent prognosis. Malignant tumours require chemo and radiation therapy.

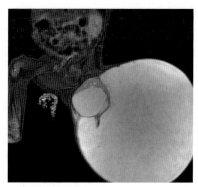

Fig. 4.43 Sagittal T2WI shows a large predominantly high signal cystic lesion arising from the sacrum in a newborn. There is an area of mixed signal intensity more proximally.

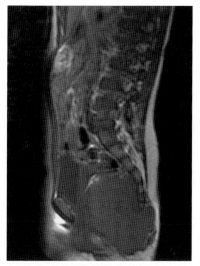

Fig. 4.44 In another child a sagittal T1WI demonstrating the midline location of the teratoma. The lesion is of low signal intensity.

Neuroblastoma

Malignant tumour of primitive neural crest cells, which can arise anywhere along the sympathetic chain, from the cervical region to the inferior pelvis. Commonest sites are the adrenal medulla, retroperitoneum and posterior mediastinum. It can metastasize. Commonest extra cranial solid malignancy in children. Typically presents by 2yrs, with younger children having a better prognosis.

Clinical presentation

A painless abdominal mass, associated with general malaise, irritability, weight loss, opsoclonus-myoclonus (abnormal movement of the eyes and extremities), cerebellar ataxia and hypertension. Over 90% of neuroblastomas are associated with elevated levels of catecholamines in the urine (vanillylmandelic acid [VMA]).

A subtype of the disease, the 4S, presents in children <1yr with metastatic disease confined to the skin, liver and bone with near 100% survival and spontaneous remission.

Imaging

Radiographs

- Non-specific soft tissue mass.
- ►Calcifications(30%)
- Widening of the para-spinal tissues and intervertebral foramina with paraspinal tumours.
- Bone metastases can be lucent/sclerotic or mixed lesions.
- Pathological fractures.

Ultrasound

- Large echogenic suprarenal mass.
- Areas of mixed echogenicity due to haemorrhage and necrosis.
- Calcification with acoustic shadowing.
- Increased vascularity on Doppler ultrasound.
- Encasement and displacement of vessels.
- Extension across the midline.
- Liver lesions are of low echogenicity.

CT

- Heterogeneous suprarenal mass with areas of mixed attenuation due to necrosis and haemorrhage.
- ►Calcification (>80%).
- ►Invasion of surrounding tissues, typically crosses the midline.
- ►Encasement of the major abdominal vessels.
- Spinal canal invasion.
- Low attenuation metastatic liver lesions.
- Lytic/sclerotic/mixed lesions in bone.

MRI

- ►Suprarenal mass with heterogeneous signal characteristics depending on haemorrhage, calcification and tissue necrosis.
- Often high signal on T2WI and low signal on T1WI.
- Encasement of vessels.
- Spinal cord extension with widening of the intravertebral foramen.
- Liver metastases.

Nuclear medicine
Meta-idobenzylguanidine (MIBG)
- Uptake by tissues with catecholamine production.
- Will detect metastatic skeletal disease.
- Detecting extent of MIBG uptake in tumours.
- 30% tumours may not show any uptake.

^{99m}Tc-MDP bone scan
- Uptake seen in bone metastases, including some that do not take up MIBG.
- Calcified mass can undertake uptake.

Differential diagnosis
- Wilms' tumour (displacement of tissue, less calcification).
- Neonatal adrenal haemorrhage (regression over time).
- Phaeochromocytoma.

Management
Prognosis depends on staging. Confined to a single region is stage 1, 90% survival. Stage 2 is extension within the organ but not crossing the midline. Extension crossing the midline, 30%, distal metastases 10%, 4S as discussed. Chemotherapy, surgical resection and bone marrow transplantation. Stage 4S may require no treatment with spontaneous resolution.

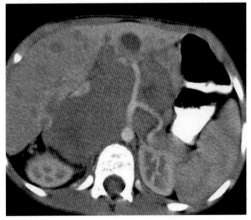

Fig. 4.45 Abdominal mass lesion encasing the aorta and its branches.

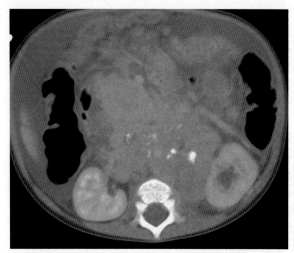

Fig. 4.46 Abdominal mass with irregular calcification within it.

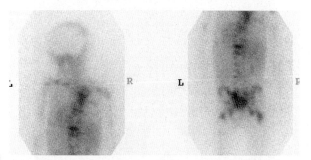

Fig. 4.47 MIBG scan showing uptake through out the spine due to metastatic deposits.

Neonatal adrenal haemorrhage

Bleeding into a normal adrenal gland in the perinatal period, associated with perinatal stress factors including asphyxia, infection, traumatic delivery and coagulopathies. Commoner in full-term, large babies, and on the right, but can be bilateral (10%).

Clinical presentation

Newborn child with anaemia, falling haematocrit, jaundice or adrenal insufficiency.

Imaging

Radiographs

- ▶In the acute period radiographs are normal.
- Calcification can occur after weeks or longer.

Ultrasound

- In the acute phase an echogenic mass replacing or expanding the adrenal gland.
- Doppler studies show the mass is avascular.
- ▶Follow-up sonography shows the blood products liquefying and forming a mixed echogenic mass and eventually the adrenal gland returns to its normal size.
- It can calcify.
- If ultrasound shows the mass is enlarging then the diagnosis needs to be reconsidered and a neuroblastoma excluded.

MRI

- Suprarenal mass.
- Signal intensity on T1 WI and T2 WI will vary depending on the age of the blood products and will change as the blood evolves.
- Gradient echo sequences most sensitive for haemosiderin detection.
- Useful when neuroblastoma is suspected.

Differential diagnosis

- ▶Neuroblastoma (no decrease in size, increased vascularity, elevated VMAs).
- Congenital adrenal hyperplasia, typically bilateral.
- Wolman's disease.

Management and prognosis

Serial ultrasound and observation. Important to exclude a neuroblastoma.

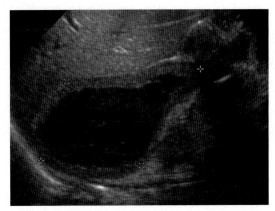

Fig. 4.48 Large mixed echogenic lesion in the position of the right adrenal gland. There is some displacement of the kidney at the liver edge. The haemorrhage has a thickened outer wall with a mixed echogenic centre.

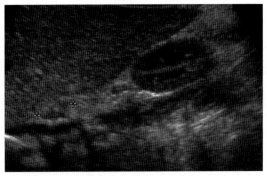

Fig. 4.49 Follow-up imaging of the same patient shows over a two-week period that the large cystic area has almost completely disappeared and there is a small mixed echogenic area in the region of the right adrenal gland.

Hepatobiliary
Clinical presentations and role of imaging

Karl Johnson

Jaundice

In the newborn, a prompt diagnosis is necessary as biliary atresia needs urgent treatment. In the older child, appropriate drug history, family history of metabolic disorders and infective screen are important. Cholestasis is obstruction to biliary flow from the liver to the duodenum.

Neonatal cholestasis

- Extra-hepatic:
  - Cholelithiasis.
  - Choledochal cyst (📖 p. 278).
  - Perforation.
  - Duodenal duplication.
  - Pancreatic haemangioma.
- Extra- and intra-hepatic:
  - Biliary atresia (📖 p. 276).
- Intra-hepatic:
  - Sclerosing cholangitis.
  - Transient neonatal cholestasis.
  - Alagille's syndrome.
  - Alpha-1 antitrypsin deficiency.
  - Infections.
  - Cystic fibrosis (📖 p. 66).
  - Parenteral nutrition.
  - Niemann–Pick disease.
  - Tyrosinaemia.
  - Galactosaemia.
  - Mitochondrial respiratory chain disorders.

Childhood cholestasis

- Extra-hepatic:
  - Cholelithiasis (gallstones).
  - Choledochal cyst (📖 p. 278).
  - Tumoural compression.
  - Portal vein obstruction.
  - Post-surgical stenosis.
  - Liver trauma.
- Extra- and intra-hepatic:
  - Sclerosing cholangitis.
- Intra-hepatic:
  - Viral hepatitis.
  - Drug-induced hepatitis.
  - Benign recurrent cholestasis.
  - Alpha-1 antitrypsin deficiency.
  - Cystic fibrosis (📖 p. 66).
  - Alagille's syndrome.

Role of imaging

Radiographs
- Limited role.
- Not routinely indicated.
- Alagille's syndrome is associated with spinal anomalies.

Ultrasound
Investigation of choice.
- Neonate:
  - Biliary dilatation.
  - Presence of the gallbladder does not exclude biliary atresia.
  - Altered liver texture and focal liver abnormalities.
  - Splenomegaly.
  - Gallstones.
  - Choledochal cysts.
- Older child:
  - Biliary dilatation and obstruction.
  - Gallstones.
  - Altered liver texture.
  - Focal liver lesions.
  - Ascites.
  - Varices.
  - Splenomegaly.
  - Choledochal cysts.

MRI
Magnetic resonance cholangiopancreatography (MRCP).
- Biliary dilatation and obstruction.
- Choledochal cyst.
- Gallstones.

Nuclear medicine
^{99m}Tc: label derivatives of iminodiacetic acid (IDA) derivatives.
- Liver uptake.
- Biliary excretion (▶activity seen within the bowel excludes biliary atresia).

Haematemesis

Appropriate history to exclude trauma, foreign bodies, bleeding disorders and drug ingestion.

Causes

- Swallowed blood.
- Repeated vomiting.
- Oesophageal/gastric ulceration:
  - Foreign body.
  - Drugs.
  - Gastro-esophageal reflux (📖 p. 186).
- Oesophageal varices due to portal hypertension:
  - Portal vein thrombosis.
  - Hepatic fibrosis.
  - Hepatic vein thrombosis.
  - Cirrhosis.
  - Veno-occlusive disease.
- Bleeding disorders.
- Vascular malformations.

Role of imaging

Ultrasound

- Oesophageal and periportal varices.
- Vascular malformations.
- Indicators of chronic liver disease (echogenic small liver and ascites).
- Splenomegaly.

Fluoroscopy

- May not be required if endoscopy is available.
- Swallowed foreign bodies.
- Varices.
- Hiatus hernia.

Hepatobiliary
Differential diagnosis

Karl Johnson

Hepatosplenomegaly

Causes

Neonate
- Cardiac failure.
- Infection.
- Metabolic disorders.
- Nutritional abnormalities.
- Storage disorders.
- Malignancy(neuroblastoma).
- Biliary atresia (📖 p. 276).

Older child
- Infection:
  - Hepatitis.
  - Infectious mononucleosis.
  - Malaria.
- Malignancy:
  - Leukaemia.
  - Neuroblastoma (📖 p. 260).
  - Lymphoma.
- Portal hypertension.
- Storage disorders.
- Polycystic liver disease.
- Haematological disorders.

Role of imaging

Radiographs
- Insensitive investigation.
- Distorted soft tissue planes.
- Displaced bowel gas.

Ultrasound
- Dilated veins due to cardiac failure.
- Focal liver lesions.
- Increased echogenicity.
- Ascites.

Increased periportal echoes in neonates

- Acute hepatitis.
- Cytomegalovirus infection.
- Biliary atresia (📖 p. 276).
- Idiopathic neonatal jaundice.
- Alpha-1 antitrypsin deficiency.
- Nesidioblastosis.

Diffuse increase in liver echogenicity

- Normal variant.
- Fatty infiltration.
- Cirrhosis.
- Diffuse infiltration, e.g. glycogen storage disease.
- Miliary granulomata.
- Malignant infiltration.
- Infectious mononucleosis.
- Portal tract fibrosis.
- Severe viral or other hepatitis.
- Malnutrition.
- Brucellosis.
- Reye's syndrome.
- Tyrosinaemia.
- Steroid therapy, particularly in conjunction with cytotoxic agents.
- Radiotherapy.

Gallstones in children

- Haemolysis.
- Totalparenteral nutrition (TPN).
- Cystic fibrosis (📖 p. 66).
- Bowel resection and terminal ileum anomalies.
- Malabsorption.
- Hepatitis.
- Congenital biliary anomalies (📖 p. 276).
- Frusemide therapy.

Hepatobiliary
Disorders

Karl Johnson

Biliary atresia

This is an absent, or a severely deficient, extrahepatic biliary tree. There may be associated congenital anomalies of the heart, abdomen, spine and genitourinary tract. It is graded on the level of disease extent: type I (common bile duct atresia); type II (common hepatic duct atresia); type III (right and left hepatic duct atresia).

Clinical presentation

In the neonate with progressively worsening jaundice due to a conjugated hyperbilirubinaemia, classically accompanied by pale stools. A prompt diagnosis is essential for surgical success. Imaging findings should be correlated with clinical and histological features.

Role of imaging

Ultrasound

- Useful to exclude other causes of jaundice.
- The liver may be enlarged but with normal echotexture.
- The gallbladder may be present in 25% of cases but the common duct is not seen.
- The extrahepatic bile ducts are not visible.
- There is an echogenic triangular cord sign which is a fibrotic remnant of the common duct.
- There may be abnormality of the liver vessels.
- ▶A normal ultrasound does not exclude the diagnosis.

Fluoroscopy

- Intra-operative cholangiograms are often performed prior to surgery.

MRI

- MRCP has been used with limited success.

Nuclear scintigraphy

- ^{99m}Tc–labelled derivatives of iminodiacetic acid (e.g. diisopropyl iminodiacetic acid [DISIDA] or trimethylbromo iminodiacetic acid [TBIDA]) are used. They have a high hepatic extraction rate with a prompt hepatobiliary transit time.
- The child should be pre-treated with phenobarbitone to stimulate liver enzymes.
- ▶Lack of excretion into the small bowel within 24hrs is suggestive, but not diagnostic, of biliary atresia.
- ▶Excretion into the gut excludes biliary atresia.
- Nuclear scintigraphy has 100% sensitivity but only 90% specificity.

Differential diagnosis

- Any cause of a conjugated hyperbilirubinaemia in a jaundiced neonate:
  - Neonatal hepatitis (raised viral titres).
  - Total parenteral nutrition.
  - Biliary hypoplasia/Alagille's syndrome.
  - Choledochal malformation.
  - Cystic fibrosis.

Management and prognosis

Kasai porto-enterostomy is performed where the intestine is anastomosed to the dissected surface of the porta hepatis, its success is increased if performed within the first 2 months of life. Some cases may require liver transplantation later in life.

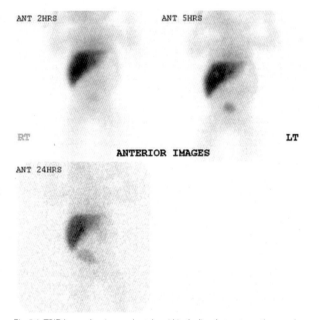

Fig. 5.1 TBIDA scan showing good uptake within the liver but no excretion, consistent with biliary atresia. The small amount of activity seen in the pelvis is within the bladder.

Choledochal cyst and Caroli's disease

This is a spectrum of cystic malformations of the extra- and intra-hepatic bile ducts. There is a classification system (Todani) based on the severity of disease:

- Type I: segmental or fusiform dilatation of the common bile duct (over 75% of cases).
- Type II: diverticulum of the lateral wall of the bile duct.
- Type III: cystic dilatation that protrudes into the duodenal wall.
- Type IV: multiple extra-hepatic bile duct cysts.
- Type V: cystic dilatation of the intra-hepatic bile duct.

Low-grade biliary obstruction may develop which can result in cirrhosis and portal hypertension, with an increased risk of bile duct perforation, stone formation, cholangitis and adenocarcinoma. Caroli's syndrome has an increased risk of cholangiocarcinoma.

Clinical presentation

In the infant, there may jaundice with acholic (pale) stools, abdominal pain and hepatomegaly. Presentation may be delayed into adulthood with a history of abdominal pain, cholangitis, pancreatitis and jaundice.

Role of imaging

Ultrasound

- ▶Dilatation of the biliary tree which may involve both intra- and extra-hepatic ducts.
- A bile duct dilated >10mm in childhood is a sensitive indicator of choledochal malformation.
- The presence and location of the cysts will help define the type of the disorder.

MRI

- ▶MR cholangiogram (MRCP) is able to demonstrate fluid-filled ducts and the location of the cystic abnormalities.
- The location of the pancreatic duct can be determined.

Differential diagnosis

- Chronic cholangitis.
- Obstructive cholelithiasis (typically a stone is seen).
- Pancreatic pseudocyst (history of pancreatitis).
- Hydatid cyst (history of exposure).
- Caroli's disease.

Management and prognosis

Surgical excision and a biliary drainage procedure is standard treatment. The extent and complexity of the surgery would increase with the grading of the disorder. In severe disease, liver failure may develop and transplantation may be necessary.

Caroli's disease

This is also classified as a Type V choledochal cyst. It is a congenital disorder, causing multifocal, saccular, non-obstructive dilatation of the intra-hepatic bile duct. It may be segmental or diffuse within the liver. Caroli's syndrome is Caroli's disease with congenital hepatic fibrosis. Fibrosis can cause portal hypertension, hepatosplenomegaly, and lead to liver failure. Increased risk of cholangiocarcinoma and renal cystic abnormalities.

Clinical presentation

Jaundice, right upper quadrant pain and cholangitis.

Role of imaging

Ultrasound
- ►Massively dilated intra-hepatic bile ducts.
- There are echogenic septae transversing the dilated ducts.
- There is the impression that the hepatic veins are surrounded by dilated ducts.
- Renal cysts.

MRI
- Multiple small saccular dilatations of the intra-hepatic bile duct (hyperintense on T2WI).
- With gadolinium, there is central dot enhancement of the portal vessel surrounded by dilated biliary tree.
- Cysts within the kidneys.

MRCP
- Multiple hyperintense oval-shaped structures within the liver.
- Bulbous dilatation of the intra-hepatic bile ducts.
- Signal void of the portal veins.

Differential diagnosis
- Polycystic liver disease (cysts with no communication with the biliary tract).
- Choledochal cyst.
- Primary sclerosing cholangitis.
- Ascending cholangitis.

Management and prognosis

If the disease is localized, surgical resection is possible. Ursodeoxycholic acid is useful to help to reduce biliary sludge. Decompression of the biliary tract may be effective. Liver transplantation for severe disease.

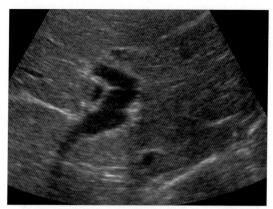

Fig. 5.2 An ultrasound image showing dilatation of the common duct.

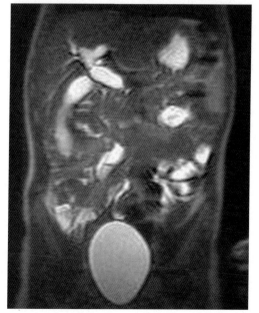

Fig. 5.3 Coronal MRCP image showing fusiform dilatation of the common duct.

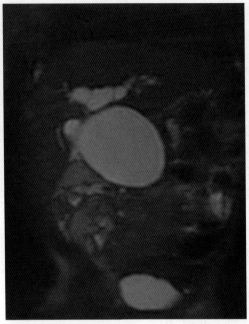

Fig. 5.4 Coronal MRCP image showing large choledochal cyst.

Mesenchymal hamartoma

This is a benign, developmental cystic liver tumour which usually presents <2yrs, M>F. The lesion can be very large at diagnosis (>15cm). The right lobe is more commonly affected than the left, but can involve both. They can be pedunculated.

Clinical presentation

Asymptomatic increase in abdominal size, a palpable right upper quadrant mass, vomiting, bowel disturbance and respiratory distress (due to diaphragmatic splinting).

Ultrasound

- ▶Multiple well-defined cysts.
- Cysts are variable in size with internal septations.
- 'Swiss-cheese' appearance.
- No calcification or haemorrhage.

CT

- Low attenuation multicystic liver lesion.
- Multiple septations.
- The septations and surrounding tissue may enhance.
- No calcification.

MRI

- T2WI: the cysts are hyperintense, the surrounding septations are hypointense.
- T1WI: typically low signal intensity.
- T1WI +C: enhancement of the septa.

Differential diagnosis

- Hepatoblastoma (alpha-feta protein and calcification).
- Haemangioendothelioma (contrast enhancement).
- Neuroblastoma metastases.

Management and prognosis

Some cases will regress spontaneously. Surgical removal is standard treatment as there is an increased incidence of malignant change. Partial hepatectomy is performed for larger lesions.

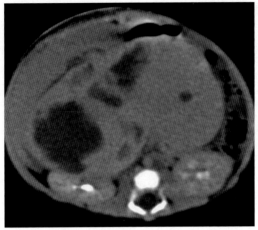

Fig. 5.5 Axial CT with partially cystic, partially solid lesion within the liver.

Hepatoblastoma

This is a malignant embryonic hepatic tumour of childhood and can present at birth up to 15yrs, commonest in infancy, M>F. More commonly located in the right lobe of the liver and often large at presentation (>10cm). Serum alpha-feta protein levels are elevated in 90% of cases.

Clinical presentation

A painless abdominal mass or hepatomegaly, may be associated with weight loss, nausea and vomiting and failure to thrive. It can be a cause of precocious puberty.

Role of imaging

Imaging is required to confirm the diagnosis and define the anatomic extent of disease (in particular vascular involvement) for pre-operative planning and chemotherapy response.

Radiographs

- Heterogeneous soft tissue mass in the right upper quadrant.
- Bowel displaced.
- Dense calcification.

Ultrasound

- ▶Well-defined heterogeneous predominately solid mass which is typically hypervascular.
- Lobulated or multifocal.
- Can involve the IVC.
- A 'spoke-wheel' appearance due to fibrous septa radiating from a central hub.
- Acoustic shadowing due to calcification.

CT

- ▶Well-defined heterogeneous low attenuation mass.
- Calcification is seen in about 50% of cases.
- Areas of haemorrhage and cystic change within the lesion.
- Enhancement is heterogeneous and less than liver parenchyma.
- Metastatic disease is seen in the lungs, para-aortic nodes and brain.

MRI

- T1WI and T2WI: signal change can be variable due to the presence of haemorrhage and necrosis.
- Typically high on T2WI but fibrous bands are hypointense.
- T1WI +C: heterogeneous enhancement.

Differential diagnosis

- Haemangioendothelioma (negative serum alpha-feta protein).
- Mesenchymal hamartoma (usually more cystic).
- Hepatocellular carcinoma (rare <3yrs, commoner >5yrs).
- Neuroblastoma metastases.

Management and prognosis

Chemotherapy and surgical resection are the mainstay treatment (with pre-surgical embolization). Liver transplantation for non-resectable disease.

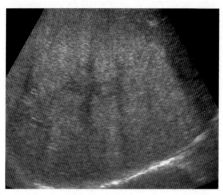

Fig. 5.6 Ultrasound shows a large well-defined mass with heterogeneous echogenicity.

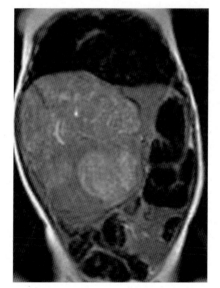

Fig. 5.7 Coronal MR image, T1W, following gadolinium shows a well-defined mass displacing adjacent structures. There is variable enhancement.

Haemangioendothelioma (infantile cavernous haemangioma)

Heterogeneous vascular mass of the liver, with 85% cases presenting before 6mths; F>M. Due to endothelial cell proliferation, typically the tumour undergoes an involutional phase and becomes smaller (disappears). When proliferating, the mass may be well-defined or diffusely infiltrates the liver, it may be solitary or multiple. It causes arteriovenous shunting.

Clinical presentation

Palpable mass with bruit over the liver, can cause high output cardiac failure (due to shunting of blood) or a consumptive coagulopathy (Kasabach–Merritt syndrome), associated cutaneous haemangiomas.

Role of imaging

Ultrasound

- Well-defined or infiltrative hypoechoic mass.
- Prominent dilated vessels with high flow.
- Calcification can occur.
- Will progressively decrease in size over time.

CT

- Low attenuation large mass on non contrasted images
- ▶Early peripheral and later central diffuse enhancement.
- Multiple lesions in the liver.
- Prominent vessels in the lesion.
- Descending aorta superior to celiac axis may be dilated due to increased blood flow.

MRI

- T1WI: low signal intensity relative to normal liver.
- T2WI: high signal intensity.
- Prominent flow voids in the lesion.
- Prominent draining veins.
- ▶Diffuse enhancement with gadolinium, initially peripheral then central.

Angiography

- Dilated hepatic arteries.
- Early filling of draining hepatic veins.
- Contrast pooling in lesions.

Differential diagnosis

- Hepatoblastoma (elevated AFP).
- Neuroblastoma metastases.
- Mesenchymal hamartoma (usually more cystic).
- Hepatocellular carcinoma (rare <3yrs, commoner >5yrs).

Management and prognosis

Lesions tend to involute spontaneously. Treatment for more severe cases include high-dose steroids, arterial embolization and surgical resection.

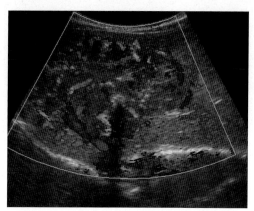

Fig. 5.8 Ultrasound image showing a homogeneous mass with prominent vascular structures.

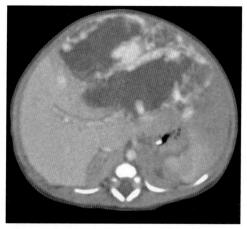

Fig. 5.9 Axial CT image following contrast shows the liver is enlarged. There is marked peripheral enhancement of a large haemangioendothelioma occupying the left lobe of the liver and low attenuation centrally.

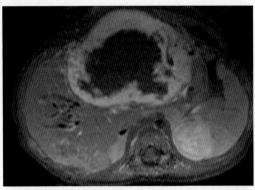

Fig. 5.10 Axial MRI (post-gadolinium T1WI) shows a large central lesion in the liver with marked peripheral enhancement.

Musculoskeletal
Clinical presentations and role of imaging

Karl Johnson

Bone pain

Bone pain may be localized or diffuse. The symptom itself is very non-specific for its causation. In children, the pain may be referred from another site and localization to any specific area may not be possible.

Causes

Skeletal

- Fracture/trauma (consider pathological or stress injuries).
- Primary tumour (benign and malignant).
- Infection.
- Dysplasia.
- Metastases (uncommon in children).
- Joint disease.

Soft tissue

- Infection.
- Trauma.
- Tumour (📖 p. 360–368).
- Juvenile dermatomyositis (JDMS) (📖 p. 358).
- Foreign body.

Role of imaging

The choice of imaging will depend on the presumed site of pain and the clinical history. For skeletal causes, radiographs should be the primary modality. For soft tissue lesions, either ultrasound or MR imaging should be considered first. All investigations are complementary.

Radiographs

- Detection of fractures.
- Bone tumours.
- ►Osteomyelitis may take over a week before any radiological changes.
- Skeletal dysplasia

Ultrasound

- Soft tissue oedema and collections.
- Can detect periosteal new bone.
- Traumatic soft tissue injuries.

CT

- Should be used only to define anatomy of known bone lesion or exclude a complication such as a pathological fracture.

MRI

►Most sensitive investigation.
- Can detect both marrow and soft tissue oedema (high signal on T2WI).
- Soft tissue injuries.
- Bone or soft tissue tumours.
- Infections.

Nuclear medicine (^{99m}Tc methylenediphosphonate)

- If pain persists with a normal radiograph.
- If the pain is multifocal.
- If there are pre-existing risk factors such as known malignant tumour.

Limping child

A child with a limp may be acute or chronic presentation. ▶With acute presentations, it is vital that sepsis either within the joint, bone or muscle is excluded promptly, as this is a treatable cause which, if inadequately managed, can result in severe long-term damage and disability. The likely cause of a limp is affected by the age of the child. The cause may be within any joint within the lower limb, the long bones, pelvis, or can be the result of an intra-abdominal, spinal or CNS lesion.

Causes

- Trauma:
  - Fractures.
  - Avulsion injuries (📖 p. 398).
  - Non-accidental injury (📖 p. 390).
  - Joint dislocation.
  - Ligamentous/tendon/muscle injury.
- Inflammatory:
  - Transient synovitis.
  - Juvenile idiopathic arthritis (📖 p. 356).
  - Juvenile dermatomyositis (📖 p. 358).
  - Henoch-Schönlein purpura.
- Infection:
  - Osteomyelitis (📖 p. 344).
  - Septic arthritis.
  - Discitis (📖 p. 378).
  - Appendicitis (📖 p. 172).
  - Psoas abscess.
- Avascular necrosis and osteochondritis:
  - Legg–Calvé–Perthes disease (📖 p. 334).
  - Osteochondritis dissecans (📖 p. 342).
  - Freiberg's disease.
  - Kohler's disease.
  - Chondromalacia patellae.
  - Idiopathic chondrolysis.
- Neoplastic:
  - Leukaemia and lymphoma (📖 p. 352).
  - Benign lesions eg: osteoid osteoma.
  - Malignant lesions, e.g. osteosarcoma. (📖 p. 362).
  - Metastasis, e.g. neuroblastoma.
- Haematological disorders:
  - Haemophilia.
  - Sickle cell disease (📖 p. 350).
- Neurological disorders:
  - Brain or spinal cord lesions.
  - Ataxia.
- Muscle disorders:
  - Muscular dystrophy.
  - Juvenile dermatomyositis (📖 p. 358).
  - Arthrogryposis.

- Bone disorders:
  - Slipped capital femoral epiphysis (📖 p. 336).
  - Leg length discrepancy.
  - Skeletal dysplasias (📖 p. 318).

Role of imaging

History and examination are important to localize the site of the limp. Pain may be referred from the hip to the knee and vice versa. ▶ A septic arthritis cannot be excluded by imaging. If sepsis is considered within a joint, aspiration and lavage are mandatory.

Radiographs
- Post-trauma.
- Detecting fractures.
- Limited value in acute joint disease, can detect more chronic conditions.
- Slipped femoral epiphysis.
- Bone tumours.

Ultrasound
- Joint effusions.
- The appearances of an effusion on ultrasound do not determine causation. Echogenic effusions may be sterile while clear effusions may be septic.
- Soft tissue oedema and abscesses.

MRI
- Excellent soft tissue and intra-articular imaging.
- Marrow disease.
- Sensitive in detecting inflammatory change within a joint.
- Assessment of intra-articular pathology.

Scoliosis/kyphosis

This is abnormal curvature of the spine in the sagittal plane which may be convex to the left or the right. Concern is raised when the curvature exceeds 10° and cannot be corrected.

Scoliosis may be structural or non-structural. Non-structural (functional) scoliosis is a mild non-progressive deformity which corrects with ipsilateral bending. Structural scoliosis shows asymmetry and loss of normal mobility of the spine.

Causes
- Idiopathic:
  - Early onset.
  - Late onset.
  - Adult.
- Neuromuscular:
  - Neuropathic.
  - Upper motor neuron (cerebral palsy, spinocerebellar degeneration, Friederich's ataxia).
  - Lower motor neuron (poliomyelitis, spinal cord injury, spinal muscular atrophy).
  - Myopathic (musculodystrophies, myopathic arthogryposis).
- Congenital.
- Osteogenic (vertebral/skeletal anomaly):
  - Abnormal bone development.
  - Failure formation (hemivertebrae, wedge vertebrae).
  - Failure of segmentation (bar and block vertebrae, fused ribs).
  - Syndromes, e.g. Klippel–Feil, spondylocostal dysostosis.
- Neuropathic:
  - Spinal cord anomaly, e.g. tethered cord, syringomyelia, diastematomyelia.
  - Spinal dysraphism, e.g. meningocele and myelomeningocele.
- Extra-vertebral abnormalities:
  - Rib fusion.
  - Sprengel deformity.
  - Hypoplastic lung.
  - Myositis ossificans progessiva.
- Developmental:
  - Skeletal dysplasia (osteogenesis imperfecta, mucopolysaccharidoses, spondyloepiphyseal dysplasia) (📖 p. 318).
  - Skeletal dysostosis (neurofibromatosis, Marfan's syndrome, Ehlers–Danlos syndrome).
- Tumour-related:
  - Vertebral (osteoid osteoma, osteoblastoma).
  - Extra-medullary (neurofibroma).
  - Intra-medullary (astrocytoma).
- Miscellaneous:
  - Post-irradiation.
  - Post-infectious (osteopathic and non-viral).
  - Post-traumatic (osteopathic).
  - Post-surgical.

- Metabolic/endocrine (osteomalacia, rickets, Cushing disease).
- Juvenile idiopathic arthritis(📖 p. 356).
- Spondylolisthesis.

Adult scoliosis presents after skeletal maturity or 20yrs old.

Kyphosis

- Vertebral malformations.
- Scheuermann's disease.
- Generalized skeletal disorders and dysmorphic syndromes.
- Infection (TB).
- Spinal cord tumours.
- Radiotherapy.
- Postural.

Role of imaging

Physical examination should assess the age of the child, neurological symptoms and the cosmetic appearance.

Radiographs

- Standing erect, PA and lateral of the entire spine.
- Assess the degree of scoliosis.
- Structural lesion within the spine.
- Assess skeletal maturity from the ossification centres of the pelvic brim.
- Surgical follow-up and post-operative complications (pneumothorax, consolidation, effusion, osteomyelitis).

CT

- Assessing vertebral anomalies.
- Assessment of rib deformity.
- Useful in post-surgical follow-up.

MRI

- Not indicated in all cases.
- Assess the integrity of the cord.
- Presence of cord lesions.
- Gadolinium enhancement if tumour suspected.

Back pain

Back pain in children is uncommon and persisting symptoms should raise concerns of significant underlying pathology. Clinical localization of the pain and aggravating and relieving factors are important.

Causes

- Muscular injuries.
- Ligament injury.
- Fractures.
- Spondylitis/spondylolisthesis.
- Discitis (📖 p. 378).
- Osteomyelitis (📖 p. 344).
- Scheuermann's disease.
- Idiopathic scoliosis.
- JIA (📖 p. 356).
- Benign neoplasms:
  - Osteoid osteoma.
  - Osteoblastoma.
  - Langerhans' cell histiocytosis (📖 p. 364).
  - Aneurysmal bone cyst.
- Malignant:
  - Ewing's sarcoma (📖 p. 360).
  - Lymphoma (📖 p. 352).
  - Leukaemia (📖 p. 352).
  - Neuroblastoma (📖 p. 260).
- Spinal cord-based lesions:
  - Cord glioma.
  - Astrocytoma (📖 p. 510).
  - Metastases.
  - Tethered cord (📖 p. 526).

Role of imaging

All the imaging modalities are complementary.

Radiographs

- Insensitive for intra-vertebral disc and cord lesions.
- The inflammatory changes of JIA may take time to appear.

CT

- Sensitive in detecting bone-based pathology.
- Poor for cord lesions.

MRI

- The most sensitive investigation in detecting the cause of back pain.
- ►STIR images sensitive in detecting marrow/disc inflammation.
- May miss spondylitis.
- Post-gadolinium sequences sensitive in detecting synovial inflammation.

Nuclear medicine

- Useful for bone-based lesions.
- High radiation dose.
- Non-specific.

Swollen/painful joint

▶In the acutely swollen joint, it is important that sepsis is excluded as this can cause rapid and severe joint destruction.

Causes

- Trauma.
- Inflammatory conditions:
  - JIA (📖 p. 356).
  - Transient synovitis.
  - Reactive synovitis.
- Infections:
  - Septic arthritis.
  - Osteomyelitis (📖 p. 344).
- Neoplasm:
  - Primary bone tumours.
  - Malignant disease.
  - Leukaemia (📖 p. 352).
- Haematological disorders:
  - Rickets (📖 p. 348).
  - Scurvy.
  - Sickle cell disease (📖 p. 350).
  - Haemophilia.

Role of imaging

In all acutely painful or swollen joints, sepsis should be excluded. Imaging cannot exclude septic arthritis and this should be done either on clinical grounds or following aspiration of the joint.

Radiographs

- Trauma.
- Bone tumours.

Ultrasound

- Joint effusion.
- Synovial hypertrophy.

MRI

- Evaluation of bone tumours.
- Joint effusions.
- Synovial hypertrophy.
- Joint derangement.
- Ligament and tendon injury.
- Soft tissue injury.
- Marrow disorders.
- Fractures.

Lower limb abnormalities

In-toeing
- Feet/ankles:
  - Metatarsus adductus.
  - Talipes varus and equinovarus.
  - Pronated feet.
- Leg/knee:
  - Blount's disease (tibia vara).
  - Medial tibial torsion.
  - Tibial hypoplasia.
- Femur/hip:
  - Cerebral palsy.
  - Femoral anteversion.

Out-toeing
- Feet/ankles:
  - Pes valgus.
  - Talipes calcaneovalgus.
- Leg/knee:
  - Lateral tibial torsion.
  - Fibular hypoplasia.
- Femur/knee:
  - DDH.
  - Femoral retroversion.
  - Flaccid paralysis.
- Idiopathic juvenile osteoporosis (and other causes of a generalized reduction in bone density).

Genu valgum (knock knee)
- Physiological.
- Trauma.
- Rickets.
- Neurological: cerebral palsy, poliomyelitis, myelomeningocele.
- Bone cysts, neurofibromatosis.

Genu varum (bow legs)
- Physiological.
- Trauma.
- Rickets (📖 p. 348).
- Blount's disease.
- Multiple enchondromatosis.
- Fracture.
- Osteomyelitis (📖 p. 344).
- Hypophosphatasia.
- Tumour.
- Osteogenesis imperfecta(📖 p. 322).
- Metaphyseal dysplasia.
- Achondroplasia(📖 p. 320).

Role of imaging

Radiographs
- Exclude an underlying dysplasia.
- Measure the degree of varus and valgus angulation.
- Assess the degree of rotation.

CT
- Leg length measurement.
- Assessment of the angle of anteversion of the hips.

Limb mass/bone lesion

The age of the child, rate of growth and associated symptoms are important in the differential diagnosis.

Soft tissue mass

Causes
- Common benign lesions:
  - Lipoma.
  - Vascular malformations.
  - Haemangioma (📖 p. 374).
  - Cystic hygroma.
  - Haematoma.
  - Lymphadenopathy.
  - Plexiform neurofibroma.
  - Ganglion cyst.
  - Abscess.
  - Myositis ossificans.
- Common malignant lesions:
  - Rhabdomyosarcoma (RMS) (📖 p. 368).
  - Synovial cell sarcoma (📖 p. 370).
  - Fibrosarcoma.
  - Primitive neuroectodermal tumour (PNET).
  - Extraosseous Ewing's sarcoma (📖 p. 360).
  - Myxoid liposarcoma.
  - Malignant fibrous histiocytoma.
  - Malignant peripheral nerve sheath tumour (MPNST).

Role of imaging in soft tissue masses

Radiographs
- Foreign body.
- Bone erosion/destruction.
- Calcification.

Ultrasound
- Differentiates cystic from solid.
- Deep tissue extension can be difficult to determine.
- Vascular lesions have increased flow on Doppler.

MRI
- Fatty lesions high signal T1WI.
- Fluid-filled lesions high signal T2WI.
- Gadolinium enhancement.
- Blood products.
- Benign lesions typically have well-defined margins, single tissue compartment and uniform signal intensity.

Common primary bone neoplasms
- Osteosarcoma (📖 p. 362).
- Ewing's sarcoma (📖 p. 360).
- Leukaemia (📖 p. 352).
- Lymphoma.

Role of imaging of a potential malignant bone lesion

Radiographs
- Assessment of site.
- Marrow and cortical bone involvement.
- Pathological fractures.

MRI
▶Inclusion of the joint above and below the lesion to detect skip metastases.
- Evaluation of neurovascular, joint, epiphyseal and soft tissue involvement.
- Determine tumour size.
- Assess response to chemotherapy.

CT and nuclear medicine (^{99m}Tc MDP bone scan)
- Lung metastases.
- Distant bone metastases.

Torticollis

Causes
- Muscular/soft tissue:
  - Congenital sternomastoid 'tumour'.
  - Trauma.
  - Myositis.
  - Soft tissue tumours.
- Cervical adenitis/absce.ss.
- Psychological: spasmodic torticollis, tic.
- Subluxations:
  - Trauma.
  - Atlanto-axial rotatory fixation (AARF) (📖 p. 402).
  - Infections of pharynx.
- Ocular:
  - IV nerve palsy.
  - Brainstem tumour.
  - Nystagmus.
- Central nervous system:
  - Posterior fossa tumour (📖 p. 510).
- Congenital vertebral anomalies:
  - Klippel–Feil syndrome.
  - Sprengel's shoulder.
  - Hemivertebrae.
- Bone tumours.

Role of imaging

Radiographs
- Vertebral anomalies.
- Fracture subluxations.
- AARF (📖 p. 402).
- Bone tumours.

Ultrasound
- Lymphadenopathy.
- Abscess.
- Soft tissue tumours.

CT
- Fractures.
- AARF.
- Bone tumours.

MRI
- Soft tissue abscess.
- Bone tumours.
- Vertebral anomalies.
- CNS and spinal lesions.

Musculoskeletal
Differential diagnosis

Karl Johnson

Soft tissue calcifications

Clumped/irregular calcification

- Scleroderma.
- Haemangioma (📖 p. 374).
- Trauma (haematoma/burns/myositis ossificans).
- Synovial sarcoma.
- JIA (post joint injection).
- Tuberculosis.
- Parosteal osteosarcoma.
- Parasitic infection.
- Hyperparathyroidism.
- Ehlers–Danlos syndrome.

'Sheets' of calcification

- Myositis ossificans progressiva.
- Juvenile dermatomyositis (📖 p. 358).

Epiphyseal and metaphyseal abnormalities

Dense vertical metaphyseal lines

- Congenital rubella.
- Congenital cytomegalovirus.
- Metaphyseal injury.
- Localized infection.
- Osteopathia striata.
- Hypophosphatasia.

Fraying and/or cupping of metaphyses

- Normal.
- Rickets (📖 p. 348).
- Localized infection.
- Chronic stress/trauma.
- Bone dysplasias (📖 p. 318).
- Scurvy.
- Copper deficiency.
- Menkes' disease.
- Hypophosphatasia.

Solitary radiolucent metaphyseal band

- Normal neonate.
- Severe systemic illness.
- Metaphyseal fracture (📖 p. 391).
- Leukaemia.
- Healing rickets (📖 p. 348).
- Metastatic neuroblastoma (📖 p. 260).
- Congenital infections.

- Intrauterine perforation.
- Scurvy.

Alternating radiolucent and dense metaphyseal bands

- Growth arrest lines (Park's).
- Rickets (📖 p. 348).
- Osteopetrosis (📖 p. 354).
- Chemotherapy.
- Chronic anaemias.
- Bisphophosonate therapy.
- Treated leukaemia (📖 p. 352).

Solitary dense metaphyseal band

- Normal infants.
- Bisphophonate therapy.
- Hypervitaminosis D.
- Heavy metal poisoning.
- Osteopetrosis (📖 p. 354).
- Congenital hypothyroidism.

Irregularity of the epiphyses

- Normal.
- Avascular necrosis.
- Bone dysplasias/storage disorders:
  - Morquio's syndrome (📖 p. 324).
  - Multiple epiphyseal dysplasia.
  - Meyer dysplasia.
  - Chondrodysplasia punctata.
- Trisomy 18 and 21.
- Prenatal infections.
- Congenital hypothyroidism.
- Warfarin embryopathy.
- Zellweger syndrome.
- Fetal alcohol syndrome.

Periosteal reactions

Parallel spiculated ('hair-on-end')
- Ewing's sarcoma (□ p. 360).
- Infection.
- Infantile cortical hyperostosis (Caffey's disease).

Divergent spiculated ('sunray')
- Osteosarcoma (□ p. 362).
- Ewing's sarcoma (□ p. 360).
- Infection (TB).

Elevated Codman's triangle
- Aggressive malignant tissue extending into the soft tissues:
  - Ewings.
  - Osteosarcoma.
- Infection—occasionally.

Localized
- Traumatic.
- Infection.
- JIA (around tendon insertion).
- Leukaemia.
- Malignant tumours (primary/secondary).
- Pathological fractures.

Bilaterally asymmetrical
- Normal features (typically 1–6mths).
- Osteomyelitis (□ p. 344).
- JIA (□ p. 356).
- Traumatic:
  - Non-accidental injury (□ p. 390).
- Leukaemia (□ p. 352).
- Malignancy or metastases (neuroblastoma).
- Sickle-cell dactylitis (□ p. 350).

Bilaterally symmetrical
- Normal infants (typically 1–6mths).
- Juvenile idiopathic arthritis (□ p. 356).
- Rickets (□ p. 348).
- Leukaemia.
- Caffey's disease.
- Scurvy.
- Prostaglandin E therapy.
- Congenital syphilis.

Abnormalities of growth

Premature closure of a growth plate

- Local hyperaemia:
  - JIA.
  - Infection.
- Trauma (📖 p. 388).
- Infection.
- Vascular occlusion.
- Radiotherapy.
- Thermal injury.
- Multiple exostoses and enchondromatosis (Ollier's disease).

Limb shortening

- Trauma:
  - Physeal injury.
  - Fracture non-union.
  - Overlapping malposition of fracture.
  - Slipped capital femoral epiphysis (📖 p. 336).
  - Burns.
  - Resection of bone tumour.
- Neuromuscular disorders:
  - Hemiplegia.
  - Post-poliomyelitis.
  - Cerebral palsy.
  - Myelomeningocele.
  - Peripheral neuropathy.
- Congenital:
  - DDH (📖 p. 330).
  - Hemiatrophy.
  - Skeletal dysplasias.
  - Malformation of femur or tibia.
- Infection/inflammation:
  - Osteomyelitis (📖 p. 344).
  - Septic arthritis.
  - Tuberculosis.
  - JIA (📖 p. 356).
- Radiotherapy.
- Multiple exostoses and enchondromatosis (Ollier's disease).

Bone lesions

Epiphyseal
- Central:
  - Chondroblastoma.
  - Histiocytosis (📖 p. 364).
- Eccentric:
  - Trevor's disease.
- Soft tissue:
  - Pigmented villonodular synovitis (PVNS).

Metaphyseal
- Central:
  - Enchondroma.
  - Osteosarcoma (📖 p. 362).
  - Ewing's sarcoma (📖 p. 360).
  - Bone cyst.
  - Giant cell tumour.
- Eccentric:
  - Aneurysmal bone cyst.
  - Osteosarcoma (📖 p. 362).
  - Ewing's sarcoma (📖 p. 360).
- Cortical:
  - Osteochondroma.
  - Osteosarcoma.
  - Ewing's sarcoma.
- Periosteal:
  - Osteosarcoma.
  - Ewing's sarcoma.
- Soft tissue;
  - Osteosarcoma.
  - Ewing's sarcoma.

Metadiaphyseal
- Central:
  - Fibrous dysplasia (📖 p. 372).
  - Abscess.
- Eccentric:
  - Chondromyxoid fibroma.
- Cortical:
  - Non-ossifying fibroma (fibrous cortical defect).
  - Osteoid osteoma.
- Soft tissue:
  - Myositis ossificans.
  - Synovial sarcoma (📖 p. 370).

Diaphyseal
- Central:
  - Langerhans cell histiocytosis (📖 p. 364).
  - Ewing's sarcoma.
  - Lymphoma.
  - Fibrous dysplasia.
- Cortical:
  - Osteoid osteoma.
  - Adamantinoma.
- Soft tissue:
  - Neurofibromatosis.
  - Rhabdomyosarcoma (📖 p. 368).

Paediatric tumours that metastasize to bone

- Neuroblastoma (📖 p. 260).
- Leukaemia (📖 p. 352).
- Lymphoma.
- Soft tissue sarcoma.
- Rhabdomyosarcoma (📖 p. 368).
- Retinoblastoma (📖 p. 484).
- Ewing's sarcoma (📖 p. 360).
- Osteosarcoma (📖 p. 362).

Synovial proliferation +/− joint effusion

- Infective:
  - Septic arthritis.
  - Viral.
  - TB.
  - Lyme disease.
- Reactive.
- Traumatic (ligament/bone injury).
- Juvenile idiopathic arthritis (📖 p. 356).
- Transient synovitis (hip).
- Haemorrhage within the joint:
  - Pigmented villonodular synovitis.
  - Vascular malformation (📖 p. 374).
  - Haemophilia.
  - Trauma.
- Autoimmune disorders:
  - SLE.
  - Systemic sclerosis.
- Idiopathic chondrolysis.
- Periarticular tumours.
- Vasculitis:
  - Henoch–Schönlein purpura.
  - Kawasaki disease.
  - Polyarteritis nodosa.
- Congenital and metabolic disorders:
  - Trisomy 21.
  - Mucopolysaccharidoses (📖 p. 324).
  - Chronic infantile neurological cutaneous and articular (CINCA) syndrome.
- Epiphyseal lesions.
  - Perthes.
  - SUFE.

Vertebral body anomalies

Coronal cleft vertebral bodies

- Normal variant.
- Bone dysplasias:
  - Chondrodysplasia punctata.
  - Kniest syndrome.
  - Metatropic dwarfism.
- Acquired.

Anterior beaking

- Central:
  - Morquio's syndrome.
- Lower third:
  - Hurler's syndrome.
  - Achondroplasia (□ p. 320).
  - Pseudoachondroplasia.
  - Cretinism.
  - Neuromuscular diseases.
  - Trisomy 21.

Posterior scalloping

- Tumours in the spinal canal.
- Neurofibromatosis (□ p. 534).
- Communicating hydrocephalus.
- Syringomyelia.
- Connective tissue disorders:
  - Ehlers–Danlos syndrome.
  - Marfan's syndrome.
  - Osteogenesis imperfecta (□ p. 322).
- Storage disorders (□ p. 324):
  - Morquio's syndrome.

Anterior scalloping

- Tuberculous spondylitis.
- Lymphadenopathy.
- Delayed motor development.

Musculoskeletal
Disorders

Karl Johnson

Bone marrow

Normal bone marrow is important in producing circulating blood cells. In the newborn child, when the body's demand for new red blood cells is high, the bone contains haematopoietic (red) marrow. As the child grows, there is gradual replacement of this haematopoietic marrow with fatty (yellow) marrow.

On MR imaging, red marrow in the long bones is low to intermediate signal intensity compared with muscle on T1WI. The vertebral bodies are less intense than the discs. Fatty marrow is of higher signal intensity on T1WI compared to muscle. The vertebral bodies become isointense with the discs, as the marrow converts.

In early childhood (1–5yrs), there is red marrow in the epiphyses and diaphyses of long bones which is gradually replaced with fatty marrow. During late childhood and early adolescence, the marrow within the spine, iliac wings, and distal metaphyses becomes more fatty.

In late adolescence, there is residual haematopoietic marrow in the axial skeleton and in the proximal metaphysis of each limb. This haematopoietic marrow is of intermediate signal intensity compared with the rest of the fatty marrow, which is of high signal intensity on T1WI.

The marrow conversion around the knee can be patchy and may be confused with malignant infiltration. Normal haematopoietic marrow does not enhance following gadolinium administration.

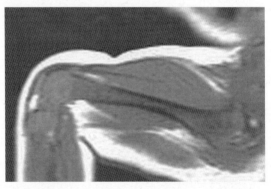

Fig. 6.1 Sagittal T1 image of the femur in a neonate. There is haemopoietic marrow throughout the femur. The marrow is of low signal intensity similar to that of the adjacent muscle.

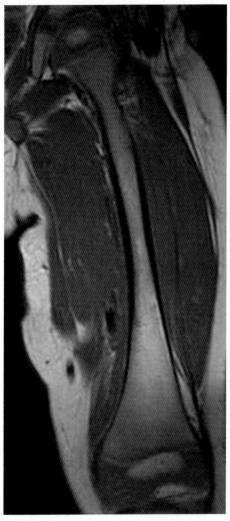

Fig. 6.2 Coronal T1W image of the femur in a 12-year-old girl. There has been conversion of the haemopoietic to fatty marrow which is of high signal and similar to that of the surrounding subcutaneous fat.

Bone dysplasias

The term bone dysplasia refers to a group of more than 150 disorders that relate to abnormalities of bone formation and development. More precisely these disorders can be divided into two broad groups: osteo-chondrodysplasias and dysostoses.

Osteochondrodysplasias are subdivided into dysplasias (abnormalities of bone and/or cartilage growth) and osteodystrophies (abnormalities of bone and cartilage textures). Dysplasias are the largest group and therefore the term 'skeletal dysplasia' is incorrectly used to describe both the osteodystrophies and dysostoses.

The dysostoses are the result of abnormalities in embryonic development of bone formation.

In all the conditions, children most commonly present with reduced stature or a reduction in limb growth. For severe conditions it can result in death during the neonatal period.

Radiological approaches to skeletal dysplasias

When clinical concern is raised about a child having a possible skeletal dysplasia the radiological approach is to perform a skeletal survey.

A skeletal survey should include the skull (AP and lateral), thoracolumbar spine (AP and lateral), chest, pelvis, one upper limb (typically the left), one lower limb and left hand (for the bone age). If it is thought that there is asymmetry of a limb then images of the contralateral side should be obtained. If the diagnosis remains uncertain, a repeat skeletal survey after at least 12mths may be appropriate.

Approach to the radiographs

It is necessary to determine the anatomical location of any abnormalities, the structure and formation of the bones, any associated complications (e.g. cardiac or renal abnormalities) and obviously whether it is performed on a live or dead child.

Anatomical location

The nomenclature of many dysplasias relates to the anatomical location of the most obvious skeletal abnormality:
- Skull—cranio, cranial;
- Face—facial;
- Mandible—mandibular;
- Clavicle—cleido;
- Ribs—costo;
- Spine—spondylo or vertebral;
- Pelvis—ischio, ilio or pubic.

If the bones of the appendicular skeleton are involved then the terms epiphyseal, metaphyseal or diaphyseal are used.

If there is shortening of the limbs then the location should be noted (rhizomelic is proximal, mesomelic is middle part or portion, such as the radius and ulna, and acromelic is distal hands and feet).

Abnormalities of the bones

When analysing the bones, it is important to determine structure, shape, size, number of bones and any soft tissue abnormalities around the bones.

The structure of the bones relates to bone density and the presence or absence of any exostoses or enchondromas.

Making the diagnosis

The skeletal survey should be reviewed to identify those characteristics which are obvious and unequivocal. The nomenclature of the dysplasia is often based upon the site of involvement (e.g. metaphyseal epiphyseal dysplasia, spondyloepiphyseal dysplasia). Within each dysplasia there are often subcategorizations, and further refinements are based on the sites of disease and other associated factors.

When determining the type of dysplasia the most obvious and unequivocal abnormalities should be recorded and used to initiate a search of suitable database which records all the known dysplasias and their radiological features. The use of computer-aided programs and electronic databases has simplified this procedure.

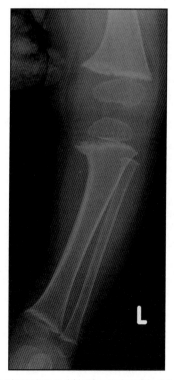

Fig. 6.3 Metaphyseal irregularity in child with metaphyseal dysplasia.

Achondroplasia

This is one of the commonest skeletal dysplasias, which classically results in a short stature and is due to a defect in chromosome 4P. It has autosomal dominant inheritance, but the majority of cases are new mutations.

Clinical presentation

Altered facies with hypoplasia of the mid face, a saddle nose and frontal bossing. There is rhizomelic (proximal) limb shortening, limited elbow extension and altered gait.

Imaging findings

Radiographs

- Skull:
  - Small skull base with narrow foramen magnum.
  - Hypoplasia of the mid face with crowding of the dentition.
  - Calvaria enlarged with frontal bossing.
  - Basal invagination.
- Spine:
  - ▶Decreased interpedicular distance which gets progressively smaller in the lower lumbar spine (opposite to normal).
  - Vertebral bodies are short, flat (bullet-shaped in early life) with loss of height. Disc spaces appear enlarged.
  - Posterior scalloping.
  - Thoraco-lumbar kyphoscoliosis and an increased lumbar lordosis.
  - Instability of the cervical spine.
- Chest:
  - Short ribs and sternum with cup-shaped anterior ends.
- Pelvis:
  - Short, wide iliac bones (tombstone appearance).
  - ▶Horizontal acetabulum.
  - Small sacroiliac notch.
- Limbs:
  - Rhizomelic shortening.
  - Flared metaphysis with large epiphysis.
  - Bowed legs.
  - Fibula longer than the tibia.
  - Trident hand: 3 components, thumb, digits 2 and 3, digits 4 and 5, with an increased gap between digits 3 and 4.

Differential diagnosis

- Hypochondroplasia (mild form of short-limbed dwarfism).
- Pseudo-achondroplasia (normal face).
- Metotropic dysplasia.

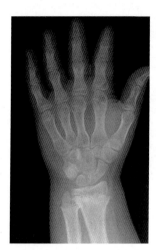

Fig. 6.4 AP radiograph of the hand. The fingers are approximately of equal length and diverge in pairs.

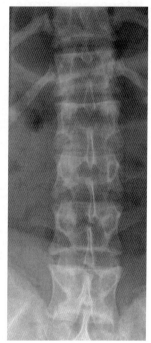

Fig. 6.5 AP lower lumbar spine. The interpedicular distance becomes narrower.

Osteogenesis imperfecta (OI)

This is an inherited disorder of collagen, resulting in abnormal bone mass, structure and strength, with other associated connective tissue abnormalities. There are a variety of subtypes of OI which vary in severity and inheritance.

Clinical presentation

Generally, the bones are osteopenic, thinned and the child is more prone to fractures with abundant callus formation when they heal. There may be bone remodelling, with bowing and deformity. The sclera tend to be blue and there are abnormal features of dentition and hearing.

Subtypes (Sillence classification)

- Type 1: (AD inheritance). Mild, may not be deforming, blue sclera, numerous fractures, less common after puberty, normal stature, marked kyphoscoliosis, dentinogenesis imperfecta.
- Type 2: (AD and AR inheritance). Severe form can cause perinatal death, blue sclera, excessive number of fractures, death due to intracranial haemorrhage, pulmonary hypoplasia and multiple rib fractures.
- Type 3: (AD and AR inheritance). Moderate/severe deformation, abnormal face, underdevelopment of the facial bones, sclera blue/grey, kyphoscoliosis, chest deformity, bowed bones, short stature.
- Type 4: (AD inheritance). Mild deformation, normal white sclera, there may be long bones and vertebral fractures, dentinogenesis imperfecta may occur but is not universal.

Imaging findings

Radiographs

- Long bones: thin cortices, overtubulated, multiple fractures, osteopenia, remodelling, exuberant callus formation.
- Following bisphosphonate therapy: multiple thin sclerotic metaphyseal bands parallel to the physis, corresponding to episodes of treatment.
- Skull: abnormal cranium with large bulk and shortened face, multiple wormian bones, frontal bossing, basilar impression/invagination.
- Spine: kyphoscoliosis, biconcave or flattened vertebral bodies, compression fractures.
- Chest: thoracic deformity, multiple rib fractures.
- Pelvis: coxa vara, protruding acetabulae.

MRI

- Basilar invagination.
- Crush fractures of vertebral bodies.
- Scoliosis/kyphosis.

Differential diagnosis

- Neurofibromatosis.
- Idiopathic juvenile osteoporosis.
- Osteomyelitis (exuberant callus formation).
- Child abuse can cause multiple fractures.

Management and prognosis

Fracture treatment. Bisphosphonate therapy.

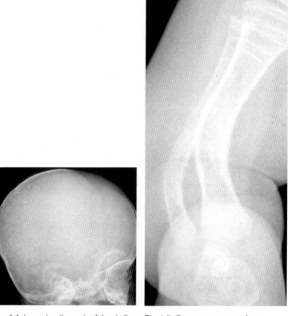

Fig. 6.6 Lateral radiograph of the skull in a child with osteogenesis imperfecta shows extensive wormian bone formation in the occiput.

Fig. 6.7 Osteogenesis imperfecta. Osteopenic bones with marked bowing deformity. The sclerotic lines around the metaphysis indicate previous biphosphonate therapy.

Mucopolysaccharidosis and dysostosis multiplex

Mucopolysaccharidoses (MPS) are a heterogeneous group of inherited disorders (all AR except MPS-2 which is X-linked), caused by deficiency of enzymes to degrade glycosoaminoglycans (mucopolysaccharides). There are nine types, the features and age of presentation are dependent upon the subtype:

- MPS 1-H: Hurlers syndrome. Onset 1–2yrs, severe dwarfism and skeletal abnormalities and neurological features.
- MPS 1-S: Scheie syndrome. Mild onset in childhood, have carpal tunnel syndrome.
- MPS 1H/S: Hurlers-Scheie syndrome.
- MPS 2: Hunter's syndrome. 2–4yrs, severe dwarfism and skeletal features, moderate neurology.
- MPS 3: Sanfilippo syndrome. Onset in childhood, severe neurological symptoms.
- MPS 4: Morquio syndrome. 1–3yrs, severe skeletal abnormalities, absent neurological features but often spinal abnormalities.
- MPS 5: now MPS 1-S.
- MPS 6: Maroteaux–Lamy syndrome. Childhood onset, severe dwarfism and skeletal abnormalities, absent neurological features.
- MPS 7: Sly syndrome. Mild to severe skeletal features, absent to severe neurology.
- MPS 8: non-existent.
- MPS 9: hydronylase deficiency.

Clinical presentation

There may be regression of speech and learning skills, mental retardation. Morphologically, there may be large head, coarse hair, hirsutism, proptosis, corneal opacification (not in Hunter's) and glaucoma, respiratory and cardiovascular abnormalities, hepatosplenomegaly, intestinal pseudo-obstruction. Generally reduced stature, scoliosis, flexion contractures and instability of the C1/C2 joint.

Dysostosis multiplex

This term refers to all the inherited storage disorders that result in a constellation of skeletal dysplasia features and includes MPS (commonest), mucolipidoses, Gaucher's disease, Niemann–Pick disease, fucosidosis, gangliodosis, mannosidosis.

Imaging findings

Radiographs

- Large head and early suture closure, J-shaped sella, thick skull base, concave or flat mandibular condyles, macroglossia.
- Thoracolumbar kyphosis with anterior beaked vertebral bodies (Morquio middle, others inferior body), vertebrae plana (flattened vertebral body), hypoplastic dens with C1/C2 and C3/C4 subluxation, dorsolumbar gibbus, posterior scalloping.
- Wide, oar-shaped ribs, short and thick clavicles.

- Abnormal pelvis, small iliac wings, tapered with steep acetabular roof and coxa valga, femoral subluxation, genu valgum.
- Thickened diaphysis of the long bones, varus humeral neck, angulated oblique growth plates of distal radius and ulna.
- Small irregular carpal bones, irregular wide metacarpals with pointed proximal ends (Trident hand).
- Cardiomyopathy.

MRI (CNS)
- Delayed myelination.
- Sulcal enlargement.
- T2WI high signal intensity of white matter due to abnormal myelin.
- Ventriculomegaly, dural thickening.
- Abnormal craniocervical junction, hypoplastic dens with mucopolysaccharide deposition around it.

Differential diagnosis
- Skeletal dysplasias (spondyloepiphyseal, multiple epiphyseal and spondylometaphyseal).
- Perthes disease.

Management and prognosis
Prevention of CNS damage through pre-natal screening. Bone marrow transplantation and enzyme replacement therapy depending on the subtype. Surgery for complications such as hydrocephalus, corneal opacity and spine stabilization.

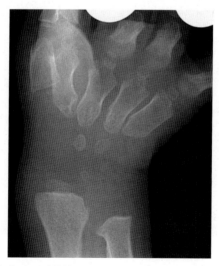

Fig. 6.8 Hand radiograph. Widened metacarpals with pointed proximal ends.

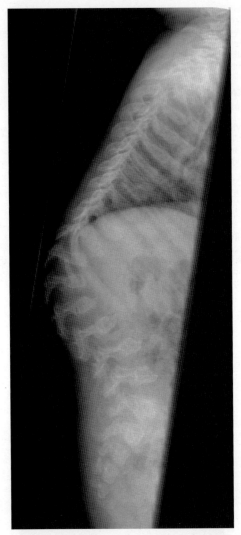

Fig. 6.9 Lateral spine radiograph showing marked anterior beaking of the inferior part. There is marked kyphosis.

Club foot (talipes equinovarus)

This is plantar flexion of the calcaneum (equinus) with inversion of the hindfoot and abduction of the forefoot (varus). It is a congenital disorder, often idiopathic, in 50% of cases bilateral. It is associated with various syndromes and cerebral palsy. The anterior tibial artery can be hypoplastic or absent in severe cases. M>F.

Clinical presentation

At birth, hindfoot in varus and equinus, forefoot in adduction. Undergrowth of lower limb with increased muscle stiffness.

Imaging findings

Radiographs

AP and lateral weight-bearing radiographs are used to measure various angles.

- AP view:
  - Talocalcaneal angle 0–10° hindfoot varus (normal 20–40°).
  - Talo-first metatarsal angle 20–40° forefoot varus (normal 0–15°).
- Lateral view
  - Talocalcaneal angle 20°– (–ve)10° (normal 35–50°).
- Lateral rotation of the talus within the ankle joint.
- Medial rotation of the calcaneum (equinus).
- Medial subluxation of the navicular at the talonavicular joint and the cuboid at the calcaneo-cuboid joint.

MRI

- Multiplanar reconstruction to show ankle and proximal joints of the forefoot.
- Proton density fast-spin echo imaging (PDFSE) fat saturated (FS) is useful to show unossified cartilage.
- Occult spinal dysraphism.

Differential diagnosis

- Congenital vertical talus.
- Rockerbottom foot.
- Amniotic band syndrome.

Management and prognosis

Non-surgical manipulation. Ponsseti method of transaction of the Achilles tendon and the serial casting of the foot as the tendon heals to achieve good anatomical positioning. Surgery for difficult cases with tendon transfers and osteotomies.

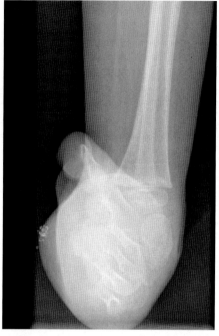

Fig. 6.10 Radiograph showing marked inversion of the plantar aspect of the foot.

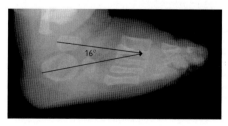

Fig. 6.11 The lateral radiograph shows a decreased talocalcaneal angle of 16° in a 6-month-old child.

Developmental dysplasia of the hip

Developmental dysplasia of the hip (DDH) or congenital dysplasia (CDH) is abnormal development of the acetabulum and proximal femoral epiphysis, resulting in superior and lateral migration of the femoral head. It is commoner in breech babies, oligiohydramnios and females and there is a familial tendency.

The normal development of the hip joint relies on the femoral head being appropriately located within the acetabulum. Disruption of this relationship between the femoral head and acetabulum will result in abnormal growth and development of all components of the hip joint.

If undiagnosed and untreated, DDH can lead to severe deformity of the hip joint, limb shortening, reduced mobility, degenerative changes and avascular necrosis.

Clinical presentation

Different neonatal screening programmes exist to detect DDH, depending on local resource and expertise, which include clinical examination and ultrasound.

In the newborn, there is an association with asymmetric skin or gluteal folds, leg length discrepancy, a palpable click on stress movements of the hip (Ortolani and Barlow manoeuvre). In an older child where the diagnosis has been delayed, there may be a history of limp, delayed walking, pain.

Imaging findings

Radiographs

- There is an abnormal shape and position of the femoral head and a shallow acetabulum.
- Subluxation to complete dislocation of the femoral head can occur.
- ▶Delayed ossification of the femoral head (usually ossified by 2–3mths), therefore it is a poor screening method in the newborn.
- Asymmetry of the proximal femoral epiphyses.
- Several lines are used for assessing location and acetabular morphology (shown in Fig. 6.13).

Ultrasound

- ▶In the neonate (up to 3mths of age), it is the modality of choice. Once the femoral epiphysis ossifies, it becomes more difficult.
- The cartilaginous component of the femoral head can be visualized along with its relationship to the acetabulum.
- Classification system developed by Graf and Harke has been used to assess hip position and function. It is based on the degree of coverage of femoral head on a true coronal image of the acetabulum, from which the acetabular roof angle (alpha angle α) is calculated.
  - Type I: normal hip, acetabular roof covers 50% of the femoral head, $\alpha > 60°$.
  - Type Ia: child <3mths of age, acetabular roof covers <50% of the head, α 50–60°.
  - Type Ib: child >3mths of age, acetabular roof covers <50% of the head, α 50–60°.

- Type Ic: critical hip subluxed and unstable, α 43–49˚.
- Type III: hip is eccentrically placed femoral head that is dislocated, α<40˚.
- Type IV: severe dysplasia, α<43˚.

MRI
- PDFSE FS. Cartilage is of high signal intensity and it is possible to differentiate between epiphyseal and articular cartilage.
- Coronal and sagittal images identify the position of the capital femoral epiphysis and the acetabulum (which is hypoplastic).
- Useful in follow-up imaging to check for location of the femoral head following surgery.

Differential diagnosis
- Cerebral palsy.
- Septic arthritis.
- Proximal focal femoral deficiency.
- Congenital coxa vara.

Management and prognosis
Initially conservative, with reduction harness and spica cast. Open reduction with varus derotational and reconstructive osteotomy. Triple osteotomy with reconstruction of the acetabulum.

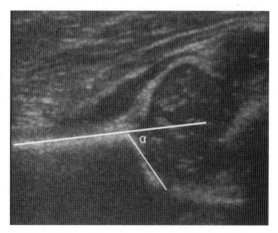

Fig. 6.12 Coronal ultrasound shows the measurement of the α angle in a normal hip.

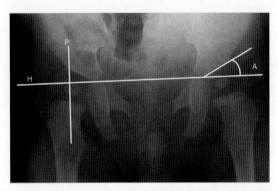

Fig. 6.13 AP radiograph of a normal child. H is the horizontal Hilgenreiner's line joining the superior points of the triradiate cartilages. P is the Perkins line from the superior lateral aspect of the acetabulum perpendicular to Hilgenreiner's line. In the normal hip the ossified epiphysis should be in the inferior medial quadrant of the intersection of these two lines. The acetabular angle is measured by a line drawn along the superior margin of the acetabulum which intersects Hilgenreiner's line.

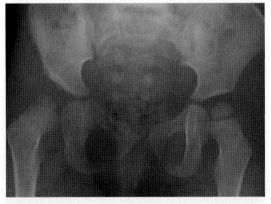

Fig. 6.14 AP radiograph showing a shallow right acetabulum and dislocated hip with a small right femoral epiphysis.

Perthes (Legg–Calvé–Perthes disease)

This is idiopathic avascular necrosis of the proximal femoral epiphysis. The infarction causes fragmentation, flattening and abnormal development of the epiphysis, femoral neck and acetabulum. M>F (5 times) (age range typically 4–10yrs). It can be bilateral in up to 15% of cases, but is rarely symmetrical. The disease is self-limiting and goes through a reparative phase with replacement of the necrotic bone. There may be long-term residual changes.

Clinical presentation

Pain in the groin or hip, often causing a limp. Pain can be referred to the knee.

Imaging findings

Radiographs

- AP and frog lateral films are indicated.
- Early features:
  - ▶Radiographs of the pelvis can initially be normal.
  - Small femoral epiphysis with widening of the joint space (best appreciated on frog lateral).
  - Subcortical lucency and fissuring (due to fracturing of the necrotic bone).
- Later features:
  - Fragmentation of the epiphysis with areas of sclerosis and lucency.
  - Loss of height of the epiphysis and subchondral lucency.
  - Widened, irregular femoral metaphysis.
  - Coxa plana and magna.
- Final stages:
  - Replacement of sclerotic bone with normal bone.
  - Epiphysis can be flattened.
  - Can be loss of congruity with the acetabulum.
- Catterall classification (groups I–IV) to grade femoral head involvement.
- Walderstrom radiographic staging (initial, fragmentation, reparative, growth and definite stages).
- Ultrasound:
  - Fragmentation and irregularity of the femoral epiphysis.
  - Synovial hypertrophy and joint effusion.

MRI

- T2WI and STIR:
  - Hyperintense joint effusion and intermediate signal synovial hypertrophy.
  - Subchondral irregularity.
- T1WI:
  - Hypointense joint effusion.
  - Linear hypointensity traversing femoral ossification centre.
  - With revascularization, the low signal necrotic epiphysis is replaced with high signal fat.

Nuclear scintigraphy
- ►Not recommended if MRI available.
- Decreased uptake secondary to the interrupted blood supply.
- Later in the disease, increased uptake may be seen as the epiphysis revascularizes.

Differential diagnosis
- Secondary avascular necrosis (e.g. steroids, sickle cell disease).
- Multiple epiphyseal dysplasia (bilateral and symmetrical while Perthes' is asymmetrical).
- Meyer's dysplasia.

Management and prognosis
Initially conservative as half of cases will improve with no treatment. Femoral and pelvic osteotomies to contain the femoral epiphysis.

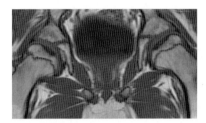

Fig. 6.15 MRI in a child with bilateral Perthes' disease. There is flattening and irregularity of the femoral epiphyses with areas of low signal within the epiphysis, indicating sclerotic ischaemic bone.

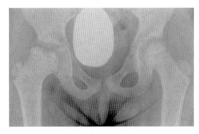

Fig. 6.16 AP radiograph of the pelvis in a 4-year-old child with Perthes' disease. There is sclerosis, flattening and irregularity of the right femoral epiphysis with sclerosis around the femoral metaphysis.

Slipped capital (upper) femoral epiphysis (SCFE/SUFE)

This is a fracture or disruption through the proximal femoral growth plate, causing posterior medial displacement of the capital femoral epiphysis. It commonly occurs between 8 and 15yrs (time of adolescent growth spurt, with a peak 13–14yrs), M>F, obese children. Association with endocrine abnormalities, rickets and previous DDH. It can be bilateral at presentation, with an increased incidence of the contralateral hip being involved within 24mths.

Clinical presentation

Onset may be acute or chronic, with limp, pain and limitation of hip movement and leg length shortening.

Imaging findings

Radiographs

▶It is imperative that both an AP and frog lateral views are taken as up to 10% of slips can be missed on the AP projection. It can present with bilateral hip involvement and caution must be used if comparisons are made between the two femoral epiphyses on a single radiograph.

There are a number of radiographic signs that demonstrate SUFE, not all of which may necessarily be present.

- Widening of the proximal femoral growth plate.
- Medial displacement of the femoral epiphysis.
- A line drawn along the superior margin of the femoral neck that is extended to the acetabulum (Klein's line) should normally intersect a small portion of the epiphysis. Failure to do so indicates a slip.
- Loss of height of the femoral epiphysis.
- Irregularity and loss of definition of the physeal growth plate.
- The metaphysis is scalloped and irregular.
- Post-treatment:
  • Irregularity and collapse of the femoral epiphysis due to avascular necrosis.
  • Loss of joint space due to chondrolysis (loss of cartilage).

MRI

- ▶Sensitive in detecting early slippage or when radiographs are equivocal.
- T2WI and STIR: high signal joint effusion, synovitis and marrow oedema.
- Physeal widening and slipped epiphysis.
- Avascular necrosis and chondrolysis in chronic cases.

Differential diagnosis

- Any cause of limp or hip pain.
- Perthes' disease.
- Infection.

Management and prognosis

Surgical fixation with fixation screws through the physis is performed. This is usually done without trying to reduce the slippage as this increases the likelihood of avascular necrosis and chondrolysis.

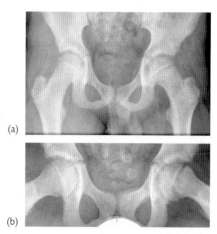

(a)

(b)

Fig. 6.17 (a) AP and (b) lateral radiographs of the femur showing slipped left upper femoral epiphysis.

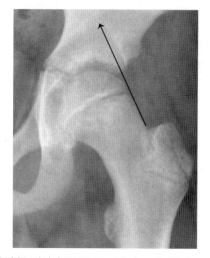

Fig. 6.18 Klein's line which does not intersect the femoral epiphysis.

Tarsal coalition

A congenital or acquired fusion of the tarsal bones, which may be osseous (synostosis), cartilaginous (synchondrosis) or fibrous (syndesmosis). Commonly involves either the calcaneonavicular or talocalcaneal joints. A fibrous coalition at birth may ossify later in life. Can be bilateral and can occur following trauma, infection, arthritis or surgery.

Clinical presentation

Asymptomatic finding, associated with pes planus (flat feet), spasticity, reduced movement and pain on activity.

Imaging findings

Radiographs

- Calcaneonavicular coalition:
  - Ossified bar connecting the calcaneum to the navicular.
  - Sclerosis and irregularity of the calcaneonavicular joint space.
  - Elongation of the anterior superior calcaneum on the lateral view (Anteater's nose sign).
  - Widening of the anterior superior calcaneum.
- Talocalcaneal:
  - Rounding of the lateral talar process.
  - Continuity of a line formed by the medial talar dome and sustentaculum tali on the lateral view (C sign).
  - Narrowing of the subtalar joints.
  - Periosteal elevation at the insertion of talocalcaneal joint.

CT

- Thin slices with multiplanar reformatting is desirable, images parallel to the talonavicular joint should be obtained.
- Osseous bar.
- Sclerosis and irregularity around the joint margins.
- Talocalcaneal coalition: abnormal downward sloping of the middle facet of the calcaneum.

MRI

- T1WI: fibrous and cartilaginous bars are low signal intensity.
- Ossific bars show continuity of marrow signal.
- T2WI: often hyperintense signal change seen around the bar.

Differential diagnosis

- JIA (📖 p. 356).
- Osteomyelitis (📖 p. 344).
- Trauma.
- Flat foot.

Management and prognosis

Conservative management with pain relief. Surgical resection or arthrodesis in severe cases.

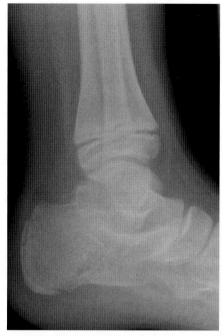

Fig. 6.19 Lateral radiograph of the foot, with prominence of the anterior end of the calcaneum due to calcaneo-navicular bar.

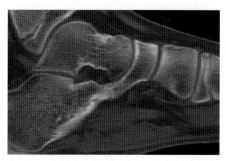

Fig. 6.20 CT reconstruction showing a calcaneo-navicular bar with a pseudoarthrosis through the bony bar.

Discoid meniscus

A discoid meniscus is a large (>13mm) congenitally abnormal meniscus which has lost its normal semilunar shape. The lateral meniscus is more commonly involved and it may be bilateral. The discoid meniscus can be a variety of shapes and sizes some which may extend into the intercondylar notch.

Clinical presentation

Often asymptomatic, can be associated with a 'snapping knee', pain, clicking, locking and effusions. It is more prone to tears and degenerative change.

Imaging findings

Radiographs

- Radiographic features are non-specific and relatively insensitive.
- High fibular head (lateral discoid).
- Hypoplastic femoral condyle, and lateral tibial spine.
- Cupping of the lateral tibial plateau.

MRI

- ▶In a normal knee, the meniscus should not occupy more than 3 consecutive sagittal images (of 4mm thickness) ('absent bow tie sign'). A discoid meniscus occupies more than 3 consecutive slices.
- Greater than 50% coverage of the lateral tibial plateau on sagittal and coronal images.
- Meniscal size greater than 13mm in cross section.
- Large meniscus with loss of the normal semilunar morphology, with no medial tapering on coronal images.
- Large pancake-like meniscus.
- Abnormal signal in the meniscus.
- Tears, degeneration and cyst formation are high signal on T2WI.

Differential diagnosis

- Bucket-handle tear: detached fragment in the intercondylar, double posterior cruciate ligament (PCL) sign.
- Flipped meniscus.
- Vacuum phenomenon (hyperextended knee, exaggerated on GRE sequences).

Management and prognosis

Conservative, arthroscopy and meniscetomy/saucerization.

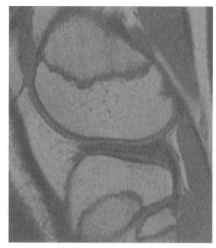

Fig. 6.21 Sagittal T1-weighted images of a knee showing discoid lateral meniscus. There is a thickened continuous meniscus with absence of the 'bowtie' appearance on multiple sagittal images.

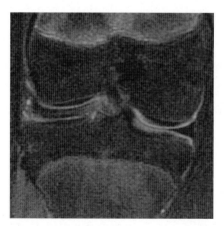

Fig. 6.22 Coronal proton-density weighted MR image shows a discoid lateral meniscus occupying the lateral compartment. There is no tapering of the margins. There is hyperintense signal within the meniscus, suggesting a degree of degenerative change.

Osteochondritis dissecans

Avascular necrosis of the subchondral bone which can affect any weight-bearing surface, common in the lateral aspect of the medial femoral condyle. Other sites: lateral femoral condyle, tibia, patella, elbow, ankle, hip, shoulder and wrist. Associated with overuse, M>F, increased incidence at 10–20yrs.

Clinical presentation

Pain aggravated by exercise, joint swelling, clicking or locking, can be asymptomatic.

Imaging findings

The role of imaging is to assess the size and stability of the lesion and to determine those lesions which can be treated conservatively and those which may need surgical intervention. MRI is the most sensitive modality for assessing stability.

Radiographs
- Lucent subchondral lesion with a sclerotic margin.
- There may be a detached fragment within the lucent area or elsewhere within the joint.

CT
- Sensitive in detecting intra-articular loose bodies.

MRI
- Possible predictors of instability:
  - >1cm displaced fragment.
  - Fluid tracking from within the joint around the bony fragment.
  - Cystic areas within the donor site.
  - Extensive oedema within the donor site.
  - Defect in the overlying cartilage.
  - Loss of continuity of the fragment with the donor site.
  - Enhancement of granulation tissue between the donor site and the fragment.
- PDFSE sequences useful in determining the integrity of the overlying cartilage.
- MR arthography:
  - Will show contrast tracking around the detached fragment in unstable lesions.
  - Outlines loose bodies.

Differential diagnosis
- Normal irregularity and development of the epiphysis.
- Avascular necrosis:
  - Injury.
  - Steroids.
  - Sickle cell disease.
- Stress insufficiency fracture.

Management and prognosis

Stabilized by rest and reduced physical activity. Drilling around the donor site may improve blood flow and vascularity. Surgical fixation for larger fragments. Cartilage transplants.

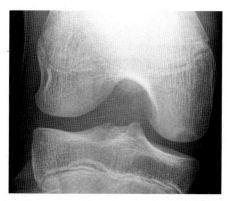

Fig. 6.23 A different patient than that shown in Fig. 6.24 shows a lytic defect in the medial femoral condyle.

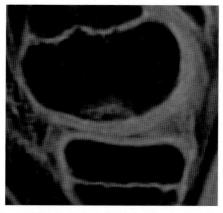

Fig. 6.24 Sagittal STIR image shows a stable OCD with surrounding oedema but intact cartilage.

Osteomyelitis

Bone marrow infection is commonly bacterial (*Staphylococcus Aureus* is the commonest) but can be fungal, viral or parasitic. Salmonella is frequently the cause in children with sickle cell disease. Spread may be haematogenous, localized or from a penetrating injury. The metaphysis of the long bones is the commonest site, with the lower limb more frequently involved. Other common sites are the humerus, femur, tibia and fibula, can occur in the skull and mandible. Neonates are at particular risk as they have vascular connection across the growth plate allowing metaphyseal to epiphyseal spread. Septic arthritis can occur.

Clinical presentation

Fever, localized pain swelling, erythema and tenderness with limitation of movement of the involved limb.
▶In the neonate, features may be non-specific with general irritability, poor feeding and mild pyrexia.

Radiographs
Acute disease
- ▶Absence of any findings does not exclude osteomyelitis as changes may take over a week to appear.
- Location is typically the metaphysis (femur, tibia, humerus, fibula, short bones, pelvis and spine).
- Epiphyseal involvement commoner in younger children who retain external blood supply.
- Earliest findings are soft tissue swelling, loss of fat planes and osteopenia.
- Subperiosteal erosions and periosteal new bone formation (may take up to 10 days to occur).
- Bony destruction is typically visible in 7–14 days (can be longer).

Chronic disease
- Sclerosis or mixed sclerotic/lucent lesions.
- Marked thickening of the outer periosteum (cloaca).
- Dead bone fragment may be seen within an abscess cavity (sequestrum).
- Sinus tracts develop.
- Skin ulceration.
- Bone abscess: intramedullary lytic lesion with well-defined geographical margin, typically in the metaphysis of the tubular bones of the lower limb (Brodie's abscess).

Imaging findings

Ultrasound
- Early soft tissue swelling.
- Soft tissue abscess formation.
- Periosteal thickening and elevation.

CT
- Bone destruction and loss of cortical margins, periosteal thickening and elevation.
- Soft tissue swelling and abscess formation.

MRI

- ▶STIR and T2W FSE FS images are the most sensitive for detecting marrow oedema and soft tissue changes which are of high signal intensity.
- Both T1WI and T2WI may show periosteal new bone and cortical disruption.
- Marrow and soft tissue enhancement post-contrast.
- Surrounding soft tissue oedema and cellulitis. Breaks in the cortex allow marrow fat to leak outside bone allowing decompression of the inflammatory tissue.
- Abscess formation is seen as peripheral enhancement with central low signal intensity on T1WI post contrast.
- Synovial enhancement in adjacent joints.

Nuclear scintigraphy

- Increased uptake in the angiographic blood pool and delayed phases.
- Area of central photopenia with intraosseous infarcts or abscess.
- There may be multiple sites of infection.

Differential diagnosis

- Langerhans cell histiocytosis (LCH).
- Neuroblastoma.
- Ewing's sarcoma.
- Lymphoma.
- Leukaemia.

Management and prognosis

Identify an infective agent with image-guided needle biopsy aspiration. Antibiotics and pain management. Surgical intervention for abscess (particularly interosseous), periosteal decompressive drilling.

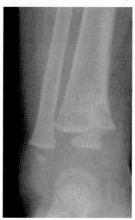

Fig. 6.25 AP radiograph of the distal tibia shows a lytic area within the medial aspect of the distal tibia with a sclerotic margin and associated periosteal reaction. The appearances are of a bone abscess.

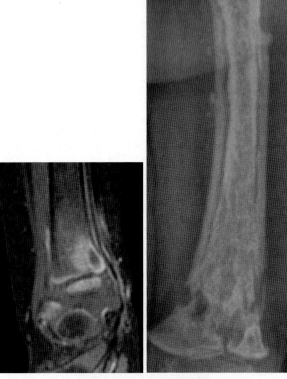

Fig. 6.26 The corresponding T1 fat-saturated post-gadolinium image shows enhancement within the marrow and a small area of low signal, indicating an abscess cavity within the bone.

Fig. 6.27 In a child with chronic osteo-myelitis, there is thickened subperiosteal new bone (cloaca). There is irregularity and fragmentation of the distal femur with a small bony fragment sequestrum.

Rickets

Rickets is failure of mineralization of the osteoid of newly formed bone in a child's skeleton. It is due to a reduced availability of either/all of calcium, phosphorus and vitamin D.

Causes
- Prematurity.
- Primary and maternal hypoparathyroidism.
- Vitamin D deficiency.
- Renal insufficiency.
- Malabsorption and poor nutrition: lack of vitamin D and calcium (Ca) in the diet.
- Inadequate exposure to sunlight.
- Liver and storage disease.
- Hypophosphatasia.

Clinical presentation

The degree of changes and deformity reflects the severity of the underlying metabolic abnormality. There is reduced stature, bowed legs, joint swelling (knees, wrists and ankles), and pathological fractures. There can be delayed closure of the anterior fontanelle, scoliosis, rachitic rosary (expanded costochondral junction) and Harrison sulci (deformity of the rib cage due to diaphragmatic pull).

Imaging findings

Radiographs
- Axial skeleton:
  - Cupping of the rib ends (rachitic rosary).
  - Scoliosis and biconcave vertebral bodies.
  - Abnormal development of the pelvis and acetabulum.
  - Frontal bossing of the skull with delayed teeth eruption.
- Appendicular skeleton:
  - ►Fraying, splaying and irregularity of the metaphysis with widening of the physis and poor outline of the epiphysis.
  - Reduced bone density with an increased trabecular pattern.
  - Subperiosteal reaction.
  - Bowing of the long bones and abnormal development around the joints (coxa vara, genu valgum, genu varum).
- Healing rickets:
  - Increased density in the zone of calcification.

MRI
- Widened physis.
- Absence of any calcification.

Differential diagnosis
- ►Leukaemia.
- Congenital syphilis.
- Non-accidental injury.
- Repetitive strain injuries.

Management and prognosis

Usually responds to vitamin D therapy and calcium supplementation.

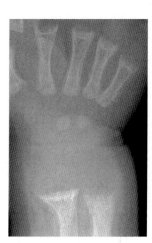

Fig. 6.28 AP radiograph of the hand shows metaphyseal widening, splaying and irregularity, and periosteal reaction. The bones are osteopenic with a coarse trabecular pattern.

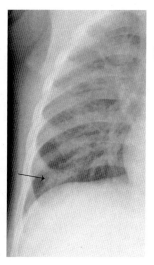

Fig. 6.29 Chest radiograph shows widening and expansion of the anterior rib ends (rachitic rosary).

Sickle cell anaemia

Autosomal recessive disorder caused by abnormal haemoglobin production (haemoglobin S). If homozygous (HbSS) it is sickle cell anaemia, the heterozygous condition (HbSA) is sickle cell trait. It may occur in combination with other haemoglobinopathies: haemoglobin C (HbSC) or β thalasaemia (HbS-thal). The defect within the haemoglobin molecule affects the shape and plasticity of the red blood cell, which under lower oxygen tension leads to increased blood flow viscosity and stasis resulting in bony infarction and necrosis (sickle crisis). In the first 6mths of life, children are protected by elevated levels of fetal haemoglobin (HbF). Sickle cell crises typically begin in the first couple of years of life. There may be progressive bone infarctions and premature arthritis.

The HbS defect does provide some protection from malaria and the majority of cases are found in people of Afro-Caribbean descent, but it can occur in Mediterranean and Middle Eastern populations.

Clinical presentation

Acutely there is a sickle cell crisis, causing bone, abdominal and chest pain due to ischaemia that can lead to infarction, infection and pyrexia. Osteomyelitis, particularly staphylococcus and salmonella, causing a generalized anaemia, jaundice, splenomegaly and growth retardation. CNS involvement may lead to stroke.

Dactylitis is a common presentation in children, causing swelling in the hands and feet and decreased range of motion.

Imaging findings

Radiographs

- Marrow hyperplasia: widening of the medullary space, thinning of the cortex, generalized osteopenia with a coarsened trabecular pattern.
- In the skull, there is a widened diploic space and decreased width of the outer table. Can create a 'hair-on-end' appearance.
- Bone infarctions within the long bones, hands and epiphyses. Vertebrae have a biconcave (fish vertebrae) appearance due to end plate infarction.
- Periosteal reaction causing a bone within a bone appearance.
- Dactylitis with periosteal thickening, bone destruction and soft tissue swelling.
- Premature epiphyseal closure can result in growth distortion.
- Cone-shaped epiphyses and widening of the metaphyses.
- Osteomyelitis.

MRI

- T1WI: generalized low signal intensity within the marrow due to replacement of fatty marrow by haemopoeitic marrow.
- T2WI: replacement of the fatty marrow causes reduced signal intensity, focal areas of increased signal intensity due to marrow infarction.
- Osteomyelitis and soft tissue infections.
- ▶Differentiating between infection and osteomyelitis may be difficult.
- Paravertebral masses due to extrahaemopoetic blood production.

Differential diagnosis

- Thalassaemia (AVN uncommon).
- Perthes disease.
- Gaucher's disease.

Management and prognosis

During a crisis, oxygen, hydration and pain management. Blood transfusions decrease the percentage of HbS but can lead to iron overload. Patient education.

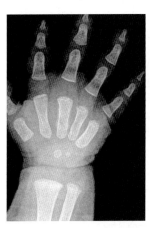

Fig. 6.30 AP radiograph in a child with sickle cell disease. There is periosteal thickening and irregularity of the metacarpal of the middle phalanges. The child presented with swelling of the digits. Appearances are of sickle cell dactylitis.

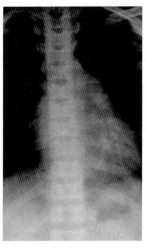

Fig. 6.31 AP thoracic radiograph showing vertebral end plate depression.

Leukaemia

A neoplastic disorder of myeloid (ML) or lymphoid (LL) white blood cells, which can be either acute (A) or chronic (C). ALL is commonest in childhood with a peak incidence between 2 and 10 years. AML accounts for 15% of childhood leukaemias, CML is a disease of adulthood.

Clinical presentation

Generalized fatigue, fever, hepatosplenomegaly, lymphadenopathy, joint effusions, recurrent infections and anaemia. Marrow involvement can cause either localized or diffuse bone pain and arthralgia.

Imaging findings

Radiographs

- ▶May be normal despite widespread marrow involvement.
- Focal areas of destruction seen with multiple well-defined lytic lesions ('moth-eaten appearance') femur>humerus>ileum>spine>tibia.
- Coarse trabecular pattern.
- Radiolucent transverse metaphyseal bands, particularly in the region of the knee and humerus with horizontal bands seen in the vertebral bodies.
- Following therapy, there can be dense metaphyseal lines.
- Generalized periostitis (smooth, lamella or sunburst pattern).
- Pathological fractures (metaphyseal similar to NAI).
- Vertebral body collapse.
- Sutural widening with prominent skull markings.

MRI

- T1WI: leukaemic infiltrates are low signal intensity, replacing the high signal intensity of marrow fat.
- STIR and T2WI: increased signal intensity of leukaemic marrow.
- Peripheral enhancement following gadolinium.

Nuclear scintigraphy

- Increased uptake of involved areas.
- Can underestimate extensive disease.

Differential diagnosis

- Metastatic disease (neuroblastoma, rhabdomyosarcoma, LCH).
- Osteomyelitis.
- Ewing's sarcoma.
- Lymphoma.
- JIA.

Management and prognosis

Chemotherapy, combined with radiotherapy and bone marrow transplantation in more severe cases. Survival is related to age and type of disease.

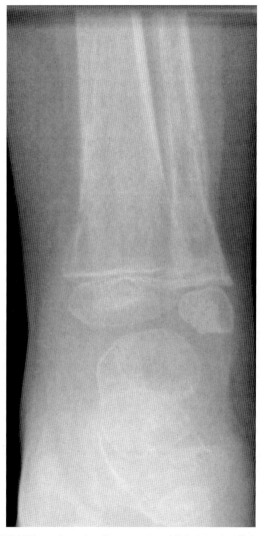

Fig. 6.32 Widespread metaphyseal lucency, periosteal thickening and a pathological fracture of the distal tibia in a child with ALL.

Osteopetrosis

A heterogeneous group of inherited disorders that cause an increase in bone mineral density due to defects in osteoclastic activity that differ in severity and inheritance pattern.

- Malignant/congenital/infantile osteopetrosis:
  - AR inheritance with a diagnosis early in life.
  - Generalized bone sclerosis, pathological fractures and infections.
  - Associated with anaemia, thrombocytopenia and granulocytopenia.
  - Cranial nerve compression leads to blindness and deafness.
  - Erlenmeyer flask deformity.
- Benign osteopetrosis:
  - AD inheritance, the diagnosis is often not made until adulthood.
  - Pathological fractures and delayed healing, particularly following tooth extraction.
  - Mild anaemia.
  - Cranial nerve compression.
  - Can be further subdivided:
  - *Type I* cranial vault involvement,
  - *Type II* sclerosis predominantly of the spine, pelvis and skull base.
- Intermediate type:
  - AR inheritance with diagnosis in first decade of life.
  - Symptoms are more severe than the benign type and include blindness, deafness and haematological symptoms.
  - Mandibular prognathism and osteomyelitis.
  - Tendency to fracture and genu valgum.
  - Hepatosplenomegaly.
- Carbonic anhydrase type II (CAII) deficiency:
  - Occurs in Mediterranean and Arab races.
  - Cause of intracranial calcification and developmental delay.

Clinical presentation

Pain, increased frequency of fractures, nerve compression (headache, blindness, deafness), osteomyelitis, abnormal dentition, an increased propensity to infection, bleeding and stroke (due to immunological abnormalities and pancytopenia).

Imaging findings

Radiographs

- Skull:
  - Macrocranium, thick dense skull base with narrow neural foramen.
  - Undeveloped or absent paranasal sinuses.
  - Abnormal dentition.
- Axial skeleton:
  - Bone within a bone appearance.
  - Either sclerotic or picture frame vertebrae.
  - Widening of the ribs.
- Appendicular skeleton:
  - ▶Dense skeleton loss of differentiation between the cortex and medulla with pathological fractures.
  - Generalized or alternate radiolucent bands in the metaphysis.

- • ▶Metaphyseal widening and flaring caused by defective tubular remodelling (Erlenmeyer flask or club-like deformity).
- • Coxa vara, bowing of the long bones.
- • Osteomyelitis.

MRI
- Absence of bone marrow.
- Extramedullary haematopoesis.
- Carpal tunnel compression.
- Ventriculomegaly and tonsillar herniation.
- Syringomyelia.
- Cervical spine compression.

Differential diagnosis
- Chronic renal failure.
- Bone dysplasias (Pyle's disease, pyknodysostosis).
- Diphosphonate induced osteopetrosis.

Management and prognosis
Bone marrow transplantation.

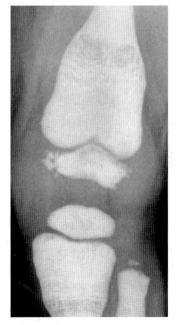

Fig. 6.33 There is loss of normal differentiation between the cortex and medulla and widening of the distal femur and proximal tibia (Erlenmeyer flask deformity).

Juvenile idiopathic arthritis

This is arthritis of unknown aetiology, lasting for more than 6 weeks in a child under 16yrs of age. Whilst it is an auto-immune disease centred around the synovial joints, it can cause significant systemic symptoms, skin rashes and uveitis. The disease is classified according to the number of joints involved, the mode of presentation and positive serology for rheumatoid factor (RhF).

Classification

- Oligoarthritis.
- Extended oligoarthritis.
- Polyarthritis (Rh+ve).
- Polyarthritis (Rh−ve).
- Psoriatic arthritis.
- Enthesitis related arthropathy.
- Systemic onset disease.

Clinical presentation

Swollen and painful joints, with restricted movement. Can be associated with uveitis, fever, rash, pericarditis, pleuritis, organomegaly and interstitial lung disease.

Imaging findings

Radiographs

- Can be normal.
- Periarticular osteopenia and soft tissue swelling.
- Growth disturbance which may initially be accelerated and then lead to early physeal fusion and restricted growth.
- Joint space narrowing.
- Periosteal reaction.
- Epiphyseal overgrowth.
- Bone remodelling.

Ultrasound

- Joint effusion.
- Synovial proliferation.
- Soft tissue swelling.

MRI

- ↑ T2 signal: joint effusion and marrow.
- Cartilage erosions (cartilage high signal on T2WI- and PD-weighted images).
- ▶Synovial thickening (>2mm) and irregularity best appreciated on post-gadolinium T1 fat-saturated or subtracted images.
- Meniscal and ligament damage.

Differential diagnosis

- Infection (need joint aspiration to exclude).
- ▶Malignancy (leukaemia, neuroblastoma).
- Reactive arthritis.
- Pigmented villonodular synovitis.

Management and prognosis
NSAIDS and steroid joint injections. Disease-modifying drugs (methotrexate).

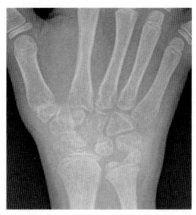

Fig. 6.34 AP radiograph of the hand shows carpal crowding and loss of normal spaces between the carpal bones, periarticular osteopenia and subcortical erosions.

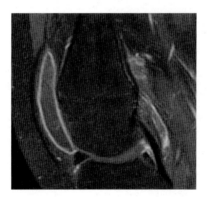

Fig. 6.35 Sagittal T1 fat-saturated image of the knee following gadolinium administration. There is widespread synovial enhancement within the joint space with low signal intensity fluid within it.

Juvenile dermatomyositis (JDMS)

An autoimmune inflammatory myopathy involving the proximal striated muscle groups and associated with systemic symptoms. Typically bilateral and symmetrical, can affect any age, commonest 5–14yrs, F>M.

Diagnostic criteria
- Symmetrical proximal muscle weakness.
- Electromyographic abnormality and muscle biopsy changes.
- Increased muscle enzymes: creatine kinase (CK) and lactic dehydrogenase (LDH).
- Biopsy-proven JDMS.
- Skin changes:
  - Heliotropic rash—violaceous/erythematous, symmetrical, periorbital swelling.
  - Goytrens papules—elevated violaceous papules: metacarpal phalangeal joint (MCP), proximal phalangeal joint (PIP) and distal interphalangeal joint (DIP), elbow and knee joints).

Clinical presentation
Proximal muscle weakness with loss of motor skills, tenderness and easily fatigued. Arthralgia, arthritis, fever, fatigue, weight loss, pericarditis, dysphagia. Respiratory compromise in severe cases.

Imaging findings
Radiographs
- Muscle, fascial and subcutaneous calcification:
  - More common in longstanding disease.
  - Can be punctate or sheet-like.
- Muscle atrophy and osteopenia.
- Milk of calcium deposition (cystic collections within the muscle).
- Interstitial lung disease.

MRI
- ▶Modality of choice.
- T2WI /STIR: hyperintense bilateral symmetrical muscle oedema.
- Thighs>pelvis>upper extremities. Anterior and lateral compartments>medial compartments.
- Can involve the neck, pharyngeal muscles and chest muscles, causing dysphagia and respiratory compromise.
- Muscle atrophy and fatty infiltration due to steroids and disuse.
- With more long-standing disease, T2WI: intermediate/high signal fluid filled milk of calcium cysts.
- Calcium deposition: low signal on all sequences.

Differential diagnosis
- Eosinophilic fasciitis.
- Infective myositis.
- Muscle injuries.
- Subcutaneous muscle nerve denervation.
- Radiation therapy.

Management and prognosis

Immunosuppression, steroids, methotrexate, intravenous gammaglobulin. Complications include calcinosis, muscle contractures, avascular necrosis.

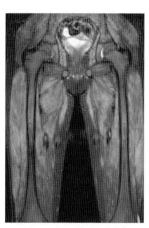

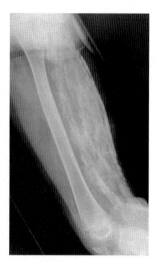

Fig. 6.36 Coronal STIR images of a child with juvenile dermatomyositis. There is widespread proximal muscle oedema seen as high signal following the direction of the striated muscle. There is relative sparing of the adductor muscles.

Fig. 6.37 Widespread sheets of calcification in a child with calcinosis secondary to juvenile dermatomyositis.

Ewing's sarcoma

This is a highly malignant round small cell sarcoma that predominantly involves bone but can be soft tissue based. Any bone can be involved but most commonly involves the diaphysis of the long bones (70%), the flat bones (25%), ribs (6%) and vertebral bodies. Involvement of the flat bones is commoner in Ewing's sarcoma than any other childhood primary bone tumour. It can metastasize to lung, bone and lymph nodes. Incidence is between 5 and 25 years of age (peak 10–15 years).

Clinical presentation

There is localized pain and a soft tissue mass, systemic systems (fever, malaise, leukocytosis) are associated. It can result in pathological fracture.

Imaging findings

Radiographs

- Aggressive-looking lesion.
- ▶Lytic intramedullary lesion with ill-defined margins and a permeative moth-eaten appearance.
- Eroded cortex with areas of sclerosis (can be predominately sclerotic).
- ▶Appearances can be similar to osteomyelitis.
- Prominent periosteal reaction which can have a layered (onion skin) or perpendicular (sunburst) pattern.
- There may be a Codman's triangle (interrupted periosteal elevation).
- Extension into the soft tissues with a large extra-osseous mass is a common feature.

CT

- Intramedullary mass with periosteal reaction, soft tissue mass.
- Chest CT to detect lung metastases.

MRI

- T1WI: the lesion is intermediate to low signal being relatively hyperintense to the surrounding bone marrow oedema.
- T2WI: high signal intensity mass compared with surrounding muscle.
- There is often a large soft tissue component and marked peri-tumoural oedema.
- ▶Post contrast images are important to help differentiate between tumour and peri-tumoural oedema.

Nuclear scintigraphy

- Intense uptake at the tumour site.
- Will detect any secondary bony deposits.

Differential diagnosis

- Osteomyelitis (symptoms are usually shorter).
- Langerhans cell histiocytosis (appearances are less aggressive).
- Osteosarcoma (usually metaphyseal in location and produces osteoid).
- Metastatic neuroblastoma (younger than 5yrs).

Management and prognosis

The appearances can be similar to osteomyelitis. Biopsy is needed and should be done in an appropriate centre. Inappropriate biopsy can lead to seeding of tumour cells. Chemotherapy followed by surgery is the treatment option of choice.

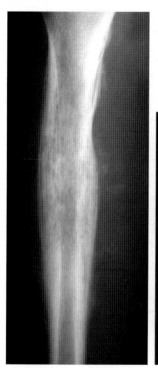

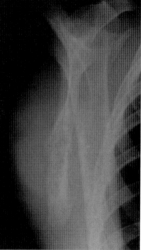

Fig. 6.38 AP radiograph of the femur. There is sunburst periosteal reaction and cortical destruction.

Fig. 6.39 Destruction and soft tissue swelling around a Ewing's sarcoma of the scapula.

Osteosarcoma

This is the commonest primary malignant bone tumour in children/young adults. It has a bimodal distribution occurring between 10 and 30yrs and after 60yrs of age. It is commoner in males. It occurs predominantly in the metaphysis of the long bones (90%) and over 75% of cases occur around the knee, with the femur more commonly involved than the tibia. It can involve the flat bones and vertebral bodies. The tumour produces osteoid and there are a variety of subtypes which include telangiectatic, paraosteal and periosteal osteosarcomas.

Clinical presentation

There is often a painful swollen mass which can result in a pathological fracture. In younger children, it can be multicentric, secondary skip lesions can occur adjacent to the primary lesion. It is associated with lung metastases and raised alkaline phosphatase. Tumours may arise from pre-existing lesions including Paget's disease, previous radiation therapy and aneurysmal bone cysts.

Imaging findings

Radiographs

- An aggressive lesion with an indistinct zone of transition.
- Areas of new bone formation and bone destruction. New bone formation will appear as sclerotic densities within the lesion.
- The tumour arises from the medullary cavity that extends to the cortex with irregular, poorly defined lucent areas and cortical destruction.
- Periosteal reaction with a Codman's triangle.
- Periosteal reaction may run perpendicular to the long axis producing a 'sunburst' pattern.
- Telangiectatic osteosarcomas are predominately lytic with multiple cystic areas within the bone which may have fluid levels within them.
- Periosteal osteosarcomas typically have no medullary involvement and are mainly diaphyseal in location. The tumour causes thickening and scalloping of the cortex.
- Paraosteal osteoid sarcomas occur in an older age group and have no medullary involvement.

CT

- Useful to detect lung metastases.

MRI

- ▶It is important to image the joint above and below the tumour to identify potential secondary skip lesions.
- T2WI and STIR images. Calcified tumours are of low signal intensity. The extensive surrounding marrow oedema is high signal intensity.
- Telangiectatic may have multiple fluid/fluid levels.
- Gadolinium uptake may be useful in discriminating between tumour and marrow oedema.

Nuclear scintigraphy

- Bone scintigraphy shows increased uptake at the tumour site.
- It is useful to detect secondary skip lesions and bone metastases.

Differential diagnosis
- Ewing's sarcoma (diaphysis of the long bones).
- Aneurysmal bone cyst may be confused with telangiectatic osteosarcomas.
- Osteomyelitis (no osteoid production).

Management and prognosis
Biopsy should be performed in a recognized centre. Chemotherapy and surgical resection.

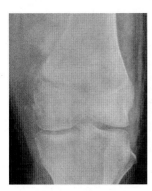

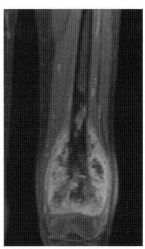

Fig. 6.40 Cortical irregularity with osteoid formation on the medial aspect of the distal femur in a patient with osteosarcoma.

Fig. 6.41 MR imaging shows a destructive lesion, periosteal reaction and soft tissue extension. The lesion is of mixed signal intensity.

Langerhans cell histiocytosis (LCH)

This disorder results from abnormal proliferation of histiocytes (Langerhan cells) within the reticular endothelial system. It is a failure of immune regulation rather than a neoplastic process, but acute dissemination can be fatal. It can occur between birth and 30 yrs (mean 5–10yrs). LCH was previously characterized in a number of ways: eosinophilic granuloma (only bone involvement and best prognosis), Hand–Schuller Christian (chronic dissemination) and Letterer–Siwe disease (acute dissemination). The present classification is based on the number of organ systems and the number of sites involved. In addition, lesions in certain organs (CNS, lungs) have special significance. The more widespread or complex the disease, the higher the staging.

Clinical presentation

Lymphadenopathy, hepatosplenomegaly, exophthalmus and diabetes inspidus. Lung involvement leads to pulmonary fibrosis. Bone lesions cause localized tenderness and pathological fractures.

Imaging findings

At diagnosis, a full skeletal survey is often necessary to delineate the extent of the disease. Flat bones are more commonly involved (70%) than long bones. Radiographs are indicated if there is local symptom change. MRI is useful if there are localized symptoms and to determine any malignant potential.

Radiographs

- Appendicular skeleton:
  - Metadiaphyseal expansile lytic lesions with ill-defined borders which may be sclerotic.
  - Endosteal scalloping and widening of the medullary cavity.
  - Typically do not cross the growth plate or articular surface.
- Axial skeleton:
  - Vertebral planar and complete collapse of the vertebral body.
  - Pelvic involvement is relatively common in younger child.
  - Permeative pattern in the ribs.
- Skull:
  - Well-defined lytic lesions with bevelled edge.
  - A sclerotic rim occurs during healing.
  - Lesions may coalesce and cause a geographic skull and cortical destruction.
  - The outer table of the skull is destroyed more than the inner table.
  - In the jaw, there is involvement of the alveolar portion of the mandible which can create a 'floating tooth' appearance.

MRI

- Lesions are of low signal intensity on T1WI and high signal intensity on T2WI.
- Marked enhancement following contrast.

Bone scintigraphy

- ▶Uptake can be variable and bone scans are a poor screening method.

Differential diagnosis
- Osteomyelitis (periosteal reaction is more common).
- Ewing's sarcoma (permeative bone destruction and periosteal reaction).
- Lymphoma.

Management and prognosis
Many lesions have a benign cause. It is important to differentiate localized from disseminated disease which has a worse prognosis.

Steroids and immunosuppression are used. In the skeleton, curettage and bone grafting is used for larger lesions at risk of fracturing. Radiotherapy for inaccessible lesions.

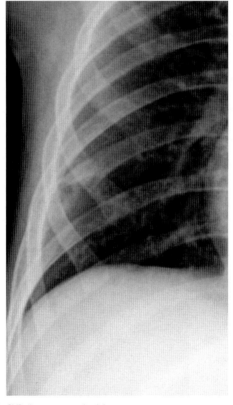

Fig. 6.42 CXR: showing expansile rib lesion.

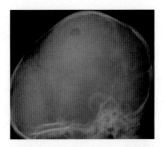

Fig. 6.43 Skull: ill-defined lytic calvarial lesion without a sclerotic margin.

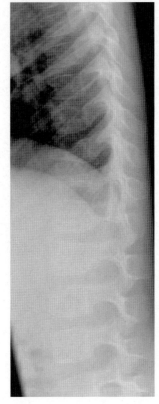

Fig. 6.44 Spine: marked vertebral collapse of the lower thoracic vertebrae.

Rhabdomyosarcoma

This is a highly malignant sarcoma arising from primitive muscle cells. It typically occurs up to 15yrs of age, with a peak incidence between 5 and 10yrs. Head, neck and orbital lesions are the commonest sites, followed by GU tract, extremities and retroperitoneum. It can metastasize to the lungs, bones, liver and lymphatics.

Clinical presentation

A soft tissue lesion which resembles muscle and causes a local mass effect. Around the orbit, it can cause exophthalmos and proptosis. Within the abdomen, there can be pain, distension and bladder outlet obstruction. Bone and joint pain can occur from osseous metastases. Systemic symptoms include anaemia and thrombocytopenia.

Imaging findings

Radiographs

- ▶A non-specific soft tissue mass with possible bone and marrow involvement.
- Bone metastases are seen as ill-defined lytic lesions.

Ultrasound

- Isoechoic to muscle.

CT

- The mass is of similar attenuation to muscle.
- Ill-defined margins and possibly local destruction of the bone.
- Extension into adjacent structures such as the nasal sinuses and intracranial cavity from an orbital lesion.
- There may be marked sclerosis and periosteal reaction in the surrounding bones.

MRI

- T1WI: the mass is isointense to muscle.
- T2WI: similar or hyperintense to muscle.
- STIR: high signal intensity.
- T1 and contrast will show heterogeneous enhancement.
- The mass has poorly defined margins.
- Local oedema, extension and destruction.

Differential diagnosis

- Neuroblastoma (calcification, elevated catecholamines).
- Neurosarcoma (extension into the soft tissue is common).
- Lymphoma/Leukaemia (lymphadenopathy).

Management and prognosis

Local resection with adjuvant chemotherapy. Prognosis depends on type and degree of malignancy. Retroperitoneal tumours have a worse prognosis. Tumours to the orbit and GU have the best prognosis. Tumour stage is based on location and spread.

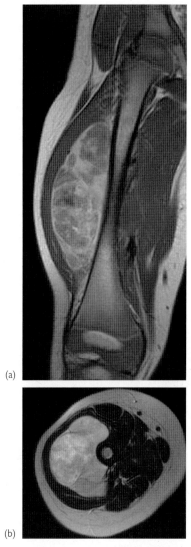

(a)

(b)

Fig. 6.45 (a) coronal T1 post-contrast images of the right thigh show a well-defined mixed signal intensity lesion which shows some enhancement occupying and involving the muscle groups at the lateral aspect of the thigh and (b) Axial T2.

Synovial sarcoma

This is a malignant tumour of mesenchymal origin. Lesions are usually well-defined, round, lobular soft tissue masses, typically <10cm in size. They occur in extra-articular regions, but within 5cm of the joint, adjacent to the synovial sheath (they can extend into the joint). Intra-articular lesions occur <10%. Lower extremities are commonest site, M>F, and occurs between 10 and 50yrs. Metastases are present at initial diagnosis in 25% of cases.

Clinical presentation

▶Slow growing, palpable soft tissue mass with a long duration of symptoms (up to 2–3yrs) and is often initially diagnosed as a benign lesion. Associated with pain and sensorimotor dysfunction.

Imaging findings

Radiographs
- Soft tissue mass close to a joint.
- Calcification ~25%.
- Bone invasion can occur (periosteal new bone formation, cortical destruction and osteoporosis).

Ultrasound
- Mixed echogenic mass.
- Either well-defined or irregular margins.

CT
- Soft tissue mass similar attenuation to muscle.
- Can contain areas of haemorrhage, necrosis, cyst formation and calcification.
- There is marked enhancement.
- CT is useful in detecting pulmonary metastases.

MRI
- T1WI: heterogeneous mass of low to intermediate signal.
- T2WI: heterogeneous mass which is hyperintense.
- There may be cystic and solid elements, with evidence of haemorrhage and fibrous tissue.
- Margins may be ill-defined.
- Marked enhancement following gadolinium.

Differential diagnosis
- Soft tissue sarcoma (proximal part of extremity, invasion into adjacent skeletal structures).
- Myositis ossificans (peripheral calcification).
- Pigmented villonodular synovitis.
- Paraosteal osteosarcoma (periosteal reaction).
- Fibromatosis.

Management and prognosis
Surgical excision and chemotherapy.

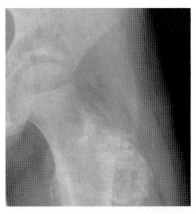

Fig. 6.46 There is an irregular calcified lesion at the lateral aspect of the left femur.

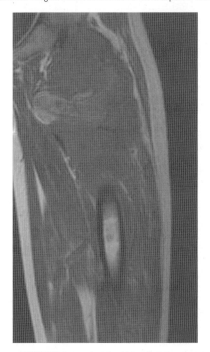

Fig. 6.47 Coronal T1WI MRI shows a low signal intensity heterogeneous mass enveloping the proximal left femur.

Fibrous dysplasia

This is a disorder of bone formation, resulting in an inability to produce mature lamellar bone. It may be monostotic (85% of cases) or polyostotic (15%) and there is a low risk of malignant change.

The polyostotic form is typically unilateral and commonly involves the skull and face (50%), pelvis and long bones. There is an association with precocious puberty (McCune–Albright's syndrome) and endocrine disorders (hyperparathyroidism, hypoparathyroidism and diabetes mellitus). Hyperpigmentation of the skin occurs at the sites of skeletal involvement (café-au-lait spots).

The monostotic form is often an incidental benign finding, but it can cause pathological fractures. Commonest in femur (40%), tibia (20%), skull, ribs and extremities.

Clinical presentation

Pathological fractures and bone remodelling. Craniofacial involvement can cause significant alteration in the child's appearance; facial and frontal bones—*leonitis ossea* (lion-like), mandible and maxillary—*cherubism*. There may be cranial nerve palsy.

Imaging findings

Radiographs

- ▶Radiolucent expansile medullary lesion which has a ground-glass appearance.
- Metadiaphysis of long bones with sparing of the epiphysis.
- Well-defined sclerotic margins and endosteal scalloping.
- No periosteal new bone formation.
- Bowing and deformity of the involved limb (this can lead to shepherd's crook deformity of the femur).
- Pseudoarthrosis can occur.
- Around the skull, mixed lytic sclerotic lesion, particularly sclerosis, involving the skull base and expansion of the calvarium, frontal bossing and facial asymmetry.

CT

- No mineralized matrix.
- No soft tissue mass.

MRI

- T1WI: homogenous low signal with thin rim of low signal sclerotic bone around the margins.
- T2WI: are of mixed signal intensity with a thin rim of low signal. Can be high signal in some cases.
- Contrast enhancement will show active lesions.

Nuclear scintigraphy

- Will determine activity and extent of lesions.
- The majority of lesions show increased uptake.
- Can be of decreased activity.

Differential diagnosis

- Neurofibromatosis.
- Paget's (adult population lesions are more sclerotic).

- Unicameral bone cyst (simple cyst with a sclerotic margin).
- Aneursymal bone cyst (expansion and fluid–fluid levels).

Management and prognosis

No treatment for asymptomatic lesions. Curettage and bone grafting for larger lesions. Bisphosphonates can be used.

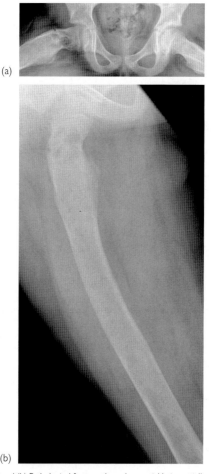

(a)

(b)

Fig. 6.48 (a) and (b) Pathological fracture through a partial lytic partially ground-glass appearing lesion in the proximal femur.

Vascular/lymphatic malformations

Congenital abnormalities due to dysplasia of small and large vascular channels. They are present at birth and can increase in size as the child grows. Unlike haemangiomas, they do not involute and are not neoplastic. M=F.

They are subcategorized based on the type of vascular channel into venous, lymphatic, capillary, arteriovenous and mixed.

Clinical presentation

May present at any time in childhood with a palpable mass, pain or limb deformity, congestive cardiac failure, steal syndrome, ulceration and bleeding. The larger the AV shunt, the earlier the presentation.

- Maffucci's syndrome: vascular malformations and multiple enchondromatosis.
- Klippel–Trelawney syndrome: vascular malformation with bone overgrowth, limb discrepancy and abnormality of the deep venous system.

Imaging findings

Radiographs

- Soft tissue mass.
- Phleboliths (venous component).
- Bone overgrowth.

Ultrasound

- Mixed echogenic lesion.
- Hypoechoic tubular and serpentine structures.
- Enlarged feeding vessels.
- Prominent draining veins.
- Increased Doppler flow (arterial component), no flow (lymphatic component).

MRI

- Multiloculated mass.
- Serpentine vessels.
- Flow voids suggest high-flow lesions (arterial component).
- No flow voids: venous stasis or lymphatic component.
- Gadolinium enhancement seen with vascular lesions. No enhancement suggests a lymphatic lesion.

Differential diagnosis

- Haemangioma.
- Lymphatic malformation.
- Soft tissue sarcoma.
- Arteriovenous fistula.

Management and prognosis

Initially conservative. Embolization and surgical excision for symptomatic lesions or rapidly enlarging lesions.

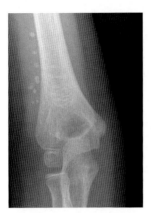

Fig. 6.49 Radiograph showing phlebo-liths in the soft tissues.

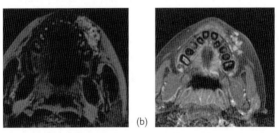

(a)　　　　　　　　(b)

Fig. 6.50 MR images of the face . There is a serpiginous heterogeneous mass in the soft with some signal flow voids, T2 images (a); and areas of enhancement (b).

Fibromatosis

A benign condition but locally aggressive with a tendency to recur. Causes localized fibrosis and infiltration of surrounding tissues which can result in significant reduction in function and morbidity. The fibrosis may be superficial (typically palm of the hand or plantar surface of the foot) or deep with involvement of muscles (shoulder, upper arm and thigh), the pelvis and abdomen. It can be multifocal.

Clinical presentation

A poorly circumscribed slow-growing mass which, if there is involvement of the surrounding muscles and tendons, can cause contractures. Tenderness is associated with nerve involvement.

Numerous descriptive terms have been applied:

- *Infantile fibromatosis/aggressive fibromatosis/extra-abdominal desmoid tumour/musculoaponeurotic fibromatosis.* Can be nodular or infiltrative, occurs in first two decades of life (infantile rarely >5yrs), can be multifocal, erosions and bowing of bone.
- *Myofibromatosis.* Commonest in infancy, increase in size and number up to 1yr than can regress, solitary or multicentric, involve bones, soft tissue and viscera, can calcify.
- *Congenital infantile fibrosarcoma.* Typically <5yrs, can erode bone.

Imaging findings

Radiographs

- Soft tissue mass with associated periosteal reaction (can calcify).
- Chronic lesions cause bone remodelling and erosions.

Ultrasound

- There is non-specific soft tissue mass with ill-defined margins.

CT

- Soft tissue mass of lower attenuation compared to the muscle.
- Proximity to bone may cause erosions and cortical destruction.

MRI

- Poorly defined mass, irregular margins and local invasion.
- T1W: typically hypo- or isointense to muscle.
- T2WI: hypointense with areas of hyperintensity and some signal heterogeneity.

Differential diagnosis

- Malignant fibrous histiocytoma.
- Synovial sarcoma.
- Rhabdomyosarcoma.
- Fibrous sarcoma.
- Venous malformation.

Management and prognosis

Surgical excision with wide margins. There may be local recurrence.

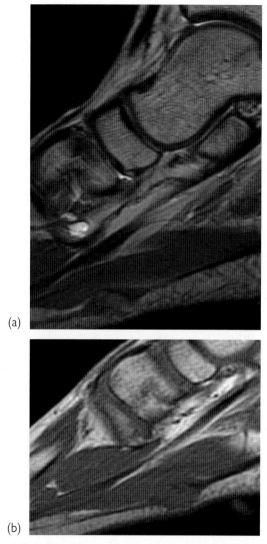

(a)

(b)

Fig. 6.51 Sagittal T1 and T2-weighted images of the foot show a hypointense mass in the plantar soft tissues involving the plantar aspect of the foot.

Discitis

This is an inflammatory process of the intervertebral disc space, most frequently seen in the lumbar region, which is due to either a bacterial, viral or unknown aetiology. Blood or tissue samples are positive in only about 30% of cases and when identified, *Staph. Aureus* is the commonest infective agent. Common between 6mths–4yrs of age.

Clinical presentation

Back pain or localized tenderness, but pain can radiate to the abdomen, hip and knee and be non-specific, which can lead to a delay in the diagnosis. Generalized fever and disability, with a refusal or inability to walk or a child who was walking starts to crawl or shuffle.

Imaging findings

Radiographs

- ▶Initial radiographs may be normal.
- ▶Disc space narrowing with irregularity and poor definition of adjacent vertebral end plates.
- Sclerosis of vertebral end plates.
- Paravertebral soft tissue mass.

MRI

- ▶The most sensitive investigation.
- Disc space narrowing, loss of signal within the vertebral body.
- With more chronic cases, there is loss of vertebral body height.
- T2WI/STIR: high signal marrow oedema in the adjacent vertebral bodies.
- Gadolinium enhancement in disc spaces, vertebral bodies and soft tissues.
- Paravertebral soft tissues, more likely with an infective (bacterial) aetiology, can be associated with abscesses (focal non-enhancing area surrounded by enhancing tissue).

Nuclear scintigraphy (bone scan)

- Increased uptake in vertebral body above and below disc.
- Typically positive from 1–2 days onset.

Differential diagnosis

- Any cause of lower back pain:
  - Muscle strains.
  - Spondylolysis.
  - Scheuermann's disease.
  - Bone tumour.
  - Osteomyelitis.

Management and prognosis

Symptomatic pain relief, antibiotics. Needle biopsy and blood cultures are often negative. Symptoms can improve spontaneously or following antibiotics. Those with proven infected cause do need antibiotics as they may develop joint destruction and spondylolysis.

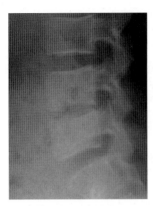

Fig. 6.52 Lateral radiograph of the spine shows irregularity of the vertebral body margins and loss of joint space at the L4/5 level.

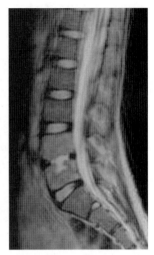

Fig. 6.53 Corresponding MR image. The T2WI shows extensive high signal marrow oedema with further areas of increase signal within the disc space. There is significant loss of the disc space.

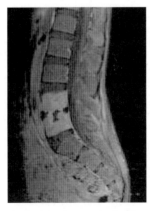

Fig. 6.54 T1WI FS postcontrast showing non-enhancing abscess in the disc space.

Assessment of the paediatric elbow

Anterior-posterior radiograph

This is taken in full extension, centred over the joint space. The olecranon is obscured by the humerus. The capitellum is lateral and articulates with the radial head. The trochlea is medial and articulates with the ulna. In normal subjects, the external humeral epicondyle lies parallel to the cortex of the humerus.

The lateral radiograph

Good-quality radiographs are vital in the assessment of the elbow joint. A lateral radiograph is taken with the elbow in 90° flexion, centred over the joint space. With a proper lateral projection, the capitellum and trochlea are superimposed. A figure of eight (or egg-timer) appearance is created from superimposed structures of the distal humerus.

Elbow ossification

Radiographs of the elbow in children will differ, depending on the age of the child. This is a consequence of the timing of the appearances of the six separate ossification centres around the joint which occur between 6mths to 12yrs of age. The exact age that each centre appears is less important than the order in which they do. The commonest sequence is: capitellum, radial head, internal (medial) humeral epicondyle, trochlea, olecranon and lateral (external humeral epicondyle). (CRITOL/CRITOE). ►While this order may vary slightly, the trochlea always ossifies after the internal epicondyle. Appreciating this sequence is important when assessing for avulsion injuries and epicondyle displacements around the joint.

Soft tissue fat pads

There are anterior and posterior extrasynovial, but intracapsular fat pads related to the distal humerus. These are seen as dark, triangular structures adjacent to the bone on a lateral radiograph. The presence of the anterior fat pad can be a normal finding. A visible posterior fat pad is abnormal and indicates an elbow effusion. ►In the presence of a posterior fat pad, a fracture must be excluded, even though it may not be visible. Absence of a fat pad does not exclude a fracture.

Anterior humeral line

In normal subjects, a line drawn along the anterior surface of the humerus should pass through the capitellum with approximately 1/3 of the capitellum lying anterior to the line. Supracondylar fractures can result in either anterior or posterior displacement of the capitellum about this line.

Radio-capitellar line

On a lateral radiograph, a line drawn along the centre of the proximal portion of the radius should intersect through the centre of the capitellum. Displacement of this line indicates that the radial head is dislocated.

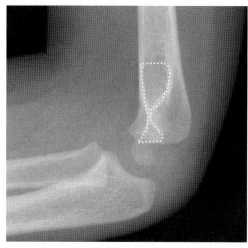

Fig. 6.55 Lateral radiograph showing the superimposition of soft tissue, producing an 'egg-timer/figure of eight' configuration of the distal humerus.

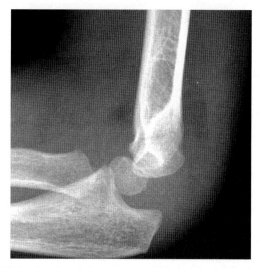

Fig. 6.56 Lateral radiograph showing elevated anterior and posterior fat pads in a child with a supracondylar fracture.

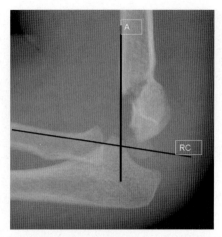

Fig. 6.57 Lateral radiograph showing the anterior humeral line and the radiocapitellar line. The capitellum lies posterior to the anterior humeral line due to the significant displacement of the supracondylar fracture.

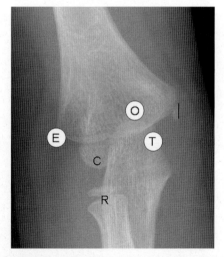

Fig. 6.58 Radiograph showing the ossification centres around the elbow joint. The capitellum, radius and internal apophysis have ossified. The markers show the site of the olecranon, trochlea and external epicondyle which are yet to ossify.

Incomplete fractures

The paediatric skeleton is considerably more pliable and elastic than the adult one. Consequently, forces applied to the bones will often cause deformity and damage to the bone without causing it to break into two fracture fragments. There are a number of different types of incomplete fractures: plastic (bowed), buckle (torus) and greenstick.

Clinical presentation

Typically a history of trauma with symptoms of pain, discomfort and a reluctance to move the injured limb. There may be associated soft tissue swelling.

Imaging findings

Radiographs

In the vast majority of cases, standard projection radiographs of the area of clinical concern are all the imaging that is required.

Buckle fractures (or torus fractures)
- A concave or convex deformity of the cortex. Typically the result of compression forces applied to the bone.
- Commonest in the distal forearm.
- The cortical deformity may be asymmetrical, with the bulging being more pronounced on the side of compression.
- ▶The defect may only be seen on single radiographic projection. It is important that two views in orthogonal planes are obtained in all cases.
- Soft tissue swelling with loss of the normal fat planes around fracture.

Plastic bowing (bending) fractures
- The bone is bent without any cortical deformity or a visible physical fracture line and they can be difficult to detect.
- Commonest in the radius, ulna and fibula.
- The defect may only be visible on a single projection.
- ▶ It is important to visualize the joints at each end of the bone because of the potential risk of associated dislocation. Deformity of the ulna can occur with radial head dislocation.
- Periosteal new bone formation may not occur during the healing process.

Greenstick fractures
- The fracture line involves one side of the cortex but does not extend across the full width of the bone.
- It may be associated with some deformity of the bone.
- When they heal, fat may prolapse into the cortical defect and may occasionally be confused with a small lytic tumour.

Differential diagnosis

Conditions associated with increased bone fragility, deformity or cortical irregularity, e.g. osteogenesis imperfecta, fibrous dysplasia, neurofibromatosis, metabolic bone disease. Clinically, the history and presentation should not cause significant concern.

Management and prognosis

Immobilization and pain relief are the standard method of treatment. Manipulation and internal fixation are rarely required.

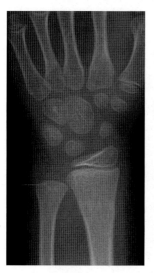

Fig. 6.59 AP radiograph of the same child as Fig. 6.60 showing cortical irregularity of the distal radius with a buckle fracture. The appearances are more obvious on the lateral radiograph, indicating the value of two views.

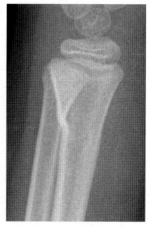

Fig. 6.60 Incomplete fractures. Lateral radiograph of the distal forearm showing a cortical bulge of the distal radius, indicating a buckle fracture.

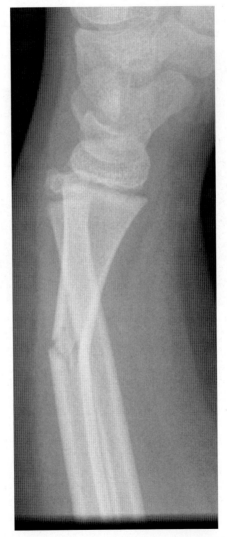

Fig. 6.61 Greenstick fracture of the distal radius. There is a cortical break on the dorsal surface with angulation of the bone, but the palmar (anterior surface of the bone) remains intact.

Physeal (growth plate) injuries

These fractures only occur in the immature skeleton (commonest 8–13 age group). The involvement of the adjacent epiphysis and/or metaphysis will characterize the fracture. The Salter–Harris (SH) classification is the most widely accepted with fractures graded I–V (refinements to this system have added additional more complex and rare fractures). Any growth plate can fracture but the upper extremity (particularly distal radius) is the commonest. Type II are the commonest and type V the rarest.

Clinical presentation

Fractures are associated with pain, swelling and reduced mobility.

Imaging findings

Radiographs

- Radiolucent fracture may extend into the growth plate.
- Widening of the physis.
- Displacement of the fractured fragments.
- Salter V fracture may initially appear normal.

CT

- It is useful to demonstrate the degree of disruption around the articular surface.
- It is most commonly used with triplane fractures of the distal tibia.

MRI

- T2WI/STIR will show marrow and soft tissue oedema.
- Demonstration of the fracture extending into unossified cartilage.
- MR imaging will identify cartilage deformity.
- Volume imaging can quantify the degree of physeal closure.

Differential diagnosis

- Triplane fracture distal tibia.
- Tillaux fracture distal tibia (SH III).
- Metaphyseal fracture (in young child consider NAI).
- Stress fracture (widening the growth plate).
- Other cause metaphyseal irregularity: rickets, mucopolysaccharidoses (MPS).

Management and prognosis

Pain relief and immobilization with open reduction and internal fixation for more severe injuries.

Complications are rare but include premature, partial or complete fusion of the physis which can lead to limb shortening, angulation and joint deformity. Prognosis is worse for types IV and V and those in the lower extremity.

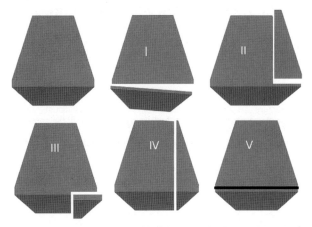

Fig. 6.62 Schematic representation of the Salter Harris classification of physeal fractures. Top left normal appearances, type I is a fracture through the growth plate, type II is a fracture through the metaphysis and growth plate, type III is through the epiphysis and growth plate, type IV is through the epiphysis, growth plate and metaphysis, type V is compression and damage to the growth plate.

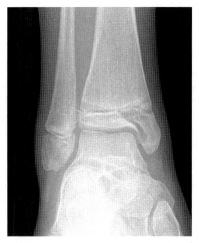

Fig. 6.63 AP radiograph of the ankle showing a Salter Harris IV fracture of the distal tibia.

Non-accidental injury: skeletal injury

Non-accidental injury (NAI) skeletal injuries forms a small part of the different forms of abuse a child may suffer (this includes shaking, burning, emotional, sexual or neglect). Skeletal NAI is the result of inappropriate forces applied by a perpetrator to a child. Skeletal injuries are commoner under the age of about 18mths, but can occur at any age.

Clinical presentation

Any fracture can either be the result of an accident or an inflicted injury. It is important that any radiological findings are assessed with the appropriate clinical history and examination.

Different types of fracture have a different level of specificity for NAI.

Fractures with low specificity for NAI
- Subperiosteal new bone formation.
- Clavicle fractures.
- Long bone shaft fractures.
- Skull fractures.

Moderate specificity for NAI
- Multiple fractures.
- Fractures of different ages.
- Epiphyseal separation injuries.
- Digital fractures.
- Complex skull fractures.
- Fractures of the vertebrae.

High specificity for NAI
- Classic metaphyseal fractures.
- Rib fractures.
- Scapula fractures.
- Sternal fractures.

Investigation of NAI

This should be a multidisciplinary approach, of which radiology forms an important part. When NAI is suspected, a full radiographic skeletal survey should be obtained. Additional investigations will depend on local protocol and resources and include repeat radiographs (after approximately 2 weeks) to identify previously occult healing fractures, skeletal scintigraphy and head CT and/or MRI.

▶Radiographs are superior in the detection of metaphyseal and skull fractures, while scintigraphy is sensitive in detecting rib fractures.

Differential diagnosis

A number of conditions may predispose an individual to fracturing because of increased bone fragility, while other conditions may mimic metaphyseal fractures:
- Osteogenesis imperfecta.
- Nutritional disorders, e.g. rickets and scurvy.
- Congenital skeletal dysplasias.

Non-accidental injury: metaphyseal fracture

Classic metaphyseal fractures (chip, corner, bucket handle), typically occur in children under 18mths of age. The fracture is in the plane of the physis and may extend into the primary spongiosa bone of the metaphysis, which is an area of relative weakness. The injury is believed to occur from a forceful twisting/pulling action or from severe shaking of the extremity. The radiographic appearances will depend on the amount of ossified bone displaced and the radiographic projection.

Imaging findings

Radiographs

- Fractures are at the metaphysis of the long bones.
- Commonest in the lower limb.
- Triangular (chip fracture) portion of bone completely separate from the metaphysis adjacent to the physis.
- Crescentic (bucket handle) portion of bone overlying the metaphysis.
- ▶Periosteal new bone may occur within about a week.
- Periosteal new bone is not a constant feature of the healing response.

Ultrasound

Ultrasound may demonstrate metaphyseal irregularity and subperiosteal haemorrhage.

Bone scintigraphy

▶Detection of metaphyseal fractures can be difficult as they occur at an area of normal increased activity, namely the growing physis.

Differential diagnosis

- Normal variations of growth (spurs).
- Rickets.
- Congenital indifference to pain.
- Menke's syndrome.
- Congenital infection.
- Scurvy.

Non-accidental injury: rib fractures

These result from severe compressive/squeezing forces applied to the chest. They can be clinically occult. Posterior rib fractures have a high specificity for NAI. Fractures at the anterior costochondral junction may heal without any callus formation.

Radiographs

- ▶Chest radiograph with oblique views of the ribs are needed to detect rib fractures.
- ▶Repeat radiographs after approximately 2 weeks will show evidence of fracture healing and detect additional 'missed' acute fractures not seen on the initial radiographs.
- Fractures are often multiple and run in a line along adjacent ribs.

Bone scintigraphy

Detection of rib fractures can be improved by the use of nuclear scintigraphy.

Differential diagnosis

- Normal compound shadowing (sternum projected over ribs).

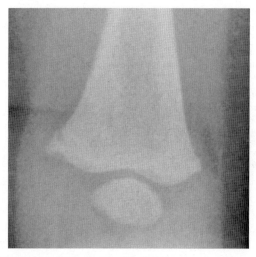

Fig. 6.64 Metaphyseal corner fracture of the distal femur.

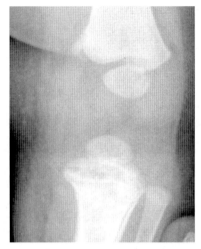

Fig. 6.65 Healing fractures of the distal femur and proximal tibia.

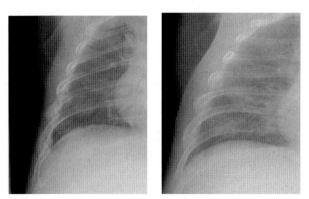

Fig. 6.66 Radiographs of the ribs taken two weeks apart showing the improved detection due to the healing response around the fractures.

Toddler's fracture

This is a spiral fracture of the distal tibia in a young (toddler) child.

Clinical presentation

Classically, the child has started to walk and then shows a reluctance to weight bear, altered gait or refusal to walk. Clinically, there is often tenderness around the distal tibia.

Similar symptoms may occur with fractures of the fibula, calcaneum and cuboid but these are less common.

Imaging findings

Radiographs

- ▶The initial radiographs may be normal or there is a hairline spiral fracture.
- Small amount of soft tissue swelling.
- Radiographs taken 7–10 days after the injury will demonstrate periosteal reaction or sclerosis around the fracture margins as a consequence of healing.
- Even if the initial radiograph is normal, routine follow-up radiographs are not indicated, unless there is clinical concern.
- Other potential fractures causing similar symptoms are buckle fractures of the tibia, fibula and tarsal bone fractures.
- Healing tarsal fractures are often seen as a sclerotic line across the bone.

MRI

- T2WI: high signal marrow oedema.
- T1WI: low signal marrow oedema.
- Fracture line low signal on all sequences.
- No soft tissue mass.

Nuclear scintigraphy (^{99m}Tc)

- Increased activity on delayed images, positive after 24hrs.

Differential diagnosis

- Osteomyelitis.
- Leukaemia or neuroblastoma (first presentation may be refusal to walk).
- Non-accidental injury (younger non-mobile child).
- Osteoid osteoma (sclerosis and cortical thickening).
- Joint disease (septic, JIA, reactive synovitis).

Management and prognosis

Conservative treatment with pain relief. Long leg cast for persisting symptoms.

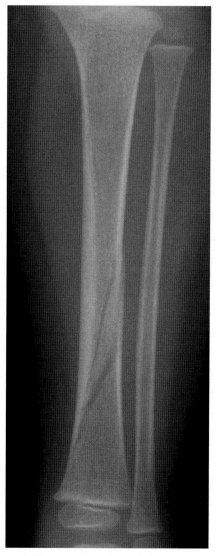

Fig. 6.67 Spiral fracture of the distal tibia in a 3-year-old child.

Humeral supracondylar fracture

This is a transverse fracture of the distal humerus at the level of the meta-diaphysis and is usually extra-articular in children. It is often the result of excessive hyperextension of the elbow joint or from a direct impact on the flexed elbow. There may be anterior or posterior displacement of the distal fracture fragment. It is a common fracture in the pre-teenage child and when seen in the non-ambulatory child should raise the suspicion of non-accidental injury.

Clinical presentation

Often it occurs from falls onto the extended outstretched hand and is associated with pain, swelling and reduced mobility. A large haematoma around the fracture site may cause compression of the brachial artery which can lead to loss of the distal radial pulse (compartment syndrome).

Imaging findings

Radiographs

- ▶On the lateral view, there is a visible posterior fat pad sign.
- ▶The anterior humeral line does not cross through the mid capitellum.
- There may be a transverse metaphyseal lucency (not seen in up to 25% of cases).
- A grading system (I–III) based on the degree of displacement has been described.

MRI

- Usually not required.
- On T2WI and STIR images high signal intensity due to marrow oedema, periarticular fluid and haematoma.
- T1WI low signal intensity due to marrow oedema.
- Low signal fracture line with cortical disruption.

Differential diagnosis

- Lateral or medial (epi)condylar fractures (fracture line does not extend across the metaphysis).
- T-condylar (supracondylar fracture with extension into the joint).
- Olecranon fracture.
- Posterior dislocation (may occur with fracture).
- Pulled elbow (effusion but no displacement of capitellum).

Management and prognosis

Minor displacement: conservative immobilization is all that is needed. With significant displacement, reduction +/– surgical fixation is necessary. Vascular and median nerve injury can occur. Cubitus varus deformity or loss of function can result from poor alignment.

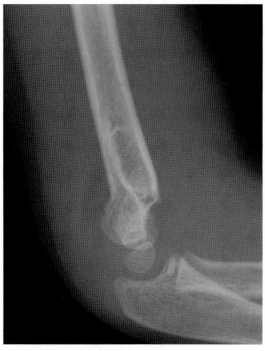

Fig. 6.68 Lateral radiograph of the elbow showing a supracondylar fracture with associated joint effusion causing elevation of the fat pads.

Pelvic avulsion injuries

This is a fracture either through bone or unossified cartilage due to forces applied by the isometric contraction of the attached muscle or tendon. Avulsion fractures account for approximately 10–15% of paediatric pelvic fractures. In adolescents, it is more likely the result of separation of an unfused apophysis. The injuries are commoner in athletic males.

The common sites for avulsion fractures correspond to the sites of the attachment of the major muscles: anterior superior iliac spine (sartorius muscle), anterior inferior iliac spine (rectus femoris—straight head), acetabular rim (rectus femoris—reflected head), ischial tuberosity (biceps femoris, semi tendonitis and semi membranosis), greater trochanter (gluteus minimus and medius), pubic bone (gracilis and abductors), iliac crest (abdominal musculature).

Clinical presentation

Acute pain or tenderness following extreme exertion. In chronic cases, there may be generalized swelling and discomfort following activity. There may be associated soft tissue swelling and haematoma formation.

Imaging findings

Radiographs

- An osseous fragment often with an irregular margin adjacent to the pelvis.
- Comparison with the contralateral side will either show presence of an avulsed fracture or increased separation of an apophysis.
- ▶If the apophysis is yet to ossify then radiographs may be normal.
- On healing, there is often exuberant callus formation around the fracture site.
- ▶In cases of chronic avulsion, there is sclerosis and irregularity which can sometimes be confused with tumours. Biopsy should be avoided.

CT

- CT will confirm the presence of an avulsed fragment and haematoma around the fracture site.

MRI

- ▶This is the most sensitive indicator of damage and can show associated damage in the muscle tendon and muscle body.
- On T2WI, there is hyperintensity and marrow oedema around the fracture site and associated tendon.
- The amount of soft tissue swelling may be extensive and there may be haemorrhage in the muscles and soft tissues.
- The involved tendon may be lax and have a slightly wavy outline.
- The avulsed osseous fragment is hypointense on T1WI.

Differential diagnosis

- ▶Bone tumours: typically, the history and location of the changes should exclude bone tumour in most cases. Muscle oedema on MRI is not typical for a tumour.
- Muscle strain: musculotendinous injuries are less common in children, muscle oedema seen on MRI.

Management and prognosis

Management is typically conservative. Localized pain relief, non-weight bearing is important. Re-injury is common if returning to activity prematurely. Surgical intervention for severely displaced avulsed fragments. If there is chronic pain, resection of bony unit and surgical reattachment.

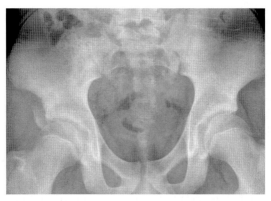

Fig. 6.69 Radiograph of the pelvis. There is an avulsion fracture of the right anterior inferior iliac spine.

Osgood–Schlatter's disease

Osgood–Schlatter's disease (OSD) is traction apophysitis of the patellar ligament at its insertion the tibial tuberosity (also called tibial osteochondrosis). It typically occurs at the onset of adolescent growth spurt, occurring at a slightly younger age in girls.

Clinical presentation

There is a slow onset of pain and tenderness over the tibial tuberosity, worsened by activity or marked flexion and extension of the knee. In severe cases where the pain is severely restricting movement, there may be wasting at the quadriceps and tightness of the hamstrings muscles.

Imaging findings

The diagnosis is essentially a clinical one and unless there are concerns about an alternative pathology, then imaging is not indicated in the majority of cases.

Radiographs

- Lateral radiographs show hypertrophy, fragmentation and irregularity of the tibial tuberosity.
- Overlying soft tissue swelling greater than 4mm.
- These findings can be normal variants.

Ultrasound

- Does not involve ionizing radiation and allows the patient to localize the site of pain.
- There is overlying soft tissue swelling, fragmentation and irregularity of the tibial tuberosity.
- ▶Ultrasound is insensitive in excluding other cases of bone pain such as an osteosarcoma.

MRI

- There is distension of the deep and superficial interpatellar bursae.
- On T2WI, high signal subchondral oedema in the tibial tuberosity and surrounding soft tissues may extend into Hoffa's fat pad.
- Thickening of the distal patellar ligament.
- Thickening, fragmentation and sclerosis of the cortex around the tibial tuberosity.

Differential diagnosis

- Patellar tendonitis: with MR imaging, signal intensity is increased in the patellar tendon.
- Sinding–Larsen–Johannson disease: traction apophysitis of the inferior pole of the patella (irregularity of the inferior pole of the patella).

Management and prognosis

Management is typically conservative with pain relief and reduction of exercise. Surgical treatment is reserved for severe cases.

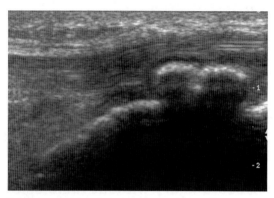

Fig. 6.70 Ultrasound showing fragmentation and irregularity of the proximal tibial plateau with thickening of the overlying tendon.

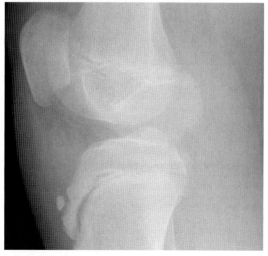

Fig. 6.71 Lateral radiograph shows fragmentation, irregularity and soft tissue swelling around the proximal tibial apophysis.

Paediatric cervical spine

Pseudosubluxation

In children, there may be a normal physiological displacement of C2 and C3 and to a lesser extent, C3 and 4, on a lateral radiograph. It is more marked in flexion. This is a physiological pseudosubluxation. It is important to differentiate from bilateral pars interarticularis fracture and facet dislocation.

If a line is drawn from the anterior aspect of the spinous process of C1 to the anterior aspect of the spinous process of C3, the anterior edges of the spinous processes of C1, 2 and 3 should all line up within 1mm of each other on both flexion and extension radiographs. If this line does not overlap the anterior aspect of C2 by 2mm or more, a true injury is present.

Spinal cord injury without radiological abnormality (SCIWORA)

The term SCIWORA was initially used to describe cord injury in the absence of plain radiographic abnormalities. With the evolution of MR imaging, two variants of the phrase have been identified:

- SCIWORA in the absence of radiographic or CT evidence of injury (but the majority of these patients demonstrate abnormality on MRI).
- SCIWORA in whom the MRI is normal despite clinical evidence of cord injury, this is the least common.

SCIWORA is more common in children than in adults due to the increased elasticity of the spinal canal, which will result in increased traction on the cord. It is commonest before 3yrs of age with a history of extension, flexion, distraction injury or cord ischaemia.

Following significant injury, MRI should ideally be performed in all children with neurological signs or symptoms.

Atlanto-axial rotatory fixation (AARF)

Also referred to as atlanto-axial rotatory subluxation and atlanto-axial rotatory dislocation. It is a cause of torticollis and a significant reduction in the range of neck rotation. The head is tilted to one side. It may be associated with spinal cord compromise.

Normal neck rotation involves cervical spine rotation at the C1/C2 (atlas–axis)articulation. The odontoid acting as a pivot for the rotation of C1. In AARF the rotation either becomes stuck in maximum physiological rotation or there may be subluxation at the C1/C2 articulation.

There are four types:

- Type 1: rotatory fixation with anterior displacement of the atlas. This is in the normal range of rotation, but it becomes fixated.
- Type 2: rotatory fixation with anterior displacement of the atlas (with respct to C2) of 3–5mm. It is associated with division of the transverse ligament.

- Type 3: AARF with anterior displacement of the atlas of more than 5mm.
- Type 4: posterior displacement of the atlas and occurs with hypoplasia of the odontoid process. This is rare.

Imaging findings

Axial CT demonstrates the C1/C2 relationship. Static CT is diagnostic for type 2 AARF, however, type 1 may be difficult to distinguish from benign torticollis. Axial CT should be performed in the presenting position, with further imaging following voluntary but maximal, ipsilateral and contralateral rotation of the head. In type 1 AARF, there is little or no rotation of the atlas.

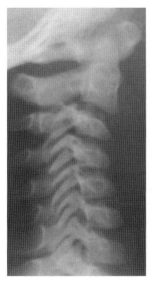

Fig. 6.72 Pseudosubluxation at the C2/C3 level.

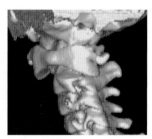

Fig. 6.73 3D CT reconstruction showing subluxation of C1 on C2.

Ear, nose and throat (ENT) and eye
Clinical presentations and role of imaging

Helen Williams

Decreased visual acuity

Visual acuity is acuteness or clearness of vision. It is measured quantitatively by the ability to identify black symbols on a white background at a standardized distance as the size of the symbols is varied. The visual acuity (VA) represents the smallest size that can be reliably identified.

Amaurosis is partial or total loss of vision, usually reserved for blindness or near blindness not caused by ocular disease.

Acute loss of vision

Cortical disease
- Hypoxia.
- Hypotension.
- Hypoglycaemia.
- Benign occipital epilepsy.
- Migraine.
- Post-traumatic: following occipital infarction or haemorrhage.
- Occipital tumour: primary lesion or metastasis.

Retinal disease
- Migraine.
- Post-traumatic, e.g. retinal detachment, interruption of vascular supply.
- Vascular occlusion (central retinal artery or vein).
- Inflammation, e.g. measles.

Optic nerve disease
- Optic neuritis, e.g. infective/inflammatory causes, demyelination, drugs, auto-immune disorders, compressive neuropathy, inherited disease.
- ▶ There is a wide differential for optic neuritis.

Miscellaneous causes
- Nutritional deficiency (causing optic neuritis): folic acid, vitamins B1, B2, B6 and B12.
- Acutely ICP, including BIH.
- Psychological (non-organic).

Progressive blindness

Lens
- Cataract formation.
- Lens dislocation.

Intraocular tumour (📖 p. 431)

Choroidoretinitis
- Congenital infection, e.g. toxoplasmosis, CMV.
- Viral or fungal disease especially in immunocompromised patients.
- Systemic non-infectious disease, e.g. JIA, vasculitis, chronic granulomatous disease.

Retinal disease
- Retinal degeneration: generally inherited disorders, e.g. retinitis pigmentosa, infantile Refsum disease.

Optic nerve and pathway disease
- Optic neuritis: wide differential.
- Tumour originating from optic nerve or pathway, e.g. optic glioma.
- Compression of optic nerve or pathway: tumour (e.g. pituitary or hypothalamic lesion, craniopharyngioma), vascular lesion, bony encroachment (e.g. osteopetrosis).

Miscellaneous causes
- Amblyopia due to squint.
- BIH.
- Glaucoma.

Role of imaging in visual loss

CT and MRI are used to identify and evaluate orbital and intracranial causes of visual loss, both acute and chronic. MRI is the modality of choice in most instances due to its superior spatial resolution and tissue characterization. Exceptions include acute trauma (e.g. detection of intracranial haemorrhage) and evaluation of bony structures (e.g. optic foraminal stenosis) where CT should be the primary imaging modality.

Ear pain and discharge

Ear pain

Pinna, external auditory canal (EAC) and tympanic membrane (TM)
- Infection, e.g. otitis externa, herpes infection, abscess/boil.
- Foreign body.
- Trauma.

Middle or inner ear, temporal bone
- Acute otitis media.
- Chronic serous otitis media ('glue ear'), pain is rare.
- Mastoiditis.
- Flying.

Referred pain
- Lower molar teeth.
- Temporomandibular joint.
- Pharynx.
- Cervical spine.
- Parotid, e.g. mumps.

Ear discharge
- Wax.
- Pus or foul-smelling: acute or chronic suppurative otitis media, otitis externa, abscess/boil, foreign body, cholesteatoma.
- Clear fluid: CSF, e.g. following temporal bone fracture or ear surgery (with defect in dura + tympanic membrane or EAC).
- Blood: trauma, foreign body.

Role of imaging in ear pain and discharge
In the majority of cases imaging is not required.

CT
- Pre-surgical assessment of middle ear/temporal bone abnormalities.
- Suspected cholesteatoma.
- Detect/evaluate complications of middle ear infection, e .g. mastoiditis and associated intracranial complications (☐ p. 472), cerebral abscess.
- Post-trauma to identify skull base or temporal bone fractures.

MRI
- Detect/evaluate intracranial complications of middle ear infection, e.g. cerebral abscess and venous sinus thrombosis.
- Post-operative evaluation, e.g. recurrent cholesteatoma.

Hearing loss

In conductive hearing loss (CHL) deafness is the result of a physical problem related to the sound collecting apparatus, i.e. abnormality in the EAC, the tympanic membrane or ossicles preventing conduction of sound to the cochlea. Sensorineural hearing loss (SNHL) is caused by abnormality of the inner ear structures e.g. hair cell destruction in the cochlea, vestibulocochlear nerve (CN VIII) or central auditory pathways in the brain. Mixed hearing loss has components of both CHL and SNHL.

Genetic causes account for approximately 30–50% of congenital deafness. They may be syndromic or non-syndromic, autosomal dominant or recessive, X-linked or sporadic.

Conductive hearing loss

EAC and tympanic membrane
- Wax, haematoma, infection or foreign body in the EAC.
- Genetic or syndromic causes, e.g. Down's, DiGeorge, Goldenhar, branchio–oto–facial syndromes.
- Congenital abnormalities of the EAC, e.g. atresia or stenosis.
- Perforated tympanic membrane, usually traumatic or infective.

Middle ear
- Chronic serous otitis media.
- Recurrent acute otitis media.
- Cholesteatoma.
- Locally destructive neoplasms, e.g. haemangioma, glomus tumours, facial nerve schwannoma, rhabdomyosarcoma.
- Congenital ossicular abnormalities, e.g. atresia, hypoplasia or fusion.
- Ossicular dissociation, e.g. post head injury or damage, e.g. following severe infection.
- Congenital absence of the oval window.
- Otosclerosis.

Sensorineural hearing loss

Inner ear abnormalities
- Congenital structural abnormalities of the cochlea, vestibule or semi-circular canals (e.g. hypoplasia, aplasia, common inner ear cavity, large endolymphatic sac anomaly/large vestibular aqueduct syndrome).
- Inflammatory/infective causes, e.g. congenital infection, meningitis or encephalitis, mumps, measles, other viral infections.
- Ototoxic drugs that damage cochlear hair cells or stria vascularis, e.g. aminoglycosides, vincristine, platinum-based chemotherapy agents, loop diuretics, salicylates.
- Unconjugated hyperbilirubinaemia: damages the cochlea.
- Noise-induced injury: rare in children.
- Vascular ischaemia of inner ear structures: including birth asphyxia.
- Trauma: temporal bone fracture with involvement of the cochlea.
- Perilymph fistula with oval or round window rupture: usually after sudden severe rise in ICP or trauma.
- Autoimmune disease (rare), e.g. Wegener's granulomatosis.

Vestibulocochlear nerve abnormalities

- Congenital absence or hypoplasia of CN VIII.
- Inflammatory/infective causes, e.g. congenital infection, meningitis or encephalitis, mumps, measles.
- Vascular ischaemia including birth asphyxia.
- Cerebellopontine angle lesions (📖 p. 428).
- Temporal bone fracture with CN VIII disruption.
- Idiopathic.

Central deafness (rare)

- Bilateral brainstem lesions in the region of the inferior colliculus, e.g. metastases.
- Auditory cortex lesions.

Role of imaging in hearing loss

Imaging has a limited role in the investigation of childhood deafness. Most causes of CHL do not require imaging but CT is the most appropriate modality in selected cases. SNHL usually requires investigation with CT and MRI, particularly if a cochlear implant is being considered.

CT

- EAC atresia: to determine bony or soft tissue aetiology pre-operatively + assessment of associated middle ear abnormalities.
- Define extent of suspected or known cholesteatoma, or other destructive middle ear lesion.
- Assessment of middle ear and ossicular abnormalities, congenital or acquired.
- Assessment of inner ear congenital structural abnormalities and acquired conditions, e.g. labyrinthine ossification.
- Post-traumatic deafness: identify temporal bone fractures or rarer causes, e.g. large vestibular aqueduct syndrome.

MRI

- Assessment of inner ear: congenital structural abnormalities and acquired conditions, e.g. labyrinthine ossification (often in combination with CT).
- Congenital abnormalities of cranial nerve (CN) VIII.
- Suspected CN VIII tumours and cerebellopontine angle lesions.
- Suspected central (brain) lesions.

Leukokoria

A white pupillary reflex usually resulting from an intra-ocular abnormality. Normal is orange/red.

Congenital

- Cataract.
- Coloboma.
- Retinal dysplasia.
- Persistent hyperplastic primary vitreous.

Inflammatory/infective

- Choroidoretinitis, e.g. congenital infection.
- Toxocariasis.

Neoplastic

- Retinoblastoma (📖 p. 484).
- Retinal astrocytoma.

Other causes

- Retinopathy of prematurity.
- Retinal detachment, e.g. Coat's disease, NAI.
- Intra-ocular foreign body.

Role of imaging in leukokoria

Clinical examination is the primary method of evaluating a child with leukokoria. Ophthalmic ultrasound may be used to assess the globe supplemented by MRI if an ocular mass, fluid collection or retinal detachment is identified. CT has a limited role in detection of calcification, particularly in association with masses.

Nasal obstruction

Congenital
- Choanal atresia or stenosis (📖 p. 448).
- Nasal piriform aperture stenosis (📖 p. 456).
- Encephalocele.
- Nasal dermoid (📖 p. 450).
- Nasal glioma.
- Deviation of the nasal septum.

Inflammatory/infective
- Acute or chronic rhinitis.
- Enlarged adenoids (📖 p. 470).
- Glandular fever.
- Nasal/antrochoanal polyp.

Neoplastic
- Nasal angiofibroma (📖 p. 482).
- Lymphoma.
- Rhabdomyosarcoma (📖 p. 486).
- Neuroblastoma.
- Lymphoepithelioma.

Trauma
- Haematoma associated with skull base or upper cervical fracture.
- Foreign body.

Miscellaneous
- Narcotic withdrawal (neonatal period).
- Maternal reserpine (neonatal period).

Role of imaging in nasal obstruction

Radiographs
- Confirmation of adenoidal hypertrophy and effect on nasopharyngeal airway.
- Detection of radio-opaque foreign bodies.
- Initial assessment of cervical spine injury.

CT
- Assessment of congenital bony nasal obstruction: choanal atresia and piriform aperture stenosis.
- Definitive assessment of skull base or cervical spine fracture.
- Staging/assessment of tumours if MRI not available or contraindicated.

MRI
- Modality of choice for assessment of congenital midline abnormalities and nasopharyngeal masses, including tumour staging.

Neck mass

Neck masses are common in children and caused by diverse conditions. Lesions may be classified according to position, nature or according to the organ affected.

Congenital

▶ Mostly cystic abnormalities.
- Thyroglossal duct cyst (📖 p. 464).
- Cystic lymphatic and vascular malformations (📖 p. 458).
- Branchial apparatus abnormalities (📖 p. 438).
- Foregut duplication cysts (📖 p. 148) and bronchogenic cysts.
- Dermoids and epidermoids.

Inflammatory/infective

- Reactive and infective cervical lymphadenopathy (📖 p. 426).
- Cellulitis.
- Cervical abscess.
- Immunological or connective tissue disorders.
- Sarcoidosis.
- Salivary gland inflammation/infection.
- Thyroid swelling (📖 p. 424).

Neoplasia

- Lymphoma.
- Rhabdomyosarcoma (📖 p. 486).
- Neuroblastoma.
- Leukaemia.
- Thyroid tumours.
- Salivary gland tumours.
- Castleman's disease: benign lymphoproliferative disorder of unknown aetiology.

Miscellaneous

- Fibromatosis coli (📖 p. 476).

Role of imaging in paediatric neck masses

Ultrasound is the primary imaging modality for children as it is quick, inexpensive, and provides immediate information about the location and nature of a lesion without using ionizing radiation, sedation or anaesthesia. Ultrasound can also be used to guide needle aspiration or biopsy.

Main disadvantages of ultrasound: it provides poor information about deep structures and ultrasound findings are non-specific. MRI and CT may require sedation or general anaesthetic (GA) in young children. A multi-modality approach may be required in some instances.

▶ The ultimate aim of imaging is to determine the nature and extent of a lesion, including its involvement of other structures.

Table 7.1 Advantages and disadvantages of the cross-sectional imaging modalities

Modality	Advantages*	Disadvantages/limitations*
Ultrasound	Non-ionizing Inexpensive Quick Immediate information on nature of lesion Identifies blood flow Guides biopsy/aspiration	Imaging characteristics are non-specific Poor visualization of deep tissues Unable to visualize skull base or mediastinal involvement Unable to assess other bony involvement
CT	Visualization of deep structures and spine Optimum bony detail Good soft tissue contrast with iv enhancement (less than MRI) Multiplanar reconstructions	Ionising radiation Requires iv access May require sedation or GA
MRI	Visualization of deep structures and spine Optimum soft tissue contrast Good visualization of bone involvement Multiplanar capability	Requires i.v. access in most instances May require sedation or GA Long procedure Patient-specific contraindications, e.g. cochlear implants, pacemaker (availability may be limited)

*With particular reference to neck masses in children.

Nystagmus

An involuntary, periodic, rhythmic oscillation of the eyes. The oscillations may be sinusoidal with approximately equal amplitude and velocity (*pendular nystagmus*) or more commonly having a slow initiating phase and a fast corrective phase (*jerk nystagmus*). *Physiological nystagmus* is a high-frequency low-amplitude, pendular oscillation occurring normally when lateral gaze is sustained to the point of fatigue.

Congenital or infantile (presenting <6mths of age) nystagmus may take many different forms. Involuntary, rhythmic eye movements are characteristic but the waveform, amplitude, and frequency can vary with changes in focal distance, direction of gaze, and under monocular or binocular viewing conditions. A disorder affecting any of the three mechanisms that control eye movements; fixation, the vestibulo-ocular reflex, and the neural integrator may result in nystagmus. The cerebellum, ascending vestibular pathways, and oculomotor nuclei are important components of the neural integrator.

Congenital or infantile nystagmus

- Idiopathic or familial oculomotor abnormality.
- Visual impairment or blindness.
- Associated with albinism.
- Latent and manifest latent nystagmus.
- Spasmus nutans (onset from 4mths to 3yrs of age).

Acquired nystagmus

- Disorders affecting the vestibular system, e.g. infection, tumour.
- Unilateral hemispheric lesions, e.g. infarction.
- Optic nerve or chiasm lesions.
- Brainstem lesions (e.g. tumour, infarct, haemorrhage, demyelination).
- Cerebellar lesions.
- Malformations of the craniocervical junction, e.g. Chiari I malformation.
- Spasmus nutans.
- Drugs, e.g. antidepressants, anticonvulsants, alcohol, tranquillizers.
- Ictal nystagmus.

Role of imaging in nystagmus

MRI is the modality of choice in selected cases when an underlying CNS abnormality is suspected.

Orbital swelling and proptosis

Proptosis is the abnormal forward protrusion of an organ, e.g. the eyeball (globe), also called exophthalmos.

Congenital
- Craniosynostosis including syndromic types ([book] p. 532).
- Orbital encephalocele.
- Intra-orbital vascular or lymphatic malformation.

Inflammatory/infective
- Orbital cellulitis ([book] p. 474).
- Ethmoiditis.
- Paranasal sinus mucocele.
- Cavernous sinus thrombosis.
- Inflammatory pseudotumour.
- Thyroid ophthalmopathy.

Neoplasia
- Optic nerve glioma.
- Retinoblastoma ([book] p. 484).
- Neuroblastoma.
- Lymphoma.
- Rhabdomyosarcoma ([book] p. 486).
- Haemangioma of infancy ([book] p. 480).
- LCH.
- Dermoids and teratoma.

Trauma
- Skull base or orbital fracture with haematoma.
- Also coagulopathy with intra-orbital haematoma ± history of trauma.

Role of imaging in orbital swelling and proptosis

Radiographs
- Initial assessment of suspected facial/orbital fracture.
- Initial assessment of craniosynostoses: major sutures.

Ultrasound
- Assessment of ocular mass.

CT
- Suspected skull base or orbital fracture.
- Orbital cellulitis: modality of choice to determine extent of infection and detect associated collections.
- Sinus disease: pre-operative evaluation and detect associated complications.
- Suspected intracranial venous sinus thrombosis.
- Pre-operative assessment of craniosynostosis.
- Detection of calcification in ocular masses.

MRI

- Modality of choice for assessment of ocular and extra-ocular masses including tumours and vascular lesions.
- Orbital cellulitis: determine extent of infection and detect associated collections.
- Evaluate intracranial complications of orbital or sinus infection.
- Suspected intracranial venous sinus thrombosis.

Stridor

A harsh, high-pitched, rasping, crowing or musical sound produced by turbulent air flow through a partially obstructed airway. It may be inspiratory, expiratory or biphasic.

Inspiratory stridor is associated with an extrathoracic lesion affecting the nasal airway, pharynx or larynx: expiratory stridor implies an intrathoracic lesion (tracheal or bronchial) and biphasic stridor is associated with glottic or subglottic pathology.

Acute stridor

- Croup (laryngotracheobronchitis).
- Epiglottitis.
- Diphtheria.
- Retropharyngeal lymphadenitis or abscess.
- Laryngeal spasm, e.g. hypocalcaemia associated with rickets, tetany.
- Angioneurotic oedema.
- Smoke inhalation.
- Trauma.
- Ingestion of corrosive substance.
- Foreign body.

Chronic stridor

Supraglottic causes

- Laryngomalacia.
- Micrognathia.
- Macroglossia.
- Down's syndrome.
- Supraglottic web.
- Tonsillar enlargement (🕮 p. 470).
- Lingual, aryepiglottic, thyroglossal or laryngeal cysts.

Glottic causes

- Vocal cord paralysis: congenital or acquired.
- Laryngeal web.
- Laryngeal haemangioma, polyp or papilloma.
- Cricothyroid or cricoarytenoid dislocations.
- Foreign body.

Subglottic causes

- Congenital subglottic stenosis.
- Tracheomalacia: congenital or acquired (🕮 p. 462).
- Vascular ring.
- Tracheal obstruction or stenosis, e.g. from prolonged intubation, haemangioma.
- Mediastinal tumour.
- Foreign body.

Role of imaging in stridor

Radiographs

- Limited role in detection of radio-opaque foreign bodies.

Ultrasound
- Assessment of vocal cord movement.
- May detect glottic lesions, e.g. cysts.

Fluoroscopy
- Dynamic assessment of laryngo- or tracheo-bronchomalacia.
- Upper GI contrast study: initial assessment for suspected extrinsic lesion, e.g. vascular ring or mediastinal mass.
- Catheter angiography may be used to define mediastinal vascular anatomy, particularly if patient undergoing cardiac catheterization for other reasons.

CT
- Modality of choice for assessment of intrinsic airway lesions, e.g. fixed stenosis.
- Assessment of neck and mediastinal masses including tumour staging.
- Assessment of mediastinal vascular anatomy particularly if MRI not available or contraindicated, e.g. sick neonate.

MRI
- Modality of choice for assessment of mediastinal vascular anatomy.
- Assessment of neck and mediastinal masses including tumour staging.

Squint (strabismus)

Deviation or malalignment of the eyes; Convergent squint or esotropia is inward deviation of the eye, divergent squint or exotropia is outward deviation of the eye. Most children have *heterophoria*—a latent tendency for ocular malalignment under certain conditions, e.g. fatigue, stress, illness.

Constant ocular malalignment is called *heterotropia*. Affected individuals suppress the image from one eye to avoid diplopia. If only one eye is used for fixation, vision may be permanently lost in the other eye (strabismic amblyopia). Therefore squint should be diagnosed and treated early, referred to an ophthalmologist as soon as the squint is noticed, ideally <6mths of age. Many children with neurological disorders, e.g. cerebral palsy (CP) have *non-paralytic squint* where each eye has a full range of movement when tested separately. Non-paralytic squint may have no identifiable cause, may be familial or related to an intra-ocular abnormality. Esotropia is the most common type.

▶ A fixed squint at any age is abnormal and treatable underlying conditions must be identified.

Heterophoria
- Latent squint usually convergent.
- Often corrects by 6mths of age.

Non-paralytic strabismus (concomitant)
- Accommodation to correct far-sightedness (hypermetropia).
- Lens abnormalities, e.g. cataract, high or asymmetric refractive errors.
- Nerve weakness due to febrile illness, head injury, CP.
- Retinal, optic nerve or macular lesions, e.g. retinopathy of prematurity, retinal detachment, macular abnormalities, optic nerve atrophy.

Paralytic strabismus

Congenital
- Microcephaly.
- Hydrocephalus (📖 p. 506).
- Cranial nerve palsies including Möebius syndrome.
- Brown syndrome.
- Duane syndrome.
- Congenital ptosis.
- Myasthenia gravis.

Acquired
- Microcephaly.
- Raised ICP, e.g. hydrocephalus, tumours.
- Brainstem lesions, e.g. tumours, demyelination, vasculitis.
- Intra-ocular tumour, e.g. retinoblastoma (📖 p. 484).
- Cranial nerve lesions, e.g. tumours, inflammatory/infective causes, cavernous sinus thrombosis, skull fracture following head injury.
- Myopathies.
- Myasthenia gravis.

Role of imaging in squint

In the majority of cases the cause of a squint can be determined by clinical examination. Imaging has a limited role and is confined to those in whom an underlying CNS abnormality is suspected, e.g. tumour or demyelination. MRI is the modality of choice.

Thyroid enlargement

Diffuse enlargement

- Familial goitre.
- Acute thyroiditis.
- Grave's disease.
- Multinodular goitre.

Focal mass

- Acute suppurative thyroiditis.
- Cyst.
- Adenoma.
- Carcinoma.

Role of imaging in thyroid enlargement or masses

Ultrasound

- Modality of choice for initial assessment of generalized goitre or focal mass lesions.
- May be used to guide fine needle aspiration (FNA) or core biopsy.

CT and MRI

- Determine effect of thyroid mass on airway.
- Tumour staging.

Nuclear scintigraphy

- May help determine functional status of a thyroid nodule.

Ear, nose and throat (ENT) and eye
Differential diagnosis

Helen Williams

Cervical lymph node enlargement: acute

Reactive lymphadenopathy

- Any benign local or systemic infection, e.g. measles, mumps, rubella, varicella, adenovirus, rhinoviruses, enteroviruses.
- Immunization.
- Kawasaki disease.

Infective lymphadenitis: common organisms

- Newborn period:
  - *Staph. Aureus.*
  - Occasionally late onset group B strep.
- <5years:
  - Group A strep.
  - *Staph. Aureus.*
  - Non-tuberculous mycobacterial infection.
- School age and adolescents:
  - Epstein–Barr virus (EBV).
  - CMV.
  - Toxoplasmosis.
  - TB.

Cervical lymph node enlargement: sub-acute or chronic

Cervical lymphadenopathy without (or with minimal) signs of acute inflammation, no prodromal illness or systemic symptoms, little or no response to antibiotic treatment. The exact cause is not identified in a significant proportion.

Inflammatory/infective

- Reactive lymphadenopathy:
  - Local or systemic infection or immunization.
  - Usually resolves by 5–14d.
- Atopic eczema.
- TB or atypical mycobacterium.
- Viral infection:
  - EBV/infectious mononucleosis.
  - Toxoplasmosis.
  - CMV.
  - HIV.
- Bacterial infection:
  - Cat-scratch disease (*Bartonella henselae*).
- Fungal infection.
- Immunological or connective tissue disorders.
- Sarcoidosis.

Neoplasia

- Lymphoma.
- Leukaemia.
- Rhabdomyosarcoma (📖 p. 486).
- Neuroblastoma.
- Thyroid tumours.
- Salivary gland tumours.
- Castleman's disease: benign lymphoproliferative disorder of unknown aetiology.

Cerebellopontine (CP) angle mass

Congenital
- Arachnoid cyst.

Inflammatory/infective
- Skull base origin:
  - Malignant otitis externa.
  - Osteomyelitis of the petrous apex (Gradenigo's syndrome).

Neoplasia
- Primary tumours:
  - Acoustic schwannoma.
  - Trigeminal neuroma.
  - Epidermoid.
  - Meningioma.
  - Exophytic pontine glioma.
  - Skull base/temporal bone tumours, e.g. glomus tumour.
- Metastases:
  - Ependymoma.
  - Medulloblastoma.
  - Pineoblastoma, pineocytoma.
  - Germinoma.

Midline fronto-nasal mass

Congenital
- Encephalocele.
- Dermoid/epidermoid cyst ± sinus: may have intracranial extension.
- Nasal glioma.

Inflammatory/infective
- Pott's puffy tumour: cellulitis/subgaleal abscess associated with frontal sinusitis and osteomyelitis.

Neoplasia
- Infantile haemangioma.
- Hairy or teratoid polyp.
- Fibroma.
- Lipoma.
- Lipoblastoma.
- Rarely malignancy, e.g. rhabdomyosarcoma, fibrosarcoma, PNET, granulocytic sarcoma.

Nasopharyngeal mass

Congenital
- Encephalocele.

Inflammatory/infective
- Adenoids: enlargement is normal between 1–7yrs of age (📖 p. 470).
- Antrochoanal polyp.
- Acute or chronic enlargement ± suppuration of deep/retropharyngeal lymph nodes.

Neoplasia
- Nasal angiofibroma (📖 p. 482): usually adolescents.
- Lymphoma.
- Rhabdomyosarcoma (📖 p. 486).
- Neuroblastoma.
- Lymphoepithelioma.

Trauma
- Haematoma associated with skull base or upper cervical fracture.
- Foreign body.

Ocular mass

Mass within or involving the globe.

Congenital

- Persistent hyperplastic primary vitreous.
- Retinal dysplasia.

Infection

- Toxocariasis.

Neoplasia

- Retinoblastoma (📖 p. 484).
- Retinal astrocytoma: benign tumour associated with tuberous sclerosis (TS), neurofibromastosis type 1 (NF-1), retinitis pigmentosa.
- Choroidal melanoma.

Retinal detachment

- Chronic.
- Associated with Coat's disease.

Extra-ocular orbital mass

Within the muscle cone (intraconal)
- Vascular lesions: infantile haemangioma (📖 p. 480), venous or arterio-venous malformations (📖 p. 458).
- Inflammatory pseudotumour.
- Optic nerve glioma.
- Lymphoma.
- Metastases, e.g. neuroblastoma.
- Haematoma.

Arising from the muscle cone
- Inflammatory pseudotumour.
- Thyroid ophthalmopathy.
- Rhabdomyosarcoma (📖 p. 486).

Outside the muscle cone (extraconal)
- Lymphatic malformations (📖 p. 458).
- Orbital cellulitis and abscess (📖 p. 474).
- LCH.
- Dermoids and teratoma (📖 p. 450).
- Lymphoma.
- Metastases, e.g. neuroblastoma.
- Secondary involvement by tumours involving the paranasal sinuses.

Orbital calcification

Within the globe

- Cataract.
- Retinopathy of prematurity, may calcify in older children.
- Retinoblastoma (📖 p. 484).
- Vitreous calcification following trauma or infection.
- Retinal astrocytoma.
- Optic drusen: calcification on or near the surface of the optic disc.
- Scleral calcification in association with hypercalcaemia, e.g. hyperparathyroidism, chronic renal disease.

Outside the globe

- Phleboliths: in venous or arteriovenous malformations.
- In tumours: rarely seen in optic glioma and orbital teratomas.

Pre-vertebral soft tissue swelling/ retro-pharyngeal mass (on lateral neck radiograph)

Spurious or non-pathological
- Increased soft tissue width with neck flexion or in expiration can occur <2yrs of age. May contain air trapped in the pharyngeal recesses.
- Ear lobe superimposed on the pharyngeal region.

Inflammatory/infective
- Acute or chronic enlargement ± suppuration of deep/retropharyngeal lymph nodes.

Benign neoplasia and other lesions
- Haemangioma of infancy (📖 p. 480).
- Vascular or lymphatic malformations (📖 p. 458).
- Plexiform neurofibroma.

Malignancy
- Lymphoma.
- Rhabdomyosarcoma (📖 p. 486).
- Neuroblastoma.

Trauma
- Haematoma associated with skull base or cervical fracture.

Temporal bone mass

Inflammatory/infective
- Apical petrositis.

Vascular
- Aneurysm of the petrous segment of the internal carotid artery.

Neoplastic
- Rhabdomyosarcoma (📖 p. 486).
- Lymphoma.
- Metastases, e.g. neuroblastoma, sarcoma.
- Cholesteatoma (📖 p. 478):
  - Of the petrous apex.
  - Extension from middle ear.
- LCH.
- Glomus tumours.
- Meningioma.

Ear, nose and throat (ENT) and eye Disorders

Helen Williams

Branchial apparatus anomalies

The branchial (pharyngeal) apparatus structures develop between the 4th and 6th weeks of gestation, consisting of six pairs of mesodermal branchial arches, separated by five paired endodermal pharyngeal pouches internally and five paired ectodermal branchial clefts externally. Anomalies of normal branchial apparatus development are thought to arise from incomplete obliteration of the embryonic structures and may give rise to cysts, sinus tracts or fistulae. Their origin can be determined according to knowledge of the embryology and which structures are formed from the arches, pouches and clefts.

Table 7.2 Normal anatomic structures formed by the branchial apparatus

	Cleft	Arch	Pouch
1st	External auditory canal	Mandible, muscles of mastication, malleus, incus, auricle, mandibular division of trigeminal nerve	Eustachian tube, tympanic cavity, mastoid air cells
2nd	Rudimentary	Muscles of facial expression, body and lesser horn of hyoid, stapes, facial and vestibulocochlear nerves	Palatine tonsil
3rd	Rudimentary	Superior constrictor muscles, internal carotid artery, greater horn and body of hyoid, glossopharyngeal nerve	Inferior parathyroid glands, thymus, piriform sinus
4th	Rudimentary	Thyroid and cuneiform cartilage, aortic arch, right subclavian artery, laryngeal muscles, vagus nerve	Superior parathyroid glands, apex of piriform sinus
5th	Rudimentary	Rudimentary	Parafollicular cells of the thyroid gland
6th	–	Arytenoids and cricoid cartilages, vagus nerve	–

The majority of branchial apparatus anomalies are cysts which can arise from a branchial cleft, arch or pouch remnant—usually the 1st, 2nd or 3rd apparatus. The most common type of anomaly is the 2nd branchial cyst.

Clinical presentation

Depends on the type of anomaly. Cysts: neck or peri-parotid mass, may be recurrent, particularly with repeated infection. Sinuses and fistulae may discharge and become infected.

Table 7.3 Characteristics of the branchial apparatus anomalies

Branchial apparatus	Incidence	Type of branchial anomaly (BA)	Location
First	8%	Cysts or sinuses (sinuses are best evaluated with MRI)	Periauricular or periparotid location Anterior or posterior to pinna Superficial or embedded within parotid May extend inferior to angle of mandible
Second	Up to 95%	Mostly cysts	Posterolateral to submandibular gland Lateral to carotid space Anteromedial to sternocleidomastoid (SCM) Type I: Superficial lesions, deep to platysma, along anterior border of sternocleidomastiod (SCM) Type II (most common): deeper lesions abutting carotid sheath. Anterior to SCM, posterior to submandibular gland and lateral to carotid sheath Type III: protrude between internal and external carotid arteries, extending inward to lateral pharyngeal wall. Occasionally extend superiorly to skull base. Type IV: adjacent to pharyngeal wall, deep to the internal and external carotid arteries
Third	Rare	Fistulae, cysts or complex anomalies e.g. DiGeorge syndrome, coloboma, heart disease, atresia of nasal choana, mental or growth retardation, genital and ear abnormalities (CHARGE) association	Along course of the 3rd branchial cleft or pouch Upper neck: Posterior triangle behind SCM, posterior to common or internal carotid artery Mid-lower neck: along anterior border of SCM Rarely in submandibular space Thymic cysts: rare remnants of the 3rd branchial pouch. Can occur anywhere along course of embryologic thymopharyngeal duct from angle of mandible to upper mediastinum Found adjacent to/within carotid sheath May splay carotid artery and jugular vein May be continuous with mediastinal thymus
Fourth	Very rare	Usually a fistula extending from left piriform sinus to anterior lower neck/ thyroid	Cysts extremely rare, occur anywhere along this tract, most commonly adjacent to/within left thyroid lobe 4th BA cysts in the larynx may simulate laryngoceles

Imaging findings of 2nd branchial apparatus cysts

Ultrasound

- Unilocular, ovoid, anechoic or hypoechoic cystic mass.
- ± Posterior acoustic enhancement.
- Following infection, contents may be echogenic ± septation.

CT

- Well-defined, ovoid cystic mass.
- ± Enhancement of the cyst wall with/post-infection.
- ± Inflammatory changes in surrounding tissues with/post-infection.

MRI

- Signal intensity on T1-WI depends on protein content: ↑ protein content → ↑T1 signal.
- Hyperintense on T2-WI.
- ± Enhancement of the cyst wall with/post-infection.

Differential diagnosis

Lymphatic and vascular malformations, neck abscess, suppurative lymphadenitis, parotid lymphoepithelial cysts.

Management

Cysts, sinuses and fistulae: complete surgical resection.

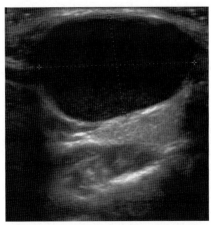

Fig. 7.1 Ultrasound of an uncomplicated second branchial cyst in a child: thin-walled, unilocular hypoechoic lesion with internal echoes/debris.

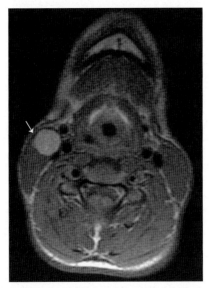

Fig. 7.2 T1-W MRI showing 2nd branchial cyst beneath anterior border of the right SCM muscle (arrow). The lesion has high signal due to proteinaceous content.

Congenital ear abnormalities

Congenital malformations of the ear constitute a large subject. Many congenital abnormalities of hearing are not associated with structural abnormalities of bone or soft tissue and therefore cannot be identified with imaging. CT and MRI are complimentary investigations and have an important role in the investigation of childhood deafness, as findings may influence management.

The temporal bone develops from two separate precursors, with development of the external and middle ear being independent of the development of the inner ear. The external and middle ear are formed from the pars branchialis originating from the 1st and 2nd branchial arches, 1st branchial groove and associated mesenchyme, whereas the inner ear develops from the pars otica arising from the auditory vesicle and adjacent mesenchyme. Because of their common embryology, significant malformations of the external ear are usually accompanied by middle ear deformities and vice versa. Inner ear abnormalities usually occur independently but nevertheless are more common in patients with other congenital ear abnormalities.

Choice of imaging modality

Radiographs
- Little role in the investigation of deafness.
- Role in assessing the electrode array of a cochlear implant: position and integrity.

CT
- Fine section, high-resolution scans optimally demonstrate temporal bone anatomy: inner and middle ear including the ossicles.
- Coronal +/− sagittal reconstructions essential.
- Soft tissue density in the middle ear cannot be reliably characterized, although may see indirect signs such as bony erosion to help determine aetiology.

MRI
- Investigation of choice for inner ear, cranial nerves and brain.
- Fine section, high resolution T2-W sequences, including 3D T2-W GRE sequences e.g. CISS, FIESTA.

▶ A sound knowledge of petrous temporal bone anatomy is essential for interpretation of imaging in congenital ear abnormalities.

External auditory canal abnormalities

The EAC may be partially or completely atretic with associated deformity (malformation/abnormal position) of the external ear (auricle). EAC stenosis usually extends from the opening to the tympanic membrane (TM), and the canal may be obliterated by bone, soft tissue or both. The EAC may also run in an abnormal direction. The TM may be present or absent. The most severe type has no identifiable EAC, absence of the tympanic bone and a bony plate where the TM is normally located, an 'atresia plate'. In affected patients the middle ear cavity and mastoid are hypoplastic with a dysplastic ossicular chain (particularly malleus and incus). In general, severity of auricular dysplasia correlates with severity of the middle ear deformity. Typically the inner ear structures are normal (90%). Usually a unilateral isolated abnormality, but may be familial or part of a craniofacial syndrome.

Clinical presentation

CHL, detectable physical abnormality. Unilateral atresia not usually treated if contralateral side is normal. Surgical reconstruction of EAC improves, but does not usually restore normal hearing. Surgical treatment of middle ear and ossicular deformities performed if possible, and may restore function to a variable degree. Dysplastic auricles are cosmetically reconstructed.

Middle ear deformities

Isolated abnormalities of the middle ear structures are much less common than those seen in association with abnormalities of the auricle and EAC. Congenital abnormalities of the middle ear include hypoplasia of the middle ear cleft which may be filled with mesenchymal tissue or contain thin bony septa.

Ossicular chain abnormalities are frequently associated, e.g. fusion of the neck of the malleus to an atresia plate, fusion of the incus and malleus, or hypoplasia/absence of the long process of the incus. Complete absence of the ossicles is unusual but absence of the stapes increases the difficulty of surgical reconstruction. Absence of the stapedius muscle or tendon may occur and the oval window may be small or atretic. The course of the facial nerve is frequently aberrant in conjunction with middle ear abnormalities, and this should be determined on imaging for pre-operative planning. Absence of the facial nerve is rare, but it may be hypoplastic. Congenital cholesteatoma of the middle ear is found in <10% of patients with middle ear deformities.

Concomitant inner ear abnormalities are rare, although the IAC may be abnormal in size or shape. Deficiency of the cochlear nerve is a surgical contraindication.

Clinical presentation

CHL. Surgical treatment/reconstruction of middle ear and ossicular deformities may improve hearing.

Inner ear deformities

Congenital abnormalities of the inner ear are diverse and have been variously classified over the years. Not all of the abnormalities detected on imaging fit neatly into a particular classification system but they are often associated with functional abnormality.

Labyrinthine aplasia: complete absence of inner ear structures (cochlea, vestibule and semicircular canals) which have failed to develop (old term Michel deformity). Very rare (<1% of all congenital ear abnormalities), with unknown aetiology. Spectrum of associated temporal bone findings: internal auditory canal (IAC) small to absent, petrous apex hypoplastic to absent, middle ear may be normal or abnormal ± ossicular fusion or absence.

Clinical presentation

SNHL from birth. Affected ear(s) will never hear, no treatment option.

Common cavity inner ear

Cochlea, vestibule and semicircular canals form common ovoid, feature-less cystic cavity of variable size. Very rare (<1% of all congenital ear abnormalities), with unknown aetiology. Semicircular canals usually absent, but may be dysplastic or normal. IAC is always abnormal and size reflects that of the common cystic cavity. Normal middle ear structures.

Clinical presentation

Usually SNHL from birth. Some patients are suitable for cochlear implantation (CI) (if bilateral abnormality), but this requires presence of a cochlear nerve.

Cochlea aplasia

Complete absence of the cochlea. Very rare (<1% of all congenital ear abnormalities). Usually associated with dysplastic (small or cystic/dilated) vestibule, semicircular canals and IAC, but they may be normal. Middle ear, EAC, vestibular aqueduct and endolymphatic duct normal.

Clinical presentation

SNHL from birth. Affected ear(s) will never hear, no treatment option.

Cystic cochleovestibular anomaly

Cystic, featureless cochlea and vestibule with figure eight configuration and no internal structures (absent cochlear turns and modiolus). Semicircular canals are abnormal and may be dilated. IAC may be dilated. Middle ear, EAC, vestibular aqueduct and endolymphatic duct normal.

Clinical presentation

SNHL from birth. Some patients may be suitable for CI.

Semicircular canal dysplasia

Malformation, hypoplasia or absence of one or more of the semicircular canals. Spectrum of abnormalities varying from dilated short lateral semicircular canal forming single cavity with the vestibule, to complete absence of all semicircular canals + small dysmorphic vestibule + oval window atresia ± cochlea abnormalities.

May be associated with labyrinthine aplasia, cochlea hypoplasia/dysplasia or common cavity abnormality, middle ear or mastoid abnormalities. Associations: CHARGE association, Allagile, Waardenburg, Crouzon and Apert syndromes.

Clinical presentation

Range of mild to profound SNHL when sporadic, CHL often present due to oval window atresia (mixed hearing loss). Syndromic types usually have profound SNHL. Some patients may be suitable for CI.

Large endolymphatic sac anomaly (LESA)

Large endolymphatic sac with variable cochlea dysplasia in >75%. Most common inner ear abnormality found with imaging. Enlarged endolymphatic sac is seen on T2-W MRI. AKA *Large vestibular aqueduct syndrome*

(LVAS), descriptive term for the CT findings in this condition (vestibular aqueduct diameter is >1.5mm in its mid-portion and larger than the posterior semicircular canal). Bilateral in >90%, associated vestibule or semicircular canal abnormalities in 50%. Cochlea is dysplastic with abnormal apical turn and deficiency of the modiolus. 'Mondini deformity' now an obsolete term with multiple alternative definitions. Associations: familial lesion with AR inheritance, Pendred syndrome.

Clinical presentation

Typically progressive SNHL with variable speed, most present <10yrs of age, often potentiated by trauma. CI used when bilateral profound SNHL develops.

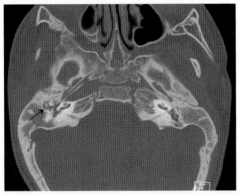

Fig. 7.3 Child with Goldenhar syndrome, complete atresia of the left EAC and right EAC stenosis. The middle ear cavity is hypoplastic bilaterally with no discernable cleft and absent ossicles on the left. Right middle ear cavity (arrow) is filled with soft tissue and the ossicles are dysplastic.

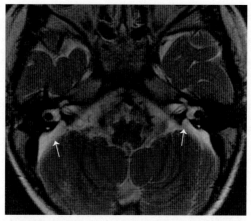

Fig. 7.4 Axial T2-W MRI of a child with bilateral SNHL showing bilateral enlargement of the endolymphatic sac and vestibular aqueduct (arrows). There is also bilateral mild cochlear dysplasia.

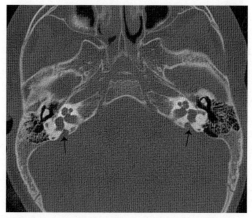

Fig. 7.5 Same patient as Fig. 7.4. Axial CT scan showing bilateral enlargement of the vestibular aqueduct and endolymphatic recesses (arrows).

Choanal atresia and stenosis

Choanal atresia is a congenital bony and/or membranous occlusion of the posterior nasal cavity at its junction with the nasopharynx, may be unilateral or bilateral. **Choanal stenosis** is narrowing without complete occlusion of the posterior nasal cavity, more common than choanal atresia.

Clinical presentation

Bilateral atresia presents at birth with severe respiratory distress (which is increased with feeding and temporarily decreased with crying), inability to pass NGT. Unilateral atresia/stenosis usually presents later in childhood, often with chronic unilateral nasal discharge ± mild nasal obstruction.

Associations: orofacial clefts, midline face/brain abnormalities. >50% patients with bilateral choanal atresia are syndromic (e.g. CHARGE, Crouzon, Di George or Treacher Collins syndrome), have chromosomal anomalies or other congenital abnormalities. Most unilateral atresias are sporadic.

▶ Bilateral choanal atresia is a surgical emergency.

Imaging findings

CT

▶ Nasal suction ± application of nasal decongestant drops recommended prior to CT scan.
- Funnel shaped, narrowed posterior nasal cavity.
- Choana <3.5mm diameter.
- Medial bowing of posterior maxilla.
- Thickened or 'split' posterior vomer ± fusion with maxilla.
- ± Bony or membranous occlusion of the choana.
- Nasal cavity filled with air, soft tissue or fluid.
- In unilateral disease nasal septum deviated towards affected side.
- ± Hypoplasia ipsilateral maxillary sinus.

Differential diagnosis

Piriform aperture stenosis, bilateral congenital dacrocystoceles, mid-face hypoplasia syndromes, e.g. Apert's, nasal cavity narrowing associated with prematurity, nasopharyngeal atresia, sphenoidal–ethmoidal encephalocele.

Management and prognosis

Bilateral choanal atresia/stenosis: establish oral airway without delay. Passage of NGT may relieve obstruction in membranous atresias. Surgical correction required for bony atresia and stenosis. Surgery performed in neonatal period for bilateral disease. Re-stenosis occurs in some patients.

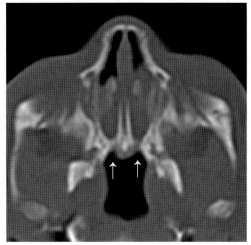

Fig. 7.6 Axial CT scan showing bilateral choanal atresia (arrows).

Dermoids and sinuses

Dermoid and epidermoid cysts are commonly located around the skull and midface. Pathogenesis uncertain, but believed to arise from persistence of ectodermal remnants at sites of suture closure, neural tube closure or diverticulation of the cerebral hemispheres during embryogenesis. Histological classification according to cell type in wall of the lesion: *epidermoid*—fibrous wall and squamous epithelium without skin appendages or connective tissue derivatives; *dermoid*—contains a variable number of skin appendages (hair, hair follicles and sebaceous glands etc.); *teratoma*—contains skin appendages and connective tissue derivatives (i.e. components of all three embryological germ layers). All types can contain proteinaceous material and therefore may appear cystic. If there is fat in the lesion the most likely diagnosis is a dermoid. Presence of fat and calcium is most suggestive of a teratoma.

Common locations of dermoids/epidermoids: orbital/peri-orbital, midline (AF, glabella, nasion, vertex, suboccipital) and frontotemporal>parietal locations. Frequently affected sutures: frontozygomatic, sphenofrontal, sphenosquamosal, squamosal, coronal, lambdoid and parietomastoid.

Nasal lesions (sinuses or cysts) occur in multiple locations from the glabella to columella. May be associated with external skin ostia or deep sinus tracts ± intracranial extension through a bony defect.

Clinical presentation

Firm, well-defined mass lesion, present from birth, typically do not change in size, but may enlarge slowly over time. Sudden enlargement following rupture. Nasal lesions may be associated with a broad nasal bridge and hypertelorism.

▶ MRI is the imaging modality of choice, particularly for midline lesions which may have intracranial extension.

Imaging findings

Radiographic signs

- Scalloped bony lucency with sclerotic margins.

Ultrasound

- Useful for simple, superficial lesions.
- Well-defined, avascular, thin-walled structure.
- May appear cystic or have variable echogenicity.

CT

- Thin-section focused CT best modality for demonstrating bony defects or scalloping, and calcification.
- Cysts have low attenuation, ± rim enhancement.
- Bifid/V-shaped crista galli or enlarged foramen cecum (of the frontal bone) seen with midline lesions that have intracranial extension.

MRI

- Cysts: well-defined, thin-walled structure, ± rim enhancement.
- Epidermoid: low/intermediate signal on T1-WI, high signal on T2-WI, restricted diffusion on DWI.

- Dermoid: intermediate/high signal on T1-WI (may contain fat), variable signal on T2-WI, variable signal on DWI.
- Bifid/V-shaped crista galli or enlarged foramen cecum (of the frontal bone) seen with midline lesions that have intracranial extension.
- Dermal sinus tracts: subcutaneous linear hypointensity on T1-WI, typically hyperintense on T2-WI (especially with fat-suppression).

Differential diagnosis

Midline lesions: congenital anterior encephalocele, nasal glioma, infantile haemangioma, hairy/teratoid polyp, fibroma, lipoma, lipoblastoma, malignant lesions, e.g. rhabdomyosarcoma. Other locations: vascular and lymphatic malformations, infantile haemangioma, dacrocystocele, branchial anomalies, lymph nodes, rhabdomyosarcoma.

Management and prognosis

Complete surgical excision.

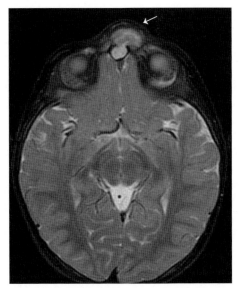

Fig. 7.7 Nasal dermoid: axial T2-W MRI with fat suppression showing a high signal soft tissue mass over the nasal bridge (arrow). The lesion extends into a bony defect in the skull vault but not intracranially.

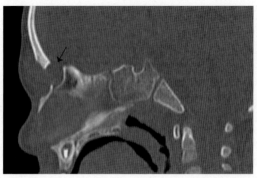

Fig. 7.8 CT scan (sagittal reconstruction) of the patient in Fig. 7.7 optimally demonstrates the midline bony defect (arrow).

Nasolacrimal duct dacrocystocele

Congenital dilatation of the nasolacrimal apparatus secondary to proximal and/or distal duct obstruction. AKA nasolacrimal duct mucocele. Most common abnormality of the nasolacrimal apparatus in infants, typically presenting from 4 days–10 weeks of age. Abnormalities in the normal embryological development of the nasolacrimal system may be responsible. Proximal obstruction → dilatation of nasolacrimal sac. Distal obstruction → dilatation of nasolacrimal sac and duct. Cystic expansion of the distal nasolacrimal duct creates cyst in inferior meatus or nasal airway. May cause airway obstruction, especially if bilateral. Most occur sporadically and are not associated with other congenital abnormalities, occasionally familial. Initial unilateral lesions may become bilateral.

Clinical presentation

- Proximal obstruction: typically small, round, bluish mass at medial canthus discovered shortly after birth.
- Distal obstruction: submucosal nasal cavity mass.
- Nasal obstruction: excessive tear production, inflammatory changes, preseptal oedema, abscess formation.

▶ Best imaging modality: thin section axial CT with coronal reconstructions for lesions not responding to initial management. Also excludes other causes of nasal obstruction.

Imaging findings

CT

- Well-defined, thin-walled, cystic medial canthus mass + enlarged bony nasolacrimal duct.
- ± Inferior meatal cyst: may displace inferior turbinate and/or nasal septum.
- Absent/minimal wall enhancement, unless infected.
- Infection → thick rim enhancement ± fluid-fluid levels.

MRI

- Thin-walled, cystic medial canthus mass.
- Hypointense on T1-WI, but may have ↑ signal with proteinaceous content or infection.
- Hyperintense on T2-WI.
- Absent/minimal wall enhancement, unless infected.
- Infection → thick rim enhancement ± fluid–fluid levels.

Differential diagnosis

Dermoid or epidermoid at medial canthus, naso-orbital encephalocele. Other causes of nasal obstruction in the neonatal period, e.g. choanal atresia, piriform aperture stenosis.

Management and prognosis

Conservative treatment initially with massage and antibiotics. Probing with irrigation or stent placement may be required or even endoscopic resection and marsupialization of the duct. Early intervention recommended to prevent infection and nasal obstruction. >90% of congenital distal obstructions resolve spontaneously by 1yr of age. Occasional recurrence in adulthood.

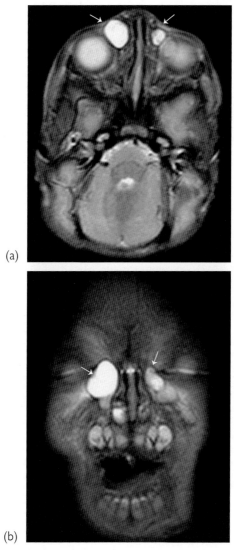

Fig. 7.9 (a) Axial and (b) coronal T2-W MRI showing bilateral dacrocystoceles (arrows) in a neonate, right side larger than left. The child also had cerebral and cardiac abnormalities.

Piriform aperture stenosis

Congenital stenosis of the anterior nasal cavity including the inlet (piriform aperture) with a patent nasal airway. Uncommon cause of upper airway obstruction in neonates. Aetiology: chromosomal abnormality in up to 50% (AD or AR, variable penetrance), teratogenic effects (maternal diabetes mellitus, alcoholism). May be associated with a single central maxillary incisor and other midline abnormalities such as holoprosencephaly and posterior pituitary ectopia.

Clinical presentation

Nasal obstruction in the neonatal period, breathing difficulty, apnoea, stridor or cyanosis, especially with feeding. Symptoms may be intermittent.

▶ MRI to identify midline cerebral abnormalities, and endocrine testing for pituitary function indicated in all patients with this diagnosis.

Imaging findings

CT
- Imaging modality of choice.
- Narrowed anterior nasal cavity:
  - Piriform aperture <8mm diameter, including nasal septum.
  - Single anterior nare width <2mm.
- ± Bony overgrowth of nasal process/medial maxilla.
- ± Hypoplastic triangular-shaped palate.
- ± Inferiorly projecting midline palatal bony ridge.
- ± Incisor abnormalities:
  - Partial fusion of both central upper incisors.
  - Single central, normal sized or mega-incisor.

MRI
- ± Holoprosencephaly.
- ± Posterior pituitary ectopia.
- ± Chiari I malformation.

Differential diagnosis

Choanal atresia or stenosis, mucosal oedema causing nasal obstruction, mid-face hypoplasia syndromes, e.g. Apert's, nasal cavity narrowing associated with prematurity.

Management and prognosis

Mild narrowing: conservative management with oxygen, nasal airway, continuous positive airway pressure (CPAP). Severe narrowing, failure of conservative management or life-threatening episodes: surgery to resect bone from inferior margin of the piriform aperture and relieve obstruction. Excellent prognosis following treatment in the absence of associated midline brain/pituitary abnormalities.

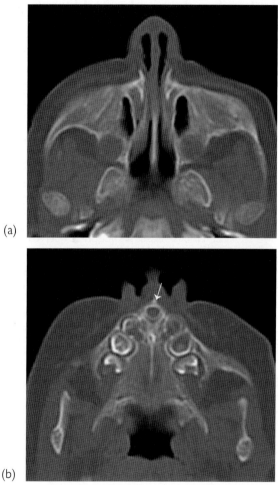

(a)

(b)

Fig. 7.10 (a) Axial CT scan showing piriform aperture stenosis in a neonate. This patient has the characteristic triangular-shaped palate and a single central incisor (b) – arrowed.

Head and neck vascular and lymphatic malformations (LM)

The head and neck are common sites for vascular malformations in children. The classification system devised by Mulliken and Glowacki based on clinical, histochemical and cellular criteria first divides vascular anomalies into two major groups: *haemangiomas* and *vascular malformations*.

Haemangiomas are true tumours consisting of rapidly dividing endothelial cells. Vascular malformations are congenital, non-proliferating anomalies, classified according to their vessel type (arteriovenous, venous, capillary, lymphatic and mixed types e.g. lymphatico–venous and capillary–lymphaticovenous) and haemodynamics (high-flow lesions and low-flow lesions). Vascular malformations can affect skin, other soft tissues or bone. They are present from birth, grow with the child and do not spontaneously involute. Some are detected antenatally, especially lymphatic malformations (LM). Venous malformations (VM) are low-flow vascular malformations, and any lesion with arterial components is classified as high-flow.

Embryologically, the lymphatic system arises from the vascular system, therefore LM are included as a subgroup of vascular malformations. Some authors separate LM into microcystic and macrocystic types according to pathologic, imaging or surgical findings which are based on the size of the cystic spaces. Microcystic LM may infiltrate the muscles and overlying skin producing tiny cutaneous vesicles but macrocystic lesions do not have cutaneous stigmata. The terms cystic hygroma and lymphangioma are obsolete.

LM are often part of a combined vascular malformation, frequently venous malformations, and are often referred to as venolymphatic or lymphaticovenous malformations (both low-flow). ↑ Incidence of LM with Turner's and Noonan's syndrome, Trisomies 21 (Down's syndrome), 13 (Patau's syndrome) and 18 (Edward's syndrome), other genetic disorders and structural abnormalities such as cardiac and neural tube defects.

▶ Head and neck vascular malformations may be complicated by haemorrhage or infection, airway, pharyngeal or oesophageal obstruction.

Clinical presentation

Depends on location and composition. Soft tissue mass: may be firm or fluctuant, overlying skin discolouration. Orbital lesions may cause proptosis. Rapid enlargement of LM can occur secondary to infection or haemorrhage within the lesion if it has vascular elements.

▶ Role of imaging: help characterise the lesion in conjunction with clinical assessment and determine extent. Best modalities: Ultrasound and MRI.

Imaging findings: LM and other low-flow lesions

Ultrasound
- Cystic, multiloculated mass.
- No evidence of high (arterial) flow on Doppler.

CT
- LM: low attenuation (cystic), trans-spatial, multiloculated mass.
- Mixed venous–lymphatic or VM may have solid components.

- ± Fluid–fluid levels/layered debris following infection or haemorrhage.
- Peripheral or heterogeneous enhancement with infection or vascular component.
- ± Adjacent bony remodelling.
- ±Phleboliths in venous malformations.

MRI
- LM: cystic, trans-spatial, multiloculated mass.
- VM: multiple serpiginous channels.
- Cystic components variable signal on T1-WI depending on protein or lipid content, haemorrhage or infection.
- Cystic and vascular components high signal on T2-WI.
- Microcystic LM, mixed venous–lymphatic or VM may have solid appearing components.
- ± Fluid–fluid levels/layered debris following infection or haemorrhage.
- Peripheral or heterogeneous enhancement with infection or vascular component.

Imaging findings: high-flow lesions

Ultrasound
- Cystic, solid or mixed lesion.
- Evidence of high (arterial) flow on Doppler.

CT
- Enhancing soft tissue mass with prominent vessels in and around the lesion.
- ↑Incidence of bony changes, e.g. remodelling, resorption, hypertrophy compared with low-flow lesions.

MRI
- Mass isointense to muscle on T1-WI, mildly hyperintense on T2-WI.
- Multiple vascular flow voids within and around the lesion.
- Enlarged draining veins.
- Intense contrast enhancement.
- ± Effects on adjacent bone.

Differential diagnosis
- Branchial apparatus anomalies.
- Infantile haemangioma.
- Teratoma.
- Plexiform neurofibroma.
- Rhabdomyosarcoma.

Management and prognosis
The need for treatment is dependent on multiple factors including cosmetic appearance, associated complications and type of malformation. Low-flow lesions in the head and neck are treated with percutaneous sclerosis ± surgical excision. Aspirin may be used to prevent thrombosis in VM. High-flow lesions are treated with transarterial embolization.

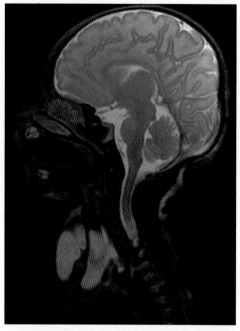

Fig. 7.11 Sagittal T2-W MRI with fat suppression of a neonate with an asymptom-atic midline lymphatic malformation in the suprasternal neck, extending into the upper mediastinum. The lesion is multiloculated with fluid signal intensity and was detected on antenatal ultrasound.

Tracheomalacia

Abnormal flaccidity of the supporting tracheal cartilage leading to collapse of the tracheal walls with associated airway narrowing. Usually a benign condition. Types of tracheomalacia: primary congenital intrinsic abnormality of the airway, or acquired secondary to abnormal extrinsic compression on the airway (e.g. vascular ring) or prolonged intubation (e.g. premature infants). Abnormality may be focal or diffuse. May be accompanied by laryngomalacia or bronchomalacia. Associated with genetic disorders or syndromes, other congenital abnormalities, e.g. CHD, OA.

Clinical presentation

Primary tracheomalacia or congenital lesions causing airway compression usually present in the neonatal period with expiratory stridor (crowing sound), which is worse in the supine position and with crying or feeding. Other symptoms: chronic cough or feeding difficulties, GOR.

▶ The normal trachea has parallel walls on all types of imaging.

Imaging findings

Radiographic signs

- Narrowing or compression of the trachea.
- ± Mass or vascular lesion causing abnormal mediastinal contour.

Fluoroscopy

- Dynamic imaging may show abnormal collapse of the trachea, >50% reduction of inspiratory AP diameter in expiration.
- Upper GI contrast study: may show indirect signs of vascular ring or detect GOR.
- Catheter angiography: may be used to define vascular ring anatomy.

CT

- Demonstrates tracheal narrowing.
- ± vascular anomalies or masses causing tracheomalacia.

MRI

- Demonstrates vascular anomalies and masses causing tracheomalacia.

▶ Sedation for MRI (or CT) is contraindicated if there is significant airway compromise.

Differential diagnosis

Laryngomalacia (alone), normal collapse of the trachea in expiration (<50% of inspiratory AP diameter in expiration), congenital tracheal stenosis (complete tracheal rings), foreign body, acute or chronic tracheal inflammation: by viral or bacterial infections, relapsing polychondritis, chronic granulomatous disease, Wegener's granulomatosis etc.

Management and prognosis

Treatment and prognosis depend on aetiology. Many children with primary disease improve by 1yr of age as tracheal cartilage matures. Conservative management: humidification of inspired air, care with feeding, control of infections. Surgery required to correct any underlying cause, e.g. vascular ring or mass. Tracheostomy occasionally required for failure of conservative management or severe disease. Surgical aortopexy widens the AP diameter of the trachea. Tracheal stenting and resection of affected segments are options but results variable.

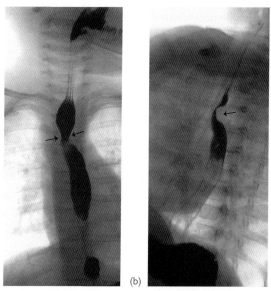

(a)   (b)

Fig. 7.12 (a) AP and (b) lateral images from a contrast swallow in a child with expiratory stridor since birth due to tracheomalacia caused by a double aortic arch. There is bilateral impression on the contrast filled upper oesophagus in AP projection (arrows), and a prominent posterior indentation in lateral projection (arrow).

Thyroglossal duct cyst (TGDC)

Most common cystic neck mass, accounting for 70–90% of all congenital neck masses in children. TGDC lie along the course of the thyroglossal duct, a normal fetal structure extending from the foramen cecum in the base of the tongue to the thyroid bed in the suprasternal lower neck. The tract normally involutes during the 5th–6th week of gestation, but persistent remnants of secretory epithelium may form a cyst. TGDC are often classified according to their position in relation to the hyoid bone, as suprahyoid (20–25%), infrahyoid (25–65%) or level with the hyoid bone (15–59%). Infrahyoid lesions are usually embedded within the strap muscles. Rarely TGDC may contain the only thyroid tissue with absence of a normal thyroid gland in the lower neck.

Clinical presentation

Small (<4cm), well-defined, non-tender, round or ovoid midline mass that moves upwards on protrusion of the tongue. In young children this sign may not be elicited. Infrahyoid lesions may be slightly off midline (para-median). Rarely TGDC are found in the base of the tongue and may present with tongue swelling following infection.

Complications: infection; malignancy (<1%), usually papillary carcinoma. Most present in adulthood but reported in children as young as 6yrs of age. Malignancy usually incidental finding on histological examination of excised specimen, but rarely can be identified as a solid mass within TGDC on pre-operative imaging.

Imaging findings

Ultrasound

- Variable sonographic appearance, even in the absence of infection.
- Anechoic, hypoechoic, pseudosolid (echogenic) or heterogeneous.
- Thin or thick-walled (especially if inflamed).
- ± posterior acoustic enhancement.
- ± internal septation.
- Tract extending to the hyoid bone may be identified.

▶ Important role of ultrasound: identification of a normal thyroid gland pre-operatively.

CT

- Low attenuation (cystic), well-defined, midline mass.
- Occasional septation.
- Peripheral enhancement with infection.
- Associated carcinoma may have eccentric solid mass ± calcification.

MRI

- Cyst usually hypointense on T1-WI, proteinaceous contents may be hyperintense.
- Hyperintense on T2-WI.
- Rim enhancement if infected.

Differential diagnosis

Lingual or sublingual thyroid, necrotic midline lymph node, dermoid or epidermoid, submandibular/sublingual space abscess, laryngocele.

Management and prognosis

Sistrunk procedure: cyst, entire tract and central portion of the hyoid bone are surgically excised. Recurrence rate is <4% thereafter.

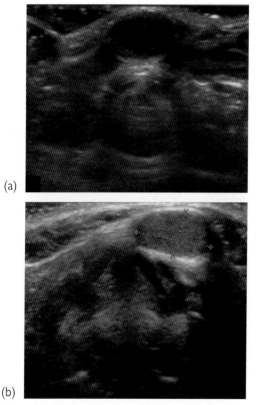

(a)

(b)

Fig. 7.13 Two examples of infrahyoid thyroglossal duct cysts on US. (a) Shows a hypoechoic, midline lesion whereas in (b) the lesion is hyperechoic and para-median (left sided).

Acute suppurative lymphadenitis

Common condition in young children. Lymph node involvement is usually secondary to bacterial URTI/oropharyngeal infection with seeding of draining lymph nodes which can → fluctuant abscess or spreading cellulitis. *Staph. Aureus.* or group A beta-haemolytic streptococci usual causative organisms. Anaerobic oral organisms and viral infection can also cause lymphadenitis. Viral infection less likely to suppurate and more often self-limiting.

Clinical presentation

Rapid unilateral enlargement of cervical lymph nodes, with warmth, erythema and tenderness, irritability, malaise and pyrexia. Associated with ↑ WCC and inflammatory markers. Typically occurs following a URTI, pharyngitis, tonsillitis or otitis media.

Imaging findings

Ultrasound

- Differentiates simple lymphadenopathy from confluent/suppurating nodes.
- Inflammatory nodes:
  - Discrete, round to oval masses.
  - ↑Flow on colour Doppler.
  - May enlarge and become confluent.
- Confluent nodal mass:
  - Mixed echogenicity mass.
  - ↑Flow on colour Doppler.
- Lymph node abscess formation:
  - Hypoechoic central part of the node/nodal mass.
  - ↓Flow centrally with ↑ peripheral vascularity on colour Doppler.

❶ Thick, echogenic fluid in abscesses can appear solid therefore abscess may be missed on ultrasound.

CT

- Thick, enhancing node wall with central low attenuation.
- Inflammatory mass with central low attenuation.
- Subcutaneous oedema and surrounding inflammatory changes.

MRI

- Central low signal intensity of nodes or mass on T1-WI.
- Diffuse or central high signal intensity on T2-WI (especially with fat suppression).
- Abscesses show marked peripheral enhancement.

Differential diagnosis

- Infected branchial apparatus abnormalities.
- TB and non-TB mycobacterial adenitis.
- Necrotic metastatic nodes.

Management and prognosis

Intravenous antibiotics for small suppurative nodes and to treat primary infection. Larger abscesses usually require incision and drainage.

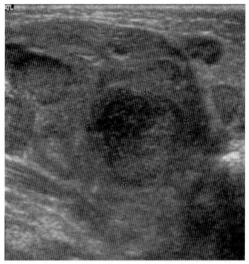

Fig. 7.14 Transverse ultrasound of an inflammatory lymph node mass in the neck with areas of suppuration/necrosis (marked by calipers).

Deep cervical infection and retropharyngeal abscess

Pyogenic nasopharyngeal and tonsil infection may involve the retropharyngeal lymph nodes which can suppurate and perforate into the parapharyngeal or retropharyngeal spaces. Bacterial lymphadenitis commonly involves the retropharyngeal space in children aged 1–5yrs and there may not be a visible or palpable cervical mass to suggest the diagnosis. Typical age 6–12mths. In most cases adenopathy extends from the neck into the retropharyngeal space → suppuration of involved nodes → abscess formation. However, cellulitis is more common than discrete abscess.

Clinical presentation

Pharyngeal pain, drooling, dysphagia, neck stiffness ± torticollis following a URTI are highly suspicious especially if the child appears toxic. Stridor or shortness of breath occurs if airway compromised.

Complications: airway compromise, septic shock, cervical fasciitis, mediastinal extension, jugular thrombosis, involvement of the carotid sheath can → arterial erosion or spasm with risk of stroke. Grisel's syndrome (Atlanto-axial subluxation secondary to ligamentous laxity following a cervical inflammatory process).

▶ Enhanced CT or MRI required to assess extent of infection, abscess formation and involvement of the carotid sheath.

Imaging findings

Radiographic signs

- Pre-vertebral soft tissue thickening ± gas.
- Loss of cervical lordosis.
- Airway displacement ± narrowing.

❶ Radiography is not imaging modality of choice and can be misleading.

CT

- Thickened retropharyngeal soft tissues ± inflamed palatine tonsil.
- Drainable collections of pus are fluid attenuation, ± enhancing rim.

MRI

- Diffuse thickening of retropharyngeal soft tissues.
- Affected tissues low signal on T1-WI, high signal on T2-WI (especially with fat suppression).
- Abscesses: central low signal intensity on T1-WI with marked peripheral enhancement post contrast.

Differential diagnosis

- Vascular or lymphatic malformations affecting the retropharyngeal space.
- TB and non-TB mycobacterial adenitis.
- Croup.
- Exudative tracheitis.
- Epiglottitis.

Management

▶ The airway is the first treatment priority, affected patients may require intubation. Particularly important if imaging under sedation required.

Intravenous antibiotics, aspiration or surgical drainage of pus collections.

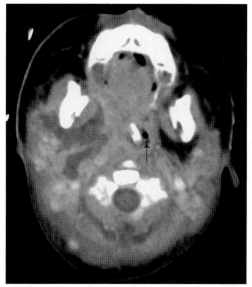

Fig. 7.15 Enhanced CT scan of a child with extensive deep abscess formation, affecting multiple fascial compartments including the right parapharyngeal, masticator and parotid spaces. Abscess extends to the carotid space but the right carotid and internal jugular are patent and of normal calibre. The airway is severely narrowed (arrow).

Enlarged tonsils and adenoids

Enlargement of the pharyngeal (palatine and adenoid) tonsils may cause medical problems either due to their effect on the airway or adjacent structures, and can act as a focus for infection. ↑Incidence in children with Down's syndrome. Rarely enlargement of the lingual tonsils may contribute to airway problems/obstructive sleep apnoea.

Adenoids vary in size with age; rarely visible on radiographs <6mths of age, proliferate rapidly in infancy and are largest between 2–10yrs of age. They gradually decrease in size from 10yrs onwards. Palatine tonsils assessed by direct visualization, size variable.

Clinical presentation

Nasal obstruction, obstructive sleep apnoea, recurrent otitis media (2° to obstruction of the eustachian tube), recurrent URTI or pharyngitis.

▶ Lateral soft tissue neck radiograph useful to confirm adenoidal enlargement and effect on the nasopharyngeal airway.

Imaging findings

Radiographic signs

- Convex soft tissue in the posterior nasopharynx.
- Variable encroachment on nasopharyngeal airway.
- Upper limit of normal adenoid size: 12mm AP diameter.
- Enlarged palatine tonsils may be identified as lobulated soft tissue densities posterior to the tongue/overlying soft palate.

MRI

- Palatine tonsils and adenoids high signal on T2-WI (especially with fat suppression).
- Lingual tonsils: masses at tongue base, high signal on T2-WI.
- Cine MRI may be used to evaluate obstructive sleep apnoea.

Differential diagnosis

Enlargement of tonsils due to lymphoma, glossoptosis, hypopharyngeal collapse associated with neuromuscular disorders.

Management and prognosis

Palatine tonsillectomy ± adenoidectomy. Indications based on clinical criteria rather than imaging findings. Recurrence of enlarged adenoids is common following surgery, although palatine tonsils tend not to recur.

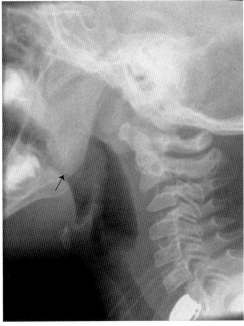

Fig. 7.16 Lateral soft tissue radiograph of a 2-year-old with nasal obstruction and frequent episodes of URTI. There is narrowing of the nasopharyngeal airway due to adenoidal enlargement and the palatine tonsils are also enlarged (arrow).

Mastoiditis

Mastoiditis develops when middle ear inflammation spreads to the mastoid air cells, resulting in infection and destruction of the mastoid bone. Occurs in all age groups including adults, but highest incidence in young children, peak age 6–13mths. Antibiotic treatment of acute or complicated otitis media has decreased the incidence of acute mastoiditis. Latent, or masked mastoiditis, refers to chronic disease which can be sub-clinical, often secondary to partial antibiotic treatment of acute otitis media.

Clinical presentation

- Acute mastoiditis: fever, otalgia and pain behind the ear, sometimes accompanied by a tender mass, history of concurrent or recent episode of acute otitis media. Typically associated with ↑ WCC and inflammatory markers.
- Latent mastoiditis: recurrent or persistent fever, pain or non-specific symptoms (especially infants), e.g. poor feeding, irritability, ± external signs of mastoid inflammation, often history of recurrent/chronic otitis media.
- Cranial nerve involvement possible with advanced disease: abducens (VI) or facial (VII) nerve palsy, pain from involvement of the ophthalmic branch of the trigeminal nerve.

Complications: meningitis, subdural empyema, epidural abscess, sigmoid or lateral sinus thrombosis, subperiosteal or soft tissue abscess formation (Bezold's abscess is beneath SCM muscle), cranial vault osteomyelitis, petrous apicitis, labyrinthitis, hearing loss, cranial nerve palsy, carotid artery spasm or arteritis.

▶ Early contrast-enhanced temporal bone CT advised in children with suspected acute mastoiditis, particularly if unresponsive to treatment.

Imaging findings

CT

- Opacification of mastoid air cells + eroded bony trabeculae (coalescence of air cells).
- Evidence of middle ear infection, e.g. fluid opacification, indrawn or perforated TM.
- Soft tissue oedema overlying mastoid process.
- ± Cortical erosion and subperiosteal abscess.
- ± Cortical erosion and soft tissue abscess.
- ± Evidence of petrous apicitis, e.g. opacification, coalescence of air cells, cortical erosion of petrous apex.
- ± Intracranial complications, e.g. subdural/epidural abscess, sigmoid or lateral sinus thrombosis.

MRI

- Low signal on T1-WI and high signal on T2-WI in mastoid air cells.
- Rim enhancement of abscesses and granulation tissue in mastoid air cells.
- Recommended for evaluation of intracranial complications detected on CT.

Differential diagnosis

LCH, rhabdomyosarcoma, involvement with cholesteatoma, lymphoma, metastatic disease.

Management and prognosis

IV antibiotics ± tympanocentesis and tympanostomy tube placement, cortical mastoidectomy, incision and drainage of abscesses, management of intracranial complications. Prognosis excellent with prompt medical and surgical treatment. Morbidity and mortality increase with intra- or extracranial complications.

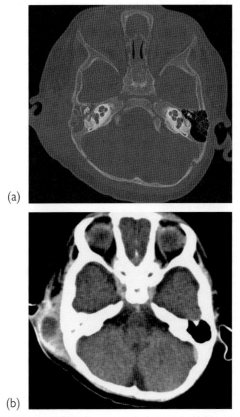

(a)

(b)

Fig. 7.17 (a) Enhanced CT scan (bone window) of a 5-month-old child with right-sided mastoiditis. There is opacification of the middle ear cleft, and mastoid air cells which are coalescent. There is also cortical erosion, with an abscess beneath the sternocleidomastoid muscle seen best on soft tissue window (b).

Orbital cellulitis

Soft tissue bacterial infection of the orbital contents frequently secondary to sinus infection, particularly ethmoiditis. Either direct spread or via venous system. All ages affected, most children are <4yrs. Common organisms <10yrs: single aerobic bacterial infection, e.g. *Strep. pneumoniae, Haemophilus influenzae, Staphylococci*; over 10yrs typically mixed organisms.

Preseptal cellulitis/peri-orbital cellulitis: inflammation anterior to orbital septum (periosteal reflection from bony orbit to tarsal plates of eyelids). Postseptal cellulitis: inflammation posterior to the orbital septum. Intraconal: within the cone formed by the extra-ocular muscles, extraconal: outside the muscle cone.

Clinical presentation

Depends on extent of infection: typically peri-orbital swelling, redness and tenderness, difficulty opening the eye, proptosis, ↓eye movements, diplopia (2° to ophthalmoplegia), ↓visual acuity.

Complications: optic neuritis or nerve ischaemia + visual loss, osteomyelitis. Intracranial complications, e.g. cavernous sinus thrombosis, meningitis, cerebritis, subdural or epidural empyema, brain abscess.

▶ Imaging modality of choice is contrast-enhanced axial CT with coronal reconstructions in patients with visual impairment or ↓ eye movements, or if peri-orbital oedema prevents adequate assessment of the eye.

Imaging findings

CT

- Peri-orbital oedema.
- Oedema and thickening of orbital soft tissues = cellulitis or phlegmon.
- ± Extra-ocular muscle swelling ± abnormal enhancement.
- ± Subperiosteal abscess.

❶ Subperiosteal abscess in the superior orbit may be missed on axial images, therefore coronal reconstructions/direct coronal scan essential.

MRI

- Best modality for evaluating intracranial complications.
- Poor at detecting bony orbital changes and intra-orbital air.

Differential diagnosis

- Orbital pseudotumour.
- Extra-ocular eye muscle myositis.
- Rhabdomyosarcoma.

Management and prognosis

IV antibiotics. Subperiosteal abscesses may need drainage but many respond to antibiotics, management of intracranial complications. Prognosis good with prompt medical and surgical treatment. Rare cause of blindness if untreated. Morbidity and mortality increase with intracranial complications.

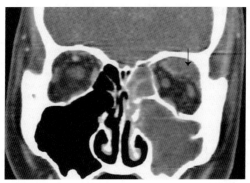

Fig. 7.18 Enhanced CT scan (coronal reconstruction) showing a left-sided superior (extraconal) subperiosteal collection (arrow) in a patient with post-septal orbital cellulitis.

Fibromatosis colli

AKA sternocleidomastoid tumour of infancy, congenital muscular torti-collis or sternomastoid pseudotumour. Only occurs in infants, most pre-senting between 2–8 weeks of age, but the process may begin prior to birth. Exact aetiology unknown, but may be related to birth trauma with haematoma formation and healing by fibrosis. History of difficult birth or an instrumental delivery frequently associated. Also associated with devel-opmental dysplasia of the hip (DDH) and tibial torsion, therefore may be related to uterine positioning.

Clinical presentation

Painless, palpable 'tumour' or mass within the SCM muscle, usually middle or lower third. Mass consists of fibrosis, collagen and fibroblasts around atrophied muscle. The SCM muscle becomes shortened as a result of these changes → torticollis in up to 20% of cases.

Complications: rare if treatment initiated without delay. Ipsilateral facial hypoplasia with skull base moulding, disturbance of visual development can occur due to persistent head tilt.

▶ Ultrasound is the imaging modality of choice.

Imaging findings

Ultrasound
- Typically 1–3cm length area of thickening or 'mass'.
- Affected SCM shorter and thicker than the contralateral muscle.
- Altered echotexture of SCM muscle: hypoechoic, echogenic or mixed echogenicity.
- May have ↑flow on colour Doppler in acute phase.
- No extension outside body of SCM.
- No calcification, lymphadenopathy or oedema.

CT
- Non-enhancing focal thickening of affected SCM muscle.

MRI
- Fusiform enlargement and shortening of affected SCM muscle.
- Variable signal intensity on T1 and T2-WI.
- Heterogeneous enhancement.

Differential diagnosis

Cervical lymphadenopathy, branchial apparatus abnormalities, congenital neuroblastoma, rhabdomyosarcoma, cervical teratoma, infantile desmoid tumour, spinal segmentation or fusion abnormalities causing torticollis.

Management and prognosis

Conservative treatment with physiotherapy motion and stretching exer-cises which force the infant to look to the opposite side. Improvement usually seen over 4–8mths. 90% full recovery with conservative treatment. Surgery to divide and/or release the SCM muscle is indicated for refrac-tory torticollis or persistent facial asymmetry >1yr of age.

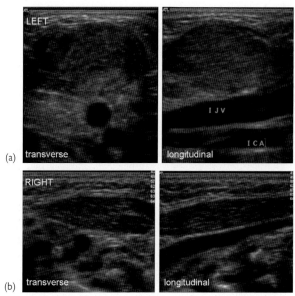

Fig. 7.19 (a) Left-sided fibromatosis colli. The left SCM muscle is diffusely enlarged and echogenic compared with the normal right side (b).

Cholesteatoma

Benign, expanding, locally aggressive lesion consisting of squamous epithelial cells and keratin trapped within the skull base (temporal bone, middle ear or mastoid). May be congenital (2–5% of total) or acquired. Erode bone through remodelling and osteolytic enzyme activity at the margin of the lesion which can ↑ with infection. Congenital lesions typically present from 6 months–5 years, located in the anterior mesotympanum/peri-eustachian tube area. Primary acquired cholesteatoma arise 2° to tympanic membrane retraction, typically from a progressively deeper medial retraction of the pars flaccida into the epitympanum. Secondary acquired cholesteatoma occur as a direct consequence of injury to the tympanic membrane, e.g. perforation 2° to acute otitis media or trauma, or post-surgical, e.g. insertion of tympanostomy tube. Middle ear most common site. Other sites: petrous apex, cerebellopontine angle, mastoid, EAC, geniculate ganglion.

Clinical presentation

Congenital lesions: avascular middle ear mass, unilateral CHL, middle ear effusion ± infection 2° to obstruction of eustachian tube. Acquired lesions: painless ear discharge, CHL, recurrent/chronic middle ear infection, foul-smelling ear discharge, vertigo, otalgia, facial nerve paralysis.

Complications: destruction of adjacent structures, e.g. ossicles, semicircular canals, facial nerve canal, tegmen tympani (with intracranial extension); facial nerve involvement, venous sinus thrombosis.

▶ Best imaging tool: unenhanced temporal bone CT, axial + coronal reconstructions.

Imaging findings

CT

- Variable size middle ear soft issue mass/opacification.
- No enhancement, but adjacent granulation tissue may enhance.
- ± Bone erosion: ossicles, scutum, middle ear wall, lateral semicircular canal, tegmen tympani, mastoid.
- Long process of incus and stapes most commonly affected.
- ± Opacification of mastoid.

MRI

- Middle ear mass, mildly hypointense on T1-WI, mildly hyperintense on T2-WI.
- No enhancement of mass, but adjacent granulation tissue or scar may enhance.
- ± Dural enhancement adjacent to defect in tegmen tympani.
- Useful for evaluation of intracranial extension or complications.

▶ Opacification of middle ear and mastoid may be due to cholesteatoma or effusion. Ossicular erosion makes cholesteatoma more likely but can occur with chronic middle ear infection.

Differential diagnosis

- For congenital lesions:
  - Acquired cholesteatoma.
  - Rhabdomyosarcoma.
  - Dehiscent jugular bulb.
  - Facial nerve schwannoma.
- For acquired lesions:
  - Congenital cholesteatoma.
  - Chronic otitis media with ossicular erosion.
  - Mastoiditis.
  - LCH.
  - Rhabdomyosarcoma.

Management and prognosis

Surgical excision ± reconstruction of ossicular chain. Prognosis depends on size and location. Smaller anterior lesions have better outcome, large lesions or lesions in posterior epitympanum or sinus tympani have up to 20% recurrence rate.

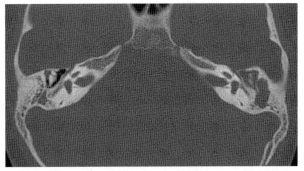

Fig. 7.20 CT of left-sided cholesteatoma. There is opacification of the entire middle ear cleft with erosion of the incus (the long process of the incus was absent, and the malleus and stapes also eroded).

Juvenile nasal angiofibroma

Rare benign, vascular, locally aggressive tumour of the nasal cavity found almost exclusively in adolescent males, but reported into third decade. Tumour centred at margin of the sphenopalatine foramen on lateral nasopharyngeal wall and spreads into the nasopharynx causing obstruction. Aetiology unknown but 25 x ↑ incidence in patients with familial adenomatous polyposis. Tumour consists of angiomatous tissue in fibrous stroma. 75% of tumours have androgen receptors.

Clinical presentation

Unilateral nasal obstruction, epistaxis, cheek pain or swelling, proptosis, anosmia, otitis media.

Imaging findings

CT

- Avidly enhancing soft tissue mass centred at sphenopalatine foramen.
- Enlargement of nasal cavity.
- Mass extends posteriorly into nasopharynx, laterally into pterygopalatine fossa, large tumours may extend into middle cranial fossa.
- Erosion or destruction of pterygoid plates.
- Displacement or destruction of maxillary sinus posterior wall.
- Enlarged feeding vessels from ECA or ICA.

MRI

- Generally isointense to muscle on T1-WI.
- Heterogeneous signal on T2-WI.
- Prominent vascular flow voids.
- Intense enhancement.
- MRA can identify vascular supply.

▶ All suspected juvenile nasopharyngeal angiofibroma should be evaluated with MRI (enhanced) + catheter angiography for surgical planning and embolization. CT best modality for assessment of bony erosion/destruction.

Differential diagnosis

- Hypervascular nasal or antrochoanal polyp.
- Lymphoma.
- Rhabdomyosarcoma.
- Germ cell tumour.
- Nasopharyngeal carcinoma.
- Fibrous dysplasia.

Management and prognosis

Surgical resection following pre-operative embolization to limit haemorrhage during surgery. Radiotherapy alone achieves up to 80% cure, also used as adjuvant treatment for unresectable lesions. Anti-androgen therapy can reduce tumour volume but generally not used in this age group. Very rarely tumours spontaneously regress. Up to 25% local recurrence following surgery.

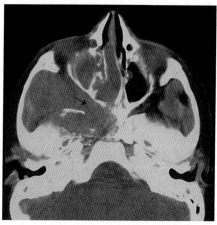

Fig. 7.21 CT scan of juvenile nasal angiofibroma in an 11-year-old boy who pre-sented with unilateral nasal obstruction. There is a large right-sided soft tissue mass centred on the sphenopalatine foramen. The mass fills and expands the right nasal cavity, and extends into the maxillary sinus, pterygopalatine fossa (which is enlarged—arrow) and right middle cranial fossa. There is associated bony erosion.

Infantile haemangioma

Benign vascular neoplasm consisting of proliferating endothelial cells: not a vascular malformation. 60% of all haemangiomas occur in the head and neck and they are the most common head and neck tumour of infancy, occurring in ~1–2% of neonates, ♀>♂ (2.5:1). Characteristic presentation in the first year of life (often shortly after birth), followed by rapid growth/proliferation to a variable size. After stabilization they enter a period of spontaneous involution with fatty replacement. A small sub-group of haemangiomas that present in the neonatal period undergo more rapid and complete involution than those occurring in infancy.

Haemangiomas in the head and neck can be single or multiple, and involve any fascial space, either superficial or deep. Most are single, superficial lesions. Haemangiomas of the parotid space are frequently bilateral and symmetrical. Multiple haemangiomas of the head and neck rarely associated with other abnormalities, the PHACES syndrome (posterior fossa and supratentorial brain malformations, haemangiomas, arterial stenosis, occlusion and aneurysm, cardiovascular and eye abnormalities, supraumbilical raphe and sternal clefts).

Clinical presentation

Proliferating lesions: enlarging, warm, red or 'strawberry-like', soft tissue mass. Deep lesions may have overlying bluish skin discolouration due to prominent draining veins. Rarely the skin may ulcerate. Orbital haemangiomas may present with proptosis. Deep lesions can encroach on the airway.

▶ Routine imaging is not required for most head and neck haemangiomas. It may be required if the diagnosis is in doubt, to determine the relationship to vital structures such as the airway, or assess response to treatment.

Imaging findings

Ultrasound

- Soft tissue mass (often echogenic) with prominent vessels.
- High flow on colour Doppler.
- Arterial and venous waveforms.

CT

- Soft tissue mass with diffuse, prominent enhancement in proliferative phase.
- Prominent vessels in and around the lesion in proliferative phase.
- Fatty infiltration in involuting phase.

MRI

- Mass isointense to muscle on T1-WI, mildly hyperintense on T2-WI.
- Vascular flow voids within and around the lesion.
- Intense contrast enhancement.
- Fat within lesion in involuting phase.

Differential diagnosis

- Arteriovenous or venous malformation.
- Rhabdomyosarcoma.
- Plexiform neurofibroma.

Management and prognosis

The majority of haemangiomas require no treatment, just observation and expectant waiting. Treatment is indicated for 'endangering' lesions that compromise vital structures such as the airway or optic nerve, compromise visual development or are associated with consumptive coagulopathy. Significant skin ulceration is also an indication for treatment. Medical management: steroids (systemic or intralesional), vincristine, α-interferon ± transcatheter embolization, laser treatment, rarely surgical excision.

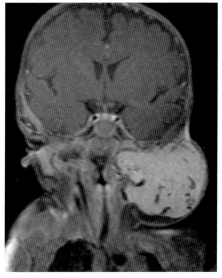

Fig. 7.22 Large, proliferating left-sided parotid haemangioma in a neonate. Coronal T1-weighted MRI, post contrast with fat suppression. The mass enhances intensely and contains multiple vascular (arterial) flow voids.

Retinoblastoma

Congenital malignant primary neoplasm arising from neuroectodermal cells of the retina. Incidence 1 in 15 000 live births. Most common intra-ocular tumour of childhood. Not usually apparent at birth. Average age at diagnosis 13mths, 90–95% diagnosed by 5yrs of age. Disease may be unilateral, bilateral, trilateral (bilateral ocular tumours + pineal or supra-sellar tumour), or quadrilateral (affecting all four sites). Leptomeningeal or haematogenous metastases rare.

Aetiology: *RB1* gene on chromosome 13 at q14 locus codes for pRB tumour-suppressor protein. Lack of both RB1 alleles → development of tumour. 60% cases sporadic, non-familial form; 40% familial hereditary form (AD) with germ line mutations or deletion of RB1 gene and spontaneous mutation of other copy. AD form responsible for all bilateral cases and multilateral disease + ~15% of unilateral disease. Slight ↑ risk in patients with Down's syndrome.

Clinical presentation

Leukokoria in 60%; squint, visual loss, inflammatory signs. Less common: anisocoria (unequal pupil sizes), heterochromia (difference in iris colour), epiphoria (watering eyes), nystagmus, glaucoma, proptosis. Screening allows earlier diagnosis in patients with ↑ risk.

▶ Children with the heritable form of retinoblastoma have ↑ risk of developing second tumours (especially after radiotherapy), e.g. osteosarcoma, soft tissue tumours, melanoma. Tumours may occur within or outside radiation field.

Imaging findings

CT
- Best modality for identification of calcification.
- Intraocular enhancing calcified retinal mass.
- ± Retinal detachment.

MRI
- Best modality for identifying extraocular extension along optic nerve and CNS disease.
- Variable intensity on T1-WI.
- Hypointense relative to vitreous on T2-WI.
- Moderate to marked enhancement.
- ± Retinal detachment.

Differential diagnosis
- Persistent hyperplastic primary vitreous.
- Retinopathy of prematurity.
- Coat's disease.
- Chronic retinal detachment.
- Toxocariasis.
- Retinal astrocytoma.
- Retinal dysplasia.
- Other causes of leukokoria.

Management and prognosis

Chemotherapy first-line treatment for low-grade intra-ocular tumours, also used in combination with other therapies to achieve cure, e.g. radiotherapy. Enucleation indicated if vision cannot be preserved due to tumour spread or retinal detachment. 90% cure for non-invasive intra-ocular disease. Prognosis correlates with degree of nerve involvement.

Extraocular disease associated with >90% mortality.

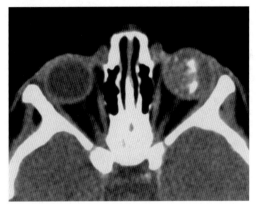

Fig. 7.23 Axial CT scan showing a calcified mass in the left eye due to retinoblastoma.

Rhabdomyosarcoma

Most common malignant soft tissue sarcoma in childhood, believed to arise from primitive striated muscle cells (rhabdomyoblasts). Over 80% occur <15yrs of age. 35–40% occur in the head and neck. Other common sites include pelvis (e.g. GU tract, bladder, prostate, vagina and testicular), extremities and trunk. Often associated with bony destruction. Head and neck rhabdomyosarcoma: orbital, parameningeal (middle ear, paranasal sinus and nasopharynx) and other sites (including cervical neck and nasal cavity). Six histological subtypes: most common *embryonal rhabdomyosarcoma* (>50% of all rhabdomyosarcoma, commonest type in head and neck and GU tract), Second most common *alveolar rhabdomyosarcoma* (especially extremities and trunk).

Clinical presentation

Depends on location:
- Orbital: proptosis, swelling or mass, decreased visual acuity.
- Nasal cavity/sinuses: nasal obstruction, facial mass, epistaxis.
- Temporal bone: otitis media, EAC or post-auricular mass.
- Neck: mass, airway compromise.

Associations: ↑incidence with NF-1, hereditary retinoblastoma, Beckwith–Wiedemann, Rubinstein–Taybi, Costello and Gorlin basal cell nevus syndromes, patients with mutations of p53 tumour suppressor gene (Li–Fraumeni syndrome). Also following treatment with alkylating agents or radiotherapy (radiation-induced second tumour).

Imaging findings

CT
- Best modality for evaluating bony changes.
- Variably enhancing mass.
- ± Necrosis.
- ± Bone destruction/erosion.

MRI
- Best modality for evaluation of peri-neural spread and intracranial extension (>50% of parameningeal tumours).
- Mass isointense to muscle on T1-WI, hyperintense on T2-WI.
- ± Necrosis.
- Variable contrast enhancement.

Differential diagnosis
- Neuroblastoma.
- Lymphoma.
- Infantile haemangioma.
- Nasopharyngeal carcinoma.
- Juvenile nasopharyngeal angiofibroma.
- Leukaemia.
- LCH.

Management and prognosis

Chemotherapy and/or radiotherapy. Surgical debulking/resection. Prognosis dependent on histological subtype and location. In the head and neck, orbital tumours have the best prognosis (80–90% disease free survival), and parameningeal tumours have the worst prognosis (40–50% disease-free survival). Embryonal rhabdomyosarcoma have a better prognosis than alveolar subtypes.

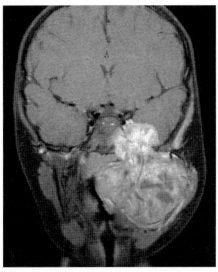

Fig. 7.24 Parameningeal rhabdomyosarcoma: coronal T1-weighted MRI, post-contrast with fat suppression. There is a large heterogeneously enhancing mass in the left side of the neck extending into the middle cranial fossa and cavernous sinus. The mass encroaches on the pharyngeal airway and there is associated bony destruction.

Neurology
Clinical presentations and role of imaging

Katharine Foster

Decreased consciousness

Decrease in consciousness can range from mild lethargy to confusion, to coma. These patients need to be assessed quickly, but a good history is essential to determine whether the cause is infectious or toxic/ischaemic. It is important that treatment of meningitis is not delayed. Trauma patients who may have an intracranial haemorrhage need imaging promtly so surgical treatment is not delayed.

- Infection:
  - Bacterial or viral meningitis (📖 p. 544).
  - Encephalitis, e.g. herpes simplex.
  - Empyema (collection of pus outside the brain secondary to mastoidts or sinusitis).
  - Intracerebral abscess.
- Haemorrhage due to trauma or a vascular malformation:
  - Intra-axial: within the brain parenchyma.
  - Extra-axial: within the skull vault, outside the brain parenchyma.
- Ischaemic:
  - Respiratory/cardiac arrest.
  - Near drowning.
  - Hypovolaemia (important to consider in trauma patients).
- Toxic:
  - Carbon monoxide poisoning.
  - Overdose.
- Metabolic:
  - Diabetic ketoacidosis.
  - Hepatic encephalopathy.
  - Renal failure.
  - Hyperammonia.
  - Mitochondrial disorders.
- Tumour (📖 p. 560–566).
- Epilepsy (post ictal state).
- Vascular:
  - Stroke (📖 p. 550).
- Demyelination: ADEM (📖 p. 546).

Role of imaging

Ultrasound

Ultrasound is a useful method of investigating for intracranial haemorrhage, particularly in neonatal patients.

CT

Useful in acutely unwell patients, to quickly exclude intracranial haemorrhage or a space occupying lesion.

MRI

MRI is useful in patients where a metabolic cause is suspected. Can be useful to show the extent or pattern of brain injury.

Headaches

The most common causes of chronic recurrent headaches in children are tension headaches and migraine. The majority of patients with headaches do not require imaging. Worrying features in the history that suggest an intracranial abnormality and require investigation include headaches that wake the child, headaches associated with bending or coughing or daily headaches that are becoming worse and worse. If the clinical examination reveals any neurological abnormality, prompt imaging is required.

- Tension.
- Migraine.
- Post-traumatic.
- Sinusitis.
- Infection:
  - Meningitis.
  - Encephalitis.
- Raised intracranial pressure:
  - Brain tumours (📖 p. 510).
  - Chiari I malformation (📖 p. 522).
  - Idiopathic intracranial hypertension.
- Hypertension.
- Intracranial haemorrhage (for example due to arteriovenous (AV) malformation (📖 p. 554).
- Venous sinus thrombosis (📖 p. 552).

Role of imaging

CT
Useful in patients who are very unwell, to exclude an intracranial haemorrhage or space-occupying lesion.

MRI
Gold standard for imaging of the brain as it gives much better anatomical detail.

Floppy infant

It is important to determine whether the infant's immobility is due to reduced level of consciousness, muscle weakness, or the child is hypotonic without major weakness (i.e. the child moves normally in the cot, but becomes floppy when handled).

Reduced level of consciousness

- Sepsis.
- Maternal drugs:
  - Inhalation anaesthetics and narcotics.
- Metabolic:
  - Hyperbilirubinaemia.
  - Hypoglycaemia.
  - Hypothyroidism.
  - Hyperammonia.
- Birth asphyxia:
  - Hypoxic ischaemic encephalopathy (📖 p. 558).

Hypotonia without major weakness

- Prematurity.
- Down's syndrome.
- Rare syndromes:
  - Prader Willi syndrome.
  - Peroxisomal disorders, e.g. Zellweger's.
  - Menkes' syndrome.
- Ligamentous laxity.

Paralytic/weakness

- Spinal cord abnormality:
  - Trauma, e.g. birth injury.
  - Spinal muscular atrophy.
- Peripheral neuropathy: rare.
- Neuromuscular junction:
  - Neonatal transitory myaesthenia gravis.
- Myopathies:
  - Myotonic dystrophy.
  - Benign congenital hypotonia.

Role of imaging

Ultrasound

Cranial ultrasound is a useful tool in neonates to exclude intracranial haemorrhage.

CT

Limited role: useful to exclude intracranial haemorrhage.

MRI

Can be useful in defining cerebral congenital abnormalities associated with rare syndromes. MRI is the best investigation to image the spinal cord.

Involuntary movements

Chorea

Continous jerky movements, randomly involving one limb to another, due to abnormality of the basal ganglia. Each movement looks like a fragment of a normal movement.

- Sydenham's chorea. Due to Group A haemolytic streptococcal throat infection. Can also cause damage to heart valves, carditis, migratory polyarthritis and erythema marginatum (rheumatic fever). ASO (anti-streptolysin-O) titre is usually raised. Imaging of the brain is usually normal, and not required if the cause is clear.
- Huntington's disease. Autosomal dominant, onset usually in young adulthood, but has been described in children. Progressive disease, with cognitive decline.
- Benign hereditary chorea: non-progressive.
- Pantothenate kinase–associated neurodegeneration (PKAN) (Hallervorden–Spatz).
- Inborn errors of metabolism:
  - Glutaric aciduria.
  - Proprionic acidaemia.
  - Phenylketonuria.
  - Homocystinuria.
  - Wilson's disease: usually present with hepatic dysfunction.
- Medication:
  - Anticholinergic drugs.
  - Anticonvulsants.
  - Antidopaminergic drugs (e.g. haloperidol, metaclopramide).

Athetosis

Slow, smooth writhing movements.

- Cerebral palsy.
- Kernicterus.

Tremor

Rythmical movement, usually of the hands.

- Benign essential tremor is usually familial (autosomal dominant).
- Anxiety.
- Thyrotoxicosis.
- Hepatic encephalopathy.
- CO_2 poisoning, solvent abuse, drug withdrawal.
- Cerebellar disease: intention tremor.

Role of imaging

MRI is the method of choice, to detect abnormalities of the basal ganglia in patients with athetosis or chorea. MRI may not be required, particularly for patients with tremor. However, if there is an intention tremor, or other signs of ataxia, MRI is indicated.

Ataxia

Ataxia is an abnormality of coordination. An ataxic gait is broad-based and unsteady. Other clinical features include limb incoordination, and intention tremor, dysarthria, involuntary eye movements (including dancing eye syndrome; opsiclonus). A full history and examination is important. A sudden, acute onset is more likely to be infectious/post-infectious or toxic. A history of gradual onset may be due to a tumour. There are a number of congenital abnormalities and inherited disorders that cause ataxia.

Acute causes of ataxia

- Infection, viral:
  - Chickenpox.
  - EBV.
- Drugs:
  - Alcohol.
- Demyelination:
  - ADEM (📖 p. 546).
  - MS.
- Haemorrhage:
  - Vascular malformations (📖 p. 554).
- Trauma:
  - Haemorrhage (📖 p. 502)
  - Vertebral artery dissection.
  - Non-accidental injury (📖 p. 390–392).
- Posterior fossa tumour (📖 p. 510).
- Neuroblastoma (opsiclonus).
- Vascular disorders:
  - Vasculitis.
  - Migraine.
- Miller–Fisher syndrome: rare variant of Guillain Barré (ataxia, ophthalmoplegia and areflexia).

Chronic causes of ataxia

- Congenital posterior fossa malformations.
  - Cerebellar hypoplasia.
  - Dandy Walker malformations (📖 p. 528).
- Ataxia telangectasia.
- Metabolic disorders:
  - Mitochondrial disorders in younger patients.
  - Wilson disease in adolescents.

Role of imaging

CT

Useful in acutely unwell, unstable patients to exclude haemorrhage, and space-occupying lesions.

MRI

Imaging method of choice.

Abnormal head size

When assessing head circumference, it is important that measurements are plotted on a centile chart. Patients who have measurements that are veering away from centiles over time are of more concern.

Macrocephaly

- Normal variation/familial.
- Hydrocephalus (📖 p. 506).
- Chronic subdural effusions.
- Neurofibromatosis (📖 p. 534).
- Achondroplasia.
- Soto's syndrome.
- Craniosynostosis of the sagittal suture causes an elongated head shape.

Microcephaly

- Normal variation/familial.
- Perinatal brain injury:
  - Hypoxic ischaemic encephalopathy (📖 p. 558).
  - Meningitis (📖 p. 544).
- Congenital infection.
- Fetal alcohol syndrome.
- Chromosomal abnormality syndromes.
- Craniosynostosis, e.g. Apert's syndrome.

Role of imaging

Plain films

May be useful to exclude craniosynostosis.

Ultrasound

A useful test in neonates and infants before closure of the anterior fontanelle. Useful to show ventricular size, periventricular leukomalacia, and intraventricular haemorrhage.

▶Limitations: 'blind spots', e.g. poor views of the subdural spaces, posterior fossa.

CT

Useful to show ventricular size. 3D reconstructions are useful to plan surgery in patients with craniosynostosis.

MRI

Gold standard investigation to evaluate the brain, and extra-axial fluid spaces.

Seizures

Seizures are one of the most common causes of admission to hospital in children. The causative organism varies with the age of the child.

Causes of seizures.

- Febrile convulsion.
- Cerebral palsy (perinatal ischaemic damage).
- Infection: bacterial meningitis, e.g. meningocccus, pneumococcus, TB, viral, e.g. herpes simplex.
- Drugs/toxins.
- Metabolic disorders.
- Tumour.
- Cortical malformations.
- Mesial temporal sclerosis.
- AV malformation.

Neonates

- Hypoxia (ischaemic encephalopathy).
- Intracranial haemorrhage (📖 p. 502).
- Metabolic, e.g. hypoglycaemia.
- Drug withrdrawal.
- Infection: TORCH, or gram –ve or Group B Streptococcus.
- Genetic: tuberous sclerosis (📖 p. 538).
- Venous sinus thrombosis (📖 p. 552).
- Cortical dysplasia (📖 p. 530).
- Non-accidental injury.

Role of imaging

Ultrasound

A useful test in neonates, to show intraventricular haemorrhage and periventricular leukomalacia.

CT

Usually the investigation of choice in acutely unwell children, to exclude a neurosurgical emergency.

MRI

The gold standard investigation to evaluate the brain. Will pick up subtle cortical malformations and mesial temporal sclerosis that are not visible on CT.

Developmental delay

The term developmental delay encompasses a huge range of symptoms and diagnoses. Taking a full history and examination is crucial. For example, delay may be secondary to poor hearing or vision.

Cerebral palsy

This term includes a range of non-degenerating neurological disabilities. Cognitive handicap is present in many patients with cerebral palsy.

Spastic diplegia usually relates to perinatal hypoxia, more common in low birth-weight or premature babies. Spastic hemiplegia usually relates to perinatal hypoxia, but can also be secondary to vascular malformations or congenital malformations. Extrapyramidal cerebral palsy causes hypotonia, choreoathetosis and dystonia. This is less common now that hyperbilirubinaemia is treated more aggressively.

Causes of cerebral palsy.
- Perinatal hypoxia (📖 p. 558).
- Perinatal hypoglycaemia.
- Neonatal hyperbilirubinaemia.
- Developmental anomalies, e.g. polymicrogyria (📖 p. 530) schizencephaly.
- Congenital infection (📖 p. 542).
- Intracerebral vascular malformations (📖 p. 554).

Regression

It is important to recognize patients who have regression, i.e. they are losing developmental milestones rather than just failing to gain them. These patients are much more likely to have a metabolic disorder, for example a mitochondrial disorder or leukodystrophy (📖 p. 516).

Role of imaging

CT
- Periventricular volume loss due to periventricular leukomalacia may be obvious if severe.
- Periventricular calcification can point to congenital infection.

MRI
- Gold standard of imaging to look for changes secondary to periventricular leukomalacia or cortical malformations (📖 p. 530).

Weak legs

Sudden onset of weakness with poor tone, and decreased reflexes
- Guillain Barré syndrome.
- Transverse myelitis.
- Cauda equina compression.

Sudden onset of weakness, with increased tone and increased reflexes
- Cord compression: tumours, fractures.
- Transverse myelitis.
- Multiple sclerosis.
- Cord infarction.

Chronic spastic weakness
- Cerebral palsy.
- Tethered cord (📖 p. 526).
- Syringomyelia (often associated with Chiari I and II malformations (📖 p. 518).

Chronic flaccid weakness
- Peripheral neuropathies:
  - Charcot–Marie–Tooth.
- Myopathies.
- Nerve trauma, e.g. Erb's palsy.
- Rare leukodystrophies, e.g. Krabbes: other neurological symptoms would be present.

Role of imaging

CT
Very useful in trauma patients to show fractures, but depicts the spinal cord poorly.

MRI
Is the best method to depict the spinal cord. IV contrast is useful in patients whom Guillain Barré syndrome is suspected: the nerve roots of the cauda equina will enhance. It should also be given to patients with a syrinx, but no underlying cause seen, to ensure there is not an underlying spinal cord tumour.

Sacral pits and patches

Skin lesions over the spine, can be markers of underlying spinal abnormalities.

Cutaneous lesions associated with congenital spinal abnormalities

- Subcutaneous mass or lipoma.
- Hairy patch.
- Dermal sinus.
- Atypical dimples: i.e. those that are deep (>5mm), or greater than 2.5cm from the anal verge.
- Vascular lesions, e.g. haemangioma.
- Skin tags.
- Scar-like lesions.

▶Imaging is not required for simple sacral dimples (<5mm deep and less than 25mm from the anal verge) or coccygeal pits.

Associated spinal abnormalities

- Tethered cord (📖 p. 526).
- Spinal dermoid or haemangioma.
- Lipomyelomeningocele.
- Diastematomyelia.
- Dermal sinuses.

▶Patients with anorectal malformations (e.g. VATER: vertebral anomalies, anorectal malformation, (o)esophageal atresia or tracheo-oesophageal atresia, and renal anomalies/radial dysplasia have an increased incidence of congenital spinal abnormalities.

Role of imaging

Ultrasound

- Best performed as early as possible. Can be difficult after 3mths as bones start to ossify.

MRI

- Gold standard investigation, but usually requires sedation or general anaesthesia in this age group.

Neurology
Differential diagnosis

Katharine Foster

Intracranial haemorrhage

CT is the best intial assessment of acute haemorrhage. Acute haemorrhage is usually hyperdense (bright) on CT. Over time the blood becomes more hypodense. Sometimes acute haemorrhage can be of mixed low and high attenuation. Intracranial haemorrhage is classified according to its position relative the to brain, and the meninges. More than one compartment can be involved at once, particularly in trauma.

Extra-axial haemorrhage (outside the brain)

Epidural haematoma
- Blood between the inner table of the skull and the dura.
- Nearly all due to trauma, and occur at the site of impact.
- Biconcave collection.

Subdural haematoma
- Crescent-shaped collection in the subdural space.
- Can spread along the falx and tentorium.

Causes
- Trauma.
- Non-accidental injury.
- Predisposing factors:
  - Atrophy.
  - Bleeding disorders.
  - Overshunting of hydrocephalus.
  - Glutaric aciduria type I.
  - Menkes'.

Subarachnoid haemorrhage
- Blood in the subarachnoid space: between the pia and arachnoid.
- When acute, seen as hyperdensity on CT within sulci, and basal cisterns.
- Usually associated with trauma.
- Aneurysms are rare in children.

Intraparenchymal haemorrhage

- Trauma can cause contusion, and large haematomas, or can cause tiny scattered haemorrhage due to shearing injury (diffuse axonal injury).
- ⚠ Spontaneous intraparenchymal haemmorhage is very rare in children, and the underyling cause should be sought.
  Can be associated with venous sinus thrombosis.
- ▶ CT:-give contrast to check that the venous sinuses are patent (📖 p. 552).
- ▶ Can be associated with arteriovenous vascular malformation (AVM, 📖 p. 554).
- CT:-give contrast to look for abnormal serpiginous vessels at site of clot.
- MRI: look for serpignous flow voids on T2 images.
- MRA.

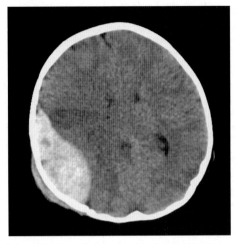

Fig. 8.1 CT scan of an infant with a large right-sided extradural haematoma causing significant mass effect.

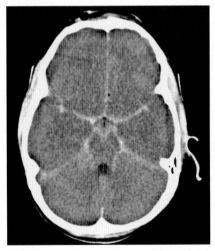

Fig. 8.2 CT scan of a teenager with acute, traumatic subarachnoid haemorrhage. There is extensive hyperintensity in the basal cisterns.

Cerebral oedema

Brain oedema is due to accumulation of water within cells, and the extra-cellular space. It can be classified into three main types:

- Vasogenic: due to leakage of fluid from vessels due to breakdown of the blood–brain barrier.
- Cytotoxic: swollen cells.
- Interstitial: excess fluid in the extracellular spaces, e.g. hydrocephalus.

Cytotoxic and vasogenic oedema often occur together, for example tumours are often surrounded by a rim of vasogenic oedema. The type of oedema can evolve over time. Cytotoxic oedema is present in acute infarction, but as the cells die, and cell membranes break down the oedema becomes vasogenic/interstitial.

CT is good at detecting both focal and diffuse areas of oedema. However, MRI is often much more sensitive, and diffusion-weighted MR imaging can distinguish cytotoxic oedema.

- Cytotoxic oedema:
  - ↑ signal on diffusion images.
  - ↓ signal on apparent diffusion coefficient (ADC) map.

Radiological signs of generalized cerebral oedema

- Poor grey white matter differentiation.
- Effacement of extra-axial fluid spaces.
- Small ventricles.
- Tonsilar herniation if severe.
- Reversal sign on CT if severe: the cerebral hemispheres are of diffusely low attenuation compared to the cerebellum.

Differential diagnosis

- Hypoxia.
- Trauma: diffuse axonal injury often cooexists with hypoxia.
- Encephalopathy.

Radiological signs of focal cerebral oedema

- CT: focal areas of low attenuation.
- MRI: focal areas of ↑T2 and FLAIR signal.

Differential diagnosis

- Infarction/ischaemia.
- Tumour.
- Infection.
- Demyelination.
- Metabolic.
- Trauma.
- Haemorrhage.
- Hydrocephalus: periventricular oedema.

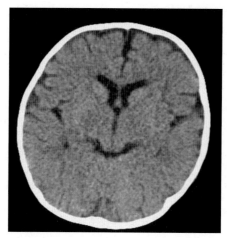

Fig. 8.3 CT of a patient without cerebral oedema. Notice how the spaces around the brain are well seen.

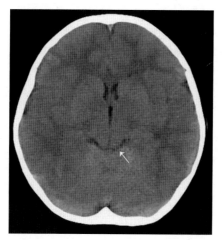

Fig. 8.4 CT of a different patient with cerebral oedema. Notice how the spaces around the brain are not well seen. The ambient cistern (white arrow) is slightly effaced. Grey/white matter differentiation is preserved in this patient.

Hydrocephalus

Hydrocephalus is an imbalance of CSF formation and absorption. This results in enlarged ventricles. It is important to examine the extra-axial fluid spaces (the fluid spaces around the brain).

Classification

1. Obstructive hydrocephalus: obstruction to CSF flow and absorption. This has two main categories.

- **Intraventricular obstruction** (non-communicating hydrocephalus)
The extra-axial fluid spaces may be effaced. There may be periventricular oedema:
  - Tumours.
  - Aqueduct stenosis: can be primary, or secondary to previous haemorrhage, or compression by a tectal plate glioma.
  - Arachnoid cysts.
  - Chiari I or II malformations: 4th ventricle can be compressed.
  - Dandy Walker malformation.
- **Extraventricular obstruction/↓absorption** (communicating hydrocephalus):
  - Past history of meningitis.
  - Intraventricular haemorrhage.
  - CSF tumour seeding (leukaemia, lymphoma, medulloblastoma).

2. Overproduction of CSF: rare.

- Choroid plexus papilloma.
- Diffuse villous hyperplasia.

Benign enlargement of the subarachnoid spaces in infants

- Other terms: benign external hydrocephalus, extraventricular obstructive hydrocephalus.
- Enlarged extra-axial CSF spaces, with normal to slightly enlarged ventricles.
- Neurologically normal children.
- May have macrocephaly: children tend to have normal/large head circumference at birth. This increases rapidly for first few months, but then normalizes at about 18mths.
- MRI is indicated to exclude hydrocephalus, and subdural haematomas.

Tonsilar herniation

Radiological signs of tonsilar herniation

- Tonsils lie greater than 5mm below foramen magnum (up to 5mm can be normal).
- Tonsils are compressed or 'peg-shaped', rather than rounded.
- Surrounding CSF spaces effaced.

Differential diagnosis

- Raised intracranial pressure:
  - Hydrocephalus.
  - Brain tumours.
  - Intracranial haemorrhage.
- Chiari malformations (☐ p. 522):
  - Can be associated with disordered CSF flow, resulting in syringomyelia and hydrocephalus.
- Intracranial hypotension 'sagging brain':
  - CSF leak from epidural/LP.
  - Can be associated with enhancing subdural collection.

Abnormal enhancement

IV contrast media can be given to help highlight pathology. In CT this is iodine-based, in MRI it is gadolinium-based. Contrast uptake is seen in areas where there is damage to the blood–brain barrier: this can be in tumours, inflammation or infarction.

Generalized gyriform enhancement
- Meningitis:
  - This may not be visible. CT is used to detect complications of meningitis, not diagnose it.
  - TB tends to involve the basal cisterns.
- CSF tumour seeding:
  - Lymphoma, leukaemia, medulloblastoma.
- Sarcoidosis:
  - Rare in children.

Focal gyriform enhancement
- Infarction.
- Encephalitis.

Linear rim enhancement over surface of the brain
- Empyema.
- Subdural haematomas: much less marked than in empyema.

Serpiginous enhancement
- Arteriovascular malformation (📖 p. 554).

Multiple cerebral enhancing lesions
- Abscesses:
  - Endocarditis.
  - Immunosuppression.
- Tumours:
  - Lymphoma.
  - Metastases (rare in children compared with adults).
  - Multiple gliomas.
- Infarction:
  - Vasculitis.
- Demyelinating plaques.
- Contusion.

Brain tumours

Tumours of the central nervous system are the second most common paediatric tumour (after leukaemia). The symptoms are very variable, depending on the age of the child and the site of the tumour. For example, posterior fossa tumours can present with ataxia, headaches or neck pain, and vomiting secondary to raised intracranial pressure.

Imaging findings

CT

- Nearly all tumours are hypodense on non-contrasted CT images (exception is medulloblastoma).

MRI

- Nearly all tumours are hyperintense on T2 images and hypointense on T1 images.
- Enhancement does not correlate with tumour grade.
- Spectroscopy is increasingly used pre-operatively to assess tumour type and grade.
- Imaging is used to guide surgical excision/biopsy. Post-operative assessement of residual tumour can be difficult initially, as there is always some enhancement, and often haemorrhage relating to surgery.
- Posterior fossa tumours, and aggressive supratentorial tumours can seed into the CSF causing 'drop metastases' in the spinal canal.

Intraparenchymal (intra-axial) tumours

Posterior fossa

Although there are 'characteristic' features for each type of tumour, there is considerable overlap in appearances.

- Medulloblastoma (📖 p. 560):
  - Usually midline, arises from the vermis (not the medulla) and often fills the 4th ventricle.
- Astrocytoma:
  - More often hemispheric, than midline.
  - May be cystic with a mural-enhancing nodule.
- Ependymoma (📖 p. 562):
  - Tends to extrude through foramen of Luschka and Magendie, and through the posterior fossa.
  - Often calcified.
- Atypical rhabdoid/teratoid tumours:
  - Aggressive tumours, similar in appearance to medulloblastoma
- Teratoma:
  - Young infants, often contain fat.
- Brainstem tumours:
  - Pontine gliomas are often quite diffuse, and tend to wrap around the basilar artery.

Supratentorial.

- Astrocytoma:
  - Variable appearance.
- Craniopharyngioma (📖 p. 564):
  - Suprasellar mass, usually with cystic component and calcification.

- Choroid plexus papilloma:
  - Lobulated, brightly enhancing intraventricular mass.
- Germinoma:
  - Enhancing lesion in suprasellar or pineal region. One of the causes of diabetes insipidus.
- DNET: Dysembryoplastic neuroepithelial tumour (📖 p. 566):
  - Benign, cortical based lesion, often with 'bubbly' appearance.
- PNET.

▶Brain metastases are rare in children. If multiple enhancing tumours are present consider lymphoma.

Extraparenchymal (extra-axial tumours)

- Epidermoid:
  - Often same signal intensity on standard MR images as CSF.
  - Bright on FLAIR and diffusion-weighted images.
- Meningioma:
  - Much less common in children than in adults.
  - Consider neurofibromatosis type II.
- Skull vault or skull base tumour:
  - Neuroblastoma.
- Diffuse meningeal tumour spread:
  - Leukaemia/lymphoma.
  - Medulloblastoma.
  - Retinoblastoma.

Pituitary abnormalities

Normal pituitary gland

- MRI is the gold standard for imaging: often other methods are inadequate.
- The posterior pituitary gland is seen as a bright structure, within the pituitary fossa on MRI T1 images.
- The pituitary gland increases in size during puberty.
- The pituitary gland and stalk normally enhance post-gadolinium.

Normal variants

- Small Rathkes' cleft cyst between the anterior and posterior pituitary. Can rarely be large and symptomatic.
- 'Empty sella': the arachnoid space protrudes into the pituitary fossa, and compresses the normal pituitary gland against the fossa floor. This can be associated with idiopathic intracranial hypertension.

Congenital abnormalities

Ectopic posterior pituitary gland

- Posterior pituitary gland lies on tuber-cinereum, or on pituitary stalk.
- Pituitary stalk absent or thin.

Hamartoma of the tuber cinereum.

- Clinical presentation: precocious puberty +/− gelastic seizures.
- Isointense nodule arising from the tuber cinereum.
- Do not enhance: if mass enhances consider astrocytoma.

Intrasellar masses

Macroadenoma

- Prolactinoma most common.
- Can be giant and invasive.
- Majority enhance.

Microadenoma

- Rare in children.
- <10mm diameter.
- Prolactinomas most common.
- Dynamic MRI can be helpful as they do enhance, but more slowly than the normal pituitary gland.

Craniopharyngioma

- Majority contain some calcification (CT can be helpful to identify this).
- Majority are mixed solid/cystic tumours.
- Cyst content signal may be high on T1 images due to high protein.

Rathkes cleft cyst

Pituitary stalk mass

Histiocytosis

- Often associated with diabetes insipidus.
- Thickened, enhancing pituitary stalk.

- Other radiological features:
  - Well-defined lucent bone lesions.
  - 'Vertebra plana', vertebral collapse.
- Germinoma.
- Lymphoma/leukaemia.
- Sarcoid (rare in children).

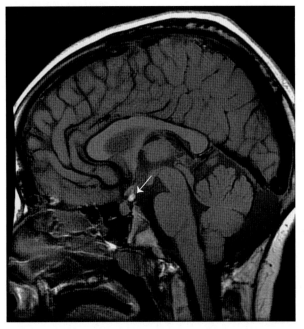

Fig. 8.5 Ectopic pituitary gland in a child with growth hormone deficiency. The posterior bright spot of the pituitary gland (white arrow) is too high. It should lie next to the anterior pituitary gland within the sella.

Intracerebral calcification

Tumours

- Craniopharyngioma: suprasellar mixed cystic and solid mass (📖 p. 564)
- Oligodendroglioma.
- Ganglioglioma.
- Choroid plexus papilloma.
- Pineal germ cell tumours.
- Astrocytoma.
- Ependymoma (📖 p. 562)
- Lipoma of the corpus callosum, may be associated with marginal calcification.

Vascular lesions

- Aneurysms: curvilinear calcification can be seen in giant aneurysms.
- Arteriovascular malformations.

Neurocutaneous syndromes

- Sturge–Weber Syndrome: gyral calcification (📖 p. 540).
- Tuberous sclerosis: subependymal nodules frequently calcify. Subependymal tubers may also calcify (📖 p. 538).
- Meningiomas: rare in children, can be associated with neurofibromatosis type II.

Infection

- Congenital cytomegalovirus infection: periventricular calcification (📖 p. 542).
- Toxoplasmosis: scattered calcification.
- Tuberculosis: granulomas calcify, particularly after treatment.
- Cystercicosis: cystic lesions, calcification follows death of scolex.

Other causes

Bilateral basal ganglia calcification

- Hypoparathyroidism and pseudohypoparathyroidism.
- Cockayne syndrome.

▶Pineal calcification is a common incidental finding.

Bilateral basal ganglia lesions

The basal ganglia consist of the globus pallidus, caudate and putamen. A large number of conditions can affect the basal ganglia, but some of these have quite a distinct radiological pattern, and MRI can help to make the diagnosis.

- Profound ischaemia:
  - Symmetrical pattern, thalami are usually also involved.
  - Neonate, predominantly affects posterior putamen, and ventrolateral thalamus.
  - Older child, predominantly affects the caudate and putamen, and thalami.
- Infection: encephalitis.
- ADEM: usually asymmetrical pattern: white matter usually also involved (📖 p. 546).
- AV malformations: can occur anywhere in the brain. Can be associated with haemorrhage, and changes associated with ischaemia due to 'vascular steal' (📖 p. 554).
- Myelinolysis: often associated with pontine oedema.
- Inborn errors of metabolism:
  - Often a very symmetrical pattern of ↑T2 signal.
  - Mitochondrial disorders.
  - GM2 gangliosidosis: basal ganglia ↑signal, thalami ↓T2 signal.
  - Glutaric aciduria I: caudate and putamen, wide sylvian fissures, subdural collections.
  - Methylmalonic and proprionic acidaemia: globus pallidus ↑T2 signal.
  - Wilson's: putamen and pons most frequent, but can also affect globus palladi, caudate and thalami.
  - Pantothenate kinase–associated neurodegeneration (PKAN) (Hallervorden–Spatz): hyperintense foci in median globus palladi on background of↓T2 signal.
  - Molybdenum cofactor deficiency, caudate and putamen, often extensive cystic white matter change.
  - L2 hydroxyglutaric aciduria: globus pallidus, often with dentate and subcortical white matter hyperintensity.
  - Huntington's: caudate and putamen ↑T2 signal.
- Kernicterus: acute T1 ↑signal globus palladi. Chronic ↑T2 signal globus palladi and dentate nuclei.
- Poisoning:
  - Carbon monoxide: globus palladi ↑T2 signal. May seen rim ↓of signal probably due to haemosiderin deposition, and periventricular white matter oedema.
- Creutzfeld-Jacob disease: caudate, putamen and thalami ↑T2 signal.

Leukodystrophy

There are multiple inborn areas of metabolism, that cause abnormal white matter. This may be due to a delay or deficiency in myelin production (hypomyelination). Some disorders cause destruction of the white matter. As a general rule, inherited metabolic white matter disorders have a symmetrical, often confluent pattern. The pattern of white matter abnormality on MRI can be very helpful in reaching a diagnosis in this diverse group of patients. Some examples are given below.

Hypomyelination

- Pelizaeus–Merzbacher: almost all are boys, classically present in first year of life with nystagmus, tremor or shaking of the head, and developmental delay. Due to lack of myelin:
  - Arrest of myelin development at a stage which is normal.
  - The white matter can appear slightly speckled or stripy.
- 18q-syndrome: patients are usually dysmorphic, short with limb abnormalities.
- Hypomyelination with atrophy of the basal ganglia and cerebellum.

Demyelination of periventricular white matter (with sparing of the subcortical U fibres)

- Metachromic leukodystrophy: confluent pattern, subcortical U fibres spared initially.
- Adrenoleukodystrophy: usually occipital predominance.
Often abnormality first appears in the splenium of the corpus callosum:
  - Leading enhancing edge predictive of active, progressive disease.
- Krabbes' disease:
  - Neonates present with seizures, irritability, blindness and hyperacusis. Basal ganglia, dentate nuclei usually affected. Thickened optic nerves. Thalami hyperintense on CT.
  - Later onset: MRI pattern mimics adrenoleukodystrophy.

Demyelination of the subcortical white matter

- Megalencephalic leukoencephalopathy with cysts.
- L2 hydroxyglutaric aciduria: globus palladi and cerebellar dentate nuclei usually involved.
- Kearns–Sayre: basal ganglia, thalami and midbrain also affected.
- Canavan's disease:
  - Peripheral white matter affected early in disease, then white matter abnormality spread centrally and becomes diffuse.
  - Globus palladi and thalami often involved.
  - Large N-acetlyaspartate (NAA) peak on spectroscopy (appears to be specific for this disorder).

Syndromes that affect other organs

- Mucopolysaccharidosis: numerous enlarged perivascular spaces.
- Lowe syndrome (occulocerebrorenal syndrome).

Abnormal skull vault

Lucent skull lesions

- Langerhans' cell histiocytosis:
  - Can be multiple or solitary.
  - Frontal bone more common, but can occur anywhere.
  - Sclerotic rim if healing.
  - May have bevelled edge.
- Osteomyelitis:
  - Can be associated with sinusitis/mastoiditis.
- Metastases:
  - Neuroblastoma, leukaemia.
- Epidermoid:
  - Common in squamous, occipital or temporal bone.
  - Scalloped appearance, sclerotic rim.
- Traumatic: leptomeningeal cyst or 'growing fracture':
  - If dura is torn, arachnoid membrane can protrude, and pulsate. CSF widens the fracture.
- Haemangioma:
  - May see radiating bony spicules.
- Meningocele:
  - Midline, usually occipital.
  - Smooth sclerotic margin, with overlying soft tissue mass.
- Burr hole.
- Normal variants: parietal foramina.

Thickened skull vault

- Normal variant.
- Chronic decreased intracranial pressure:
  - Cerebral atrophy.
  - Post shunting of hydrocephalus.
- Phenytoin therapy.
- Chronic haemolytic anaemias, 'hair on end' appearance:
  - Sickle cell disease.
  - Thalassaemia.
- Fibrous dysplasia:
  - Often has a ground-glass appearance.
- Osteopetrosis: thickening can cause encroachment of cranial nerve foramen, e.g. causing blindness.

Thinned skull vault

- Other terms copper beaten skull, lacunar skull.
- Normal variant.
- Hydrocephalus (🕮 p. 506).
- Osteogenesis imperfecta: associated with wormian bones.
- Rickets.

Spinal cord lesions

The spinal cord is best imaged with MRI. The spinal cord is usually of homogenous appearance on T1 and T2 images. The central canal should be thin. The most distal aspect of the spinal canal can be slightly dilated within the conus (ventriculus terminalis): this is a normal variant.

Syringomyelia

- Abnormal cystic spaces within the spinal canal, which may or may not connect with a dilated central spinal canal. These cystic spaces have the same signal as CSF.
- Can be secondary/associated with:
  - Chiari malformations.
  - Trauma.
  - Transverse myelitis.
  - Tumours.
▶ If no clear cause give iv contrast to exclude spinal cord tumour.

Transverse myelitis

- Acute history, of sensory deficit, usually clearly defined upper level. May have weakness in legs, incontinence.
- Swollen cord: ↑T2 signal.
- Variable enhancement.
- Usually only one lesion, which involves more than 2/3 of the cross. sectional area of the cord, and 3–4 vertebrae in length.

Spinal cord ADEM

- Multifocal lesions; brain nearly always involved (📖 p. 546).

Multiple sclerosis

- Has similar appearances to spinal ADEM and transverse myelitis.
- The brain is nearly always involved.
- History of multiple episodes is important to make diagnosis.

Spinal cord infarction

- Very acute history (less than 4hrs): usually motor signs.
- Ventral cord location: dorsal columns usually spared.

Spinal cord tumours

- Present with slow onset of pain, myelopathy, torticollis, scoliosis.

Astrocytoma

- Most common spinal cord tumour in children.
- Infiltrating tumour, often associated with syrinx above or below lesion.
- ↑T2 signal.
- Usually enhances.

Ependymoma

- Well-defined tumour.
- Location: cervical most common, followed by thoracic.
- ↑T2 signal, may contain cysts, haemorrhage.
- Usually enhances.

Neurology
Disorders

Katharine Foster

Callosal dysgenesis

The corpus callosum is the major white matter tract connecting the two cerebral hemispheres. All or part of the corpus callosum may be absent or hypoplastic. It is a relatively common congenital abnormality, and is often associated with other malformations.

Imaging findings

CT
- Parallel, widely separated ventricles.
- Dilatation of the occipital horns (colpocephaly).

MRI
- Sagittal images: gyri 'point' to 3rd ventricle due to absent cingulate gyrus.
- Coronal images:
  - Bundles of Probst (white matter tracts, which have failed to cross the midline) seen medial to the frontal horns.
  - Vertical hippocampi.
- Axial: widely spaced, parallel ventricles with dilated occipital horns.

▶Look for associated abnormalities: for example, cortical maldevelopment, inferior vermis hypoplasia, midline cysts and lipomas.

▶Look for the cingulate gyrus: if this is present the corpus callosum is usually thin/stretched rather than absent.

Differential diagnosis
- Destruction of the corpus callosum, due to previous trauma, surgery, hypoxic ischaemic encephalopathy (HIE).
- Stretched corpus callosum, due to hydrocephalus.

Management and prognosis

Prognosis can be good, from normal, to those with difficulties with cognitive tasks at school. Prognosis is worse in patients with other associated abnormalities, e.g. seizures and developmental delay.

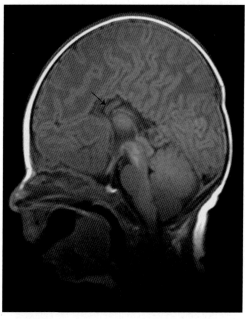

Fig. 8.6 Sagittal T1 MR of a newborn baby with dysgenesis of the corpus callosum. Only a small portion of the corpus callosum has formed (black arrow).

Chiari I malformation

This is a congenital malformation resulting in tonsilar herniation more than 5mm below the foramen magnum. The tonsils are usually 'peg-shaped' due to compression. Patients may be asymptomatic. They often have headaches which may be worse with coughing or sneezing. Other symptoms include torticollis and neck pain. Syringomyelia may cause an unsteady gait, incontinence, neuropathy, particularly in upper limbs.

Imaging findings

CT

- Tonsils protrude though the foramen magnum.
- Can demonstrate abnormality of the skull base which is seen in some patients:
  - Short, horizontal clivus.
  - Posterior tilting of the odontoid peg.
  - Can be associated craniosynostosis.

MRI

- Imaging method of choice, as can show degree of tonsilar herniation, and signal change within the tonsils.
- Compression of the 4th ventricle can cause hydrocephalus.
- Disordered CSF flow can cause syrinx formation.
- Some patients have associated tethering of the spinal cord:
  - Fat in the filum terminale.
  - Low lying conus (lower than middle of L2 vertebra).
- Flow studies may demonstrate abnormal CSF flow, and pulsatile tonsillar descent.

▶Make sure that other causes of tonsillar descent are excluded!

Treatment

- Most surgeons will operate only on symptomatic patients.
- Posterior fossa decompression +/− resection of posterior arch of C1.

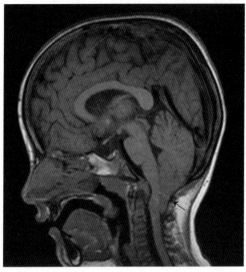

Fig. 8.7 Child with a Chiari I malformation. The cerebellar tonsils (black arrow) are peg-shaped and herniate well below the foramen magnum.

Chiari II malformation and myelomeningocele

This is a complex, posterior fossa malformation. They are nearly always associated with a neural tube closure defect, usually a myelomeningocele.

Prevention and screening

- Folate supplements to mothers before, and early after conception reduces the rate of myelomeningoceles.
- Fetal screening: ↑ alpha feto-protein.
- Fetal ultrasound: 'lemon and banana' signs of Chiari II malformation, myelomeningocele.

Imaging findings

CT

- Small crowded posterior fossa.
- 4th ventricle compressed and difficult to see.
- There is often associated hydrocephalus.
- 'Heart-shaped' incisura.
- There are often other abnormalities, e.g. dysgenesis of the corpus callosum, and the falx is often absent, resulting in gyral interdigitation.

MRI of brain and spine

- Very small posterior fossa, with herniation of medulla, cerebellum through the foramen magnum.
- Cerebellum can also herniate upwards through the incisura.
- Compressed 4th ventricle.
- Hydrocephalus.
- Elongated pons.
- Beaking of the tectal plate.
- Cervico–medullary kink.
- Associated abnormalties, e.g. dysgenesis of the corpus callosum.
- Syringomyelia.

▶A Chiari II malformation is not a 'bad Chiari I', it is a completely different entity, usually associated with a myelomeningocele.

Features of myelomeningocele

- Most common location: lumbosacral.
- CSF sac protruding through osseous spinal dysraphism.
- Low-lying cord.
- Nerve roots extend from a ventral neural placode.

Management and prognosis

- Repair of the myelomeningocele +/– ventricular shunt insertion.

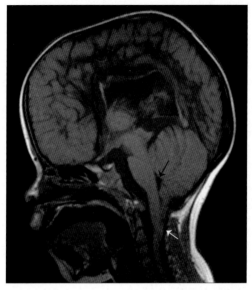

Fig. 8.8 Child with a Chiari II malformation. The tonsils (white arrow) herniate well below the foramen magnum. Notice that the 4th ventricle is also compressed (black arrow).

Tethered cord

Tethered spinal cord syndrome is a clinical diagnosis. Patients present with a spastic gait, weakness and muscular atrophy, and bladder dysfunction. Some patients have low back or leg pain.

Imaging findings

MRI is the gold standard to image the spinal cord.

MRI

- Low-lying conus: below L2.
- Thickened filum contains fat: ↑ T1 signal.
- Wide dural sac.
- Can be associated with Chiari I malformation.

Differential diagnosis

- Normal variant: asymptomatic low-lying cord.
- Spinal dysraphism: e.g. diastematomyelia.

Management and prognosis

- Symptoms are progressive without treatment.
- Outcome is better if symptoms are of short duration.
- Prophylactic treatment for asymptomatic patients is controversial.
► Cannot exclude retethering by imaging alone, this is a clinical diagnosis.

Diastematomyelia

Diastematomyelia is a split cord congenital malformation. It presents with the same clinical symptoms as tethered cord. A fibrous or bony spur splits and tethers the spinal cord into two hemicords.

Imaging findings

CT

- Best for depicting bony spur.

MRI

- Best to depict the two hemicords.
- Fibrous or osseous spur hypointense.

Common associations

- Vertebral segmentation anomalies and scoliosis.
- Spinal dysraphism (myelomeningocele/myelocele).
- Tethered cord.
- Syringomyelia.

Management and prognosis

- The prognosis is dependent on whether other abnormalities are present, e.g. kyphoscoliosis.
- Symptoms may progress if untreated.
- The majority of patients improve or stabilize following surgical untethering.

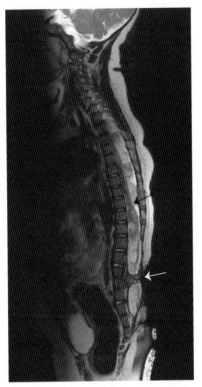

Fig. 8.9 Sagittal T2 MRI of a child with diastematomyelia. There is a prominent bony spur (white arrow). Dark flow voids are seen within the large spinal syrinx (black arrow).

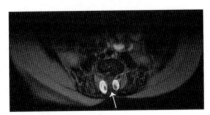

Fig. 8.10 Axial T2W MRI of the same patient. The bony spur (white arrow) is seen between the two hemicords.

Dandy Walker malformation

This is a malformation of the cerebellum and posterior fossa. They are usually detected at antenatal ultrasound screening. Clinical presentation is very variable, ranging from early mortality, seizures, developmental delay and poor motor control.

Imaging findings

CT

- Large posterior fossa cyst.

MRI

- Posterior fossa cyst which communicates with the 4th ventricle.
- Poorly formed hypoplastic cerebellar vermis rotated superiorly.
- High torcula due to enlargement of the posterior fossa by the cyst.

Differential diagnosis

- Arachnoid cyst: the 4th ventricle may be displaced or compressed.
- Congenital hypoplasia of the vermis:
  - Previously thought to be synonymous with Joubert syndrome, but is now known to be associated with many other syndromes.
  - The vermis is split, giving the mesencephalon the appearance of a 'molar tooth'.
- Dandy Walker spectrum. Previously, patients with a normal size posterior fossa, but with a hypoplastic vermis were grouped under this heading. This has led to some confusion in the literature.
- Encysted 4th ventricle.

Management and prognosis

The prognosis depends on the degree of vermian hypoplasia, and whether there are associated supratentorial abnormalities. It can be associated with hydrocephalus, which may require a shunt placed in the ventricles or the cyst.

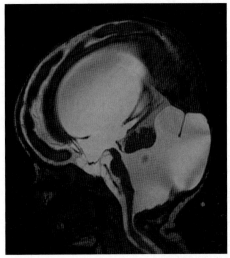

Fig. 8.11 Sagittal T2 MRI of a baby with a large posterior fossa cyst due Dandy Walker malformation. The cerebellar vermis is rotated superiorly.

Cortical malformations

At about 7 weeks gestation, the cerebral cortex begins to develop from cells lining the ventricles, called the germinal matrix. These cells *proliferate* to form neurons and glia. From about 8 weeks, neurons begin to *migrate* away from the ventricles, guided by radial glial cells which stretch from the ventricular surface to the pia. This occurs in waves, to form the cortex which has seven distinct layers of neurons. Finally the neurons form synapses with other local and distant neurons, in a process called *organization*.

This process is complex and interruptions, which can be due ischaemia, infection, toxins or genetic causes, result in cortical malformations. This can result in epilepsy, or developmental delay.

Examples of cortical malformations

Malformations due to abnormal proliferation

- Microlissencephaly (small smooth brain).
- Neurocutaneous syndromes, e.g. tuberous sclerosis.
- DNET.

Malformations due to abnormal migration

- Lissencephaly.
- Congenital muscular dystrophies.
- Subependymal heterotopia.
- Pachygyria (thickened abnormal cortex).
- Aicardi's syndrome.

Malformations due to abnormal organization

- Polymicrogyria.

Imaging findings

- MRI is the gold standard to detect abnormalities of cortical malformation. 3T magnets may be more sensitive to detect very small areas of abnormality.
- 'Gradient volume' images are useful for detailed imaging of the cortex.
- The findings depend on the type of cortical malformation present. For example, subependymal grey matter heterotopia results in focal small masses at the ventricular surface, the same signal as the normal cortical grey matter. Polymicrogyria has a crinkled appearance, with loss of the normal gyral pattern.

Management and prognosis

The prognosis depends on the type of cortical malformation, its location and its extent. For example subependymal grey matter heterotopia may be asymptomatic, but other patients may have severe developmental delay and seizures. Some are inherited disorders, so genetic counselling may be indicated for the parents and child.

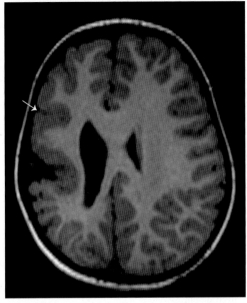

Fig. 8.12 Patient with extensive right-sided polymicrogyria (white arrow).

Craniosynostosis

Craniosynostosis describes premature fusion of the cranial sutures. This can result in distortion of the skull vault and face.
- Non syndromic: most common.
- Syndromic: e.g. Apert's syndrome.

Imaging features

Radiographs
- Loss of normal lucency due to suture fusion.
- Sclerosis at site of suture fusion.

CT
▶ Low-dose 3D CT best.
- Bony bridging across sutures.
- Abnormal skull vault shape:
  - Scaphocephaly: sagittal synostosis.
  - Frontal beaking: metopic synostosis.
  - Plagiocephaly: asymmetry due to single or assymetrical multiple synostosis.
  - Turricephaly: both coronal, or both lambdoids.
  - Brachycephaly: both coronal or both lambdoids.

MRI
- Indicated if thought to be syndromal to look for brain malformations, e.g. agenesis of the corpus callosum.
- May show tonsilar herniation.

Differential diagnosis
- Early fusion of skull sutures secondary to parenchymal loss (e.g.- perinatal hypoxia).

Management and prognosis
- Unilateral lambdoid synostosis, which causes flattening of the occiput, is common and does not usually require imaging or surgical treatment. The ear tends to be posteriorly displaced on the same side.
- Orthotic helmet if mild.
- Major craniofacial surgery:
  - Indicated to reduce raised intracranial pressure.
  - To correct craniofacial deformity if severe.

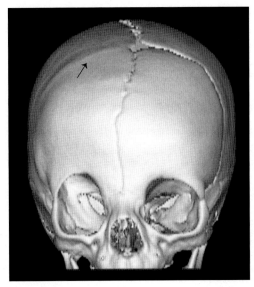

Fig. 8.13 3D-reconstructed CT scan of a patient with right coronal suture synostosis (black arrow). This has caused distortion of the metopic suture, and the shape of the right orbit.

Neurofibromatosis type I

An autosomal dominant neurocutaneous disorder, chromosomal abnormality on chromosome 17. Characterized by:
- Café-au-lait spots and axillary freckling.
- Cutaneous neurofibromas.
- Intracranial hamartomas.
- Tumours: benign and malignant.

Imaging findings of the brain

MRI
- Focal areas of signal intensity (FASI) on T2WI in both grey and white matter:
  - Are frequently seen along the optic tracts, cerebellar white matter, and basal ganglia.
  - Tend to get more prominent until the age of about 10, but have then resolved by adulthood.
  - Can cause learning difficulties.
  - Occasionally these areas can enhance, and are then difficult to differentiate from gliomas.
- Optic glioma:
  - Seen in up to 20%.
  - Range from tortuous optic nerves, to large masses.
- Other CNS tumours:
  - Astrocytomas.
  - Slightly increased risk of medulloblastoma, ependymoma.

Plexiform neurofibromas
- Can occur anywhere in the body.
- MRI: Bright on T2 images, with central dot of hypointensity 'target sign'.
- Can cause bony remodelling seen on radiographs, e.g.:
  - Harlequin orbit.
  - Ribbon ribs.

Vascular abnormalities
- Brain: stenosis and collateral vessel formation, moya moya.
- Narrowing of the abdominal aorta.
- Renal artery stenosis.

Other
- Also associated with phaeochromocytomas, and neurosarcomas.
- Dural ectasia, causing scalloping of vertebra and lateral meningoceles.
- Scoliosis.
- Tibial pseudoarthrosis.
- Some patients have learning difficulties.

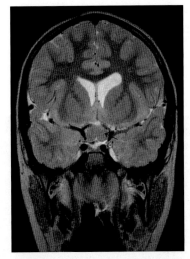

Fig. 8.14 Coronal T2 MRI of a patient with neurofibromatosis type I. This patient has an optic chiasm glioma (black arrow).

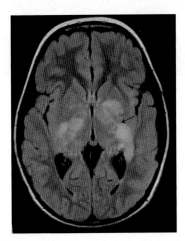

Fig. 8.15 Axial FLAIR MRI of the same patient showing extensive focal areas of hyperintensity (arrow) in the deep white matter, optic tracts and basal ganglia. This can be difficult to distinguish from optic gliomas in patients where these regions become extensive and enhance.

Neurofibromatosis type II

- Autosomal dominant: gene located on chromosome 22.
- Rare in children.
- Bilateral VIII nerve (acoustic neuromas).

Can also be associated with meningiomas, neurofibromas, and schwannomas.

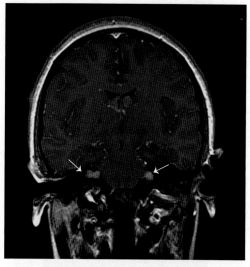

Fig. 8.16 Coronal T1 post-gadolinium MRI of a patient with neurofibromatosis type II. There are bilateral enhancing acoustic neuromas (white arrows).

Tuberous sclerosis

Tuberous sclerosis is an autosomal dominant neurocutaneous syndrome, characterized by hypopigmented skin patches (ash leaf macules). These are more obvious under UV light (Woods's lamp). Other features include:

Skin
- Facial angiofibromata.
- Periungual fibromas.
- 'Shagreen patches'.

Cardiac
- Rhabdomyomas are seen in neonates and infants: may be detected antenatally. These tend to involute over time.

Renal
- Angiomyolipoma: can grow, and haemorrhage (rare in children).
- ▶Most lesions that bleed are larger than 3.5cm in diameter.
- Cysts: common.
- Autosomal dominant polycystic kidney disease (less than 5% of patients) due to a deletion affecting the *TSC2* and *PKD1* gene on the tip of chromosome 16.
- Renal cell carcinoma: rare, occurs in less than 1% of patients with tuberous sclerosis.

Lungs
- Cystic lymphangiolyomyomatosis in young adult women.

Ocular
- Giant drusen and retinal astrocytomas (may regress).

Brain
- Seizures occur in 65–85%. These often present as infantile spasms and can be difficult to control.
- Learning difficulties are common.

Imaging findings

CT brain
- Calcified subependymal nodules.
- Subcortical tubers are more easily seen on MRI.

MRI brain
- Subependymal nodules.
- Giant cell tumours:
  - Contrast-enhancing nodule near foramen of monro.
  - Yearly surveillance recommended if incompletely calcified or enhancing as can cause hydrocephalus.
- Subcortical tubers: cortical dysplasia with balloon cells.

Differential diagnosis
- Subependymal grey matter heterotopia (do not calcify).
- Congenital CMV infection: periventricular calcification, white matter lesions and polymicrogyria (📖 p. 542).

Management and prognosis

- Vigabatrin.
- Giant cell tumours obstructing foramen of Monro need resection.
- Tuber resection may be considered if not responding to medical treatment, and seizure focus is localized to an isolated tuber.

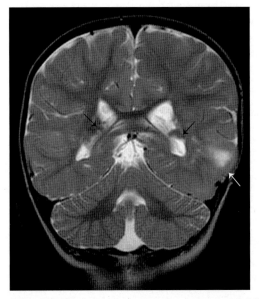

Fig. 8.17 Coronal T2 MRI of a patient with seizures due to tuberous sclerosis. This image shows bilateral subependymal nodules (black arrow), and a subcortical tuber (white arrow).

Sturge–Weber syndrome

This sporadic congenital abnormality is due to abnormal cortical vein formation. This results in venous ischaemia and infarction. Typically the abnormal veins are unilateral.

▶The majority of patients have an associated port wine stain.

Patients typically develop seizures in the first year of life. Strokes, migraine and hemiparesis may also occur.

Imaging findings

Radiographs

- 'Tram track' vascular calcification may be visible on skull X-ray.

CT

- Gyral calcification: progressive over time.
- Ipsilateral atrophy.
- Post-contrast: increased lepto-meningeal enhancement of the abnormal veins and enlargement of the ipsilateral choroid plexus.

MRI

- Ipsilateral atrophy, and gliosis.
- Ipsilateral accelerated myelin development.
- Areas of calcification are variable in appearance.
- T2* gradient: calcification low signal due to susceptibility artifact.
- Diffusion-weighted imaging: restricted diffusion in acutely ischaemic areas.
- Post-contrast: increased leptomeningeal enhancement, and enlarged ipsilateral choroid plexus.

Differential diagnosis

- Other neurocutaneous syndromes:
  - Klippel–Trenaunay–Weber: limb hypertrophy with associated vascular malformations. Features may overlap with Sturge–Weber syndrome.
  - PHACE: posterior fossa malformations, haemangiomas, arterial abnormalities, coarctation of the aorta, eye abnormalities.
  - Wyburn–Mason: facial naevus with eye/brain arteriovenous malformation.
  - Meningioangiomatosis: atrophy usually absent.
- Other causes of leptomeningeal enhancement:
  - Meningitis.
  - CNS disseminated malignancy, e.g. leukaemia, lymphoma, retinoblastoma.

Management and prognosis

- Prognosis depends on the size, and site of the abnormal cortical veins, and the extent of atrophy.
- Treatment includes medical treatment to control seizures, resection of affected lobe or hemisphere may be required if seizures are intractable.
- May be associated with eye angioma which may also need treatment to prevent glaucoma.

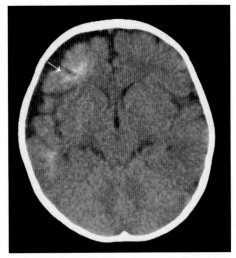

Fig. 8.18 CT of a patient with Sturge–Weber syndrome. There is atrophy of the right cerebral hemisphere with calcification (white arrow).

Congenital cytomegalovirus infection

Congenital infection due to transplacental viral transmission from the mother can cause brain abnormalities. The extent and type of abnormality depends on the gestation of the fetus at the time of infection. This is particularly true of cytomegalovirus (CMV), which is the most common cause of intrauterine infection. Congenital CMV can cause microcephaly and developmental delay, seizures, sensorineural hearing loss, hepatosplenomegaly and jaundice. The majority of infants with intrauterine CMV are asymptomatic at birth, hence the diagnosis is often delayed. The diagnosis can sometimes be made retrospectively by polymerase chain reaction (PCR) for CMV DNA from the Guthrie card.

Imaging findings

CT
- Periventricular calcification.
- Atrophy.
- Cortical malformations may be visible if extensive.

MRI
- Periventricular calcification can be difficult to detect on MRI.
- Small foci of ↑T2 signal predominantly in the parietal deep white matter.
- Ventricular dilatation due to periventricular white matter loss.
- Subcortical cysts in the anterior temporal lobes.
- Cortical malformations, e.g. polymicrogyria or agyria.

Differential diagnosis
- Toxoplasmosis: cerebral calcification often more scattered rather than periventricular.
- Congenital muscular dystrophy: associated with pontine hypoplasia and cerebellar cysts (these features are not seen in CMV).

Management and prognosis
- Antiviral agents may be considered in the small number of neonates who are symptomatic.

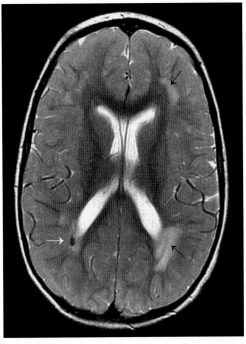

Fig. 8.19 Axial T2 MR of a child with congenital CMV. The small dark focus (white arrow) is an area of periventricular calcification. There are also foci of abnormal periventricular white matter (black arrows).

Meningitis

Meningitis, or inflammation of the meninges and CSF, can be due to bacterial or viral infection. Atypical organisms can also cause meningitis: for example TB. It is most commonly due to haematogenous spread of infection from a distant site.

Most common bacterial organisms

- Neonates: *E coli, B. haemolytic streptococci.*
- Children: *Neisseria meningitidis, Streptococcus pneumoniae.*

▶Prompt treatment can save lives.
▶Do not delay treatment waiting for imaging.

Imaging is not required in the majority of children with meningitis. Imaging can be completely normal. Subarachnoid haemorrhage can mimic the clinical picture of meningitis in adults, but this is extremely rare in children.

The major role of imaging is not making a diagnosis, but detecting complications. It can be also helpful in cases where meningitis is secondary to an underlying source, for example, mastoiditis or aggressive sinusitis. CT can show the areas of bone destruction due to osteomyelitis, and guide surgery.

Complications of meningitis

Hydrocephalus

- Intraventricular: e.g. inflammatory strands can obstruct the aqueduct.
- Extraventricular: due to impaired CSF resorption.

Encephalitis

- Focal areas of oedematous brain.
- CT: areas of low attenuation.
- MRI: areas of ↑T2 signal, ↓T1 signal, with overlying gyriform enhancement.

Empyema

- Rim-enhancing subdural collection of fluid.
- MRI: often bright on diffusion imaging.

Vasculitis and strokes

- Perivascular inflammation can cause stroke.
- CT: areas of low attenuation.
- MRI:
  - Areas of ↑T2, ↓T1 signal.
  - Areas of restricted diffusion if acute.
  - Perivascular enhancement.
  - MRA may show vascular irregularity.
  - Gyriform enhancement.

Venous sinus thrombosis (📖 p. 552).

TB meningitis

Can have a characteristic pattern, of thick meningeal enhancement on both CT and MRI, seen predominantly around the basal cisterns.

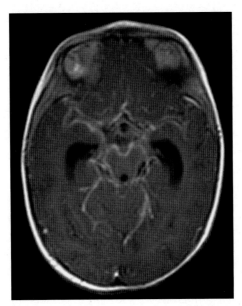

Fig. 8.20 Post-contrast MRI of a patient with TB meningitis. There is marked meningeal enhancement around the basal cisterns. This patient also had hydro-cephalus as a complication of meningitis: the temporal horns of the lateral ventricles are enlarged.

Acute demyelinating encephalopathy (ADEM)

ADEM is the most common para/post infectious disorder in children. It can be triggered 10–14 days after vaccination, or viral illness. It is usually a monophasic event, but recurrent forms can occur, raising diagnostic difficulties distinguishing from multiple sclerosis.

Imaging findings

CT
- May be normal.
- Asymmetrical low attenuation changes.

MRI
▶Pattern is usually asymmetrical.
- Much more sensitive than CT.
- Bilateral but asymmetrical signal on T2WI /FLAIR involving peripheral white matter, and grey matter.
- Lesions may or may not show restricted diffusion. Restricted diffusion suggests a worse outcome.
- Ring or punctate enhancement may occur.
- Spinal cord can also be involved.
- Imaging findings can lag behind symptoms.

Differential diagnosis

- MS: usually areas of ↑signal radiate from, and involve the corpus callosum.
- Autoimmune vasculitis.
- Posterior reversible encephalopathy: white matter oedema secondary to hypertension or immunosuppressive medication.
- Acute haemorrhagic leukoencephalopathy: a rare variant of ADEM, usually seen in infants. High mortality.
- If the pattern is very symmetrical consider a metabolic cause.

Management and prognosis

Steroids, intravenous immunoglobulin, plasmapheresis.

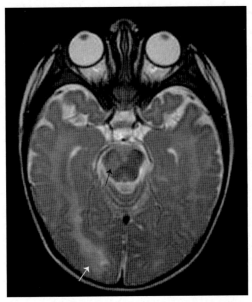

Fig. 8.21 Axial T2 image of an infant showing the patchy, asymmetrical distribution of ADEM. There is abnormal high signal in the right cerebral peduncle (black arrow) and in the right occipital lobe (white arrow).

Posterior reversible encephalopathy syndrome (PRES)

Hypertensive encephalopathy can cause headache, vomiting, confusion, seizures, and cerebral blindness. These changes are usually reversible after blood pressure has normalized. It is now known that drug toxicity can cause this clinical (and radiological) picture. It is thought to relate to auto-regulatory failure of the posterior circulation. Cyclosporin, tacrolimus, cisplatin, alpha interferon and erythropoetin have been implicated.

Imaging findings

CT

- Patchy areas of low attenuation in the posterior parietal and occipital lobes (posterior circulation distribution).

MRI

▶ Much more sensitive than CT.
- High signal on T2 and FLAIR images in the posterior parietal and occipital deep white matter and overlying cortex. Pattern is usually bilateral and symmetrical. Basal ganglia and brainstem may be involved.
- Diffusion-weighted imaging usually normal: restricted diffusion may indicate irreversible infarction.
- Post-contrast: variable patchy enhancement.

Differential diagnosis

- ADEM: does not tend to mainly involve posterior circulation distribution, and the pattern is usually asymmetrical.
- Neonatal hypoglycaemia: tends to affect the occipital lobes.
- Cerebellitis.
- Hypoperfusion/ischaemia: watershed distribution usually involve frontal lobes as well.

Management and prognosis

- Normalize blood pressure.
- Reduce dose or stop offending medication.
- Prognosis is usually good if treated promptly. Restricted diffusion may predict irreversible infarction.

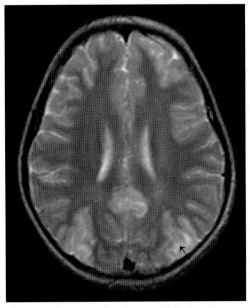

Fig. 8.22 Axial T2WI of a child with PRES. There is symmetrical high signal in the posterior aspects of both cerebral hemispheres (black arrow).

Stroke

Stroke is uncommon in children, but is probably under-recognized. The clinical symptoms depend on the area of the brain that is ischaemic/infarcted.

Causes of stroke in children

- Sickle cell disease:
  - Classically causes narrowing of the supra-clinoid region of the internal carotid arteries, and subsequent collateral vessel formation.
  - Children are now screened with MRI to detect unrecognized previous strokes, and Doppler ultrasound of the circle of Willis to detect vascular narrowing.
  - Children at risk are treated more aggressively to try and prevent further strokes.
- Vasculitis:
  - Infectious, e.g. related to varicella or meningitis.
  - Radiation.
  - Primary.
  - 'Moya moya' (means puff of smoke, and describes the small collateral vessels seen on formal angiography) can be primary, or acquired, e.g. due to sickle cell disease, neurofibromatosis and Down's syndrome.
- Embolic: e.g. through patent foramen of ovale.
- Congenital heart disease, particularly during surgery requiring cardiac bypass.
- Trauma: vertebral dissection.
- Coagulopathies: e.g. protein C and S deficiency.

Role of imaging

CT

- Focal areas, often wedge-shaped, of low attenuation.
- Clot within medium size arteries may be hyperdense.

MRI

▶Much more sensitive, particularly diffusion-weighted imaging, than CT in the early stages.

- Diffusion imaging is positive for about the first 10 days after event. The infarcted area will be bright on diffusion, and dark on the ADC map.
- Gyral swelling, blurred margin between the cortex and white matter.
- MRA can be used to detect occlusion in medium or large vessels.
- Gyral enhancement will be seen due to breakdown in the blood–brain barrier.
- MR perfusion: identifies the 'ischaemic penumbra' or brain that may be salvageable, from the area of brain that has infarcted.

Digital subtraction angiography

- May be necessary to detect abnormalities in the small cerebral vessels.

Management and prognosis
- Prognosis depends on the extent, and site of the stroke.
- Children may have better ability to recover than adults.
- Aspirin may be used for vasculopathies.
- Endovascular treatment is rarely used in children.

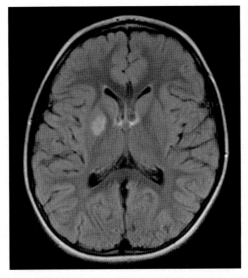

Fig. 8.23 Axial FLAIR MRI of a child with an acute infarct in the right basal ganglia.

Venous sinus thrombosis

The venous sinuses are the major pathway of venous drainage of the brain. Thrombosis results in elevated venous pressure, oedema and sometimes haemorrhage. Clinical presentation of venous sinus thrombosis is very variable, from headache and seizures, to coma.

There are a large number of causes including:

- Dehydration: particularly neonates.
- Coagulopathies.
- Infection: particularly of the mastoid, or facial sinuses which are close to the venous sinuses.
- Collagen vascular disorders: e.g. lupus.

Role of imaging

Ultrasound

- Lack of flow in the superior sagittal sinus is easy to diagnose, but the other sinuses are difficult to clearly visualize.

CT

- Non-contrast, clot is hyperdense.
- If clot involves straight sinus, bilateral thalamic oedema can cause compression of the 3rd ventricle and hydrocephalus.
- Intraparenchymal haemorrhage is hyperdense.
- Post-contrast CT:
  • Empty delta sign: enhancing dura surrounds the clot.
  • CT can be acquired as spiral scan, and then reconstructed to show extent of clot.

MRI

- Absent flow void within the sinus. Flow is normally dark on T2 images.
- MRV can help display loss of flow at site of occlusion, but beware both clot and flow can be bright on magnetic resonance venography (MRV) images. The transverse sinuses can be very small, particularly in neonates and difficult to see on MRV.
- Venous infarction:
  • Cortical swelling, poorly defined cortex.
  • Haemorrhage may be present.

Differential diagnosis

- Normal: neonatal blood is particularly hyperdense on CT (dense fetal haemoglobin, adjacent to the largely unmyelinated brain).
- Normal arachnoid granulation: small and round in shape, clots tends to be larger and 'slug-shaped'.

Management and prognosis

- Prognosis is variable, worse in the presence of venous infarction.
- Treatment is controversial: aspirin, warfarin.
- Intravascular thrombolysis may be considered in critically unwell patients.

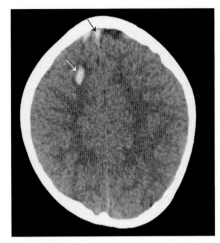

Fig. 8.24 Non-contrast CT head scan. There is acute thrombus within the sagittal sinus anteriorly (black arrow). There is a small associated region of parenchymal haemorrhage (white arrow).

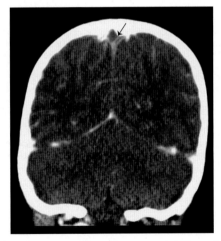

Fig. 8.25 Coronal reconstruction from a post-contrast spiral CT scan of the same patient. There is a filling defect within the superior sagittal sinus, or 'delta sign' due to venous sinus thrombosis.

Arteriovenous malformations

Excluding the perinatal period, arteriovenous malformations (AVM) are the most common cause of brain haemorrhage in children. They can occur anywhere in the brain. The majority present with haemorrhage. Epilepsy may occur with large lesions.

Imaging findings

CT
- Haemorrhage (acute haemorrhage is bright on CT scan).
- Curvilinear calcification may be present.
- Post-contrast CT: enlarged tortuous vessels close to haemorrhage.

MRI
- Dark intravascular flow voids may be visible on T2 images.
- MRA: shows feeding arteries and draining veins.

Formal angiography
- Depicts size, number and position of vessels and speed of flow, often required to plan treatment.

Differential diagnosis

- Tumour: repeat study may be required at a later date, as haemorrhage can obscure the lesion.
- Cavernoma: small popcorn-shaped, haemosiderin-lined abnormality, best seen on MRI. Gradient images are most sensitive, as emphasizes the 'blooming artefact' of haemosiderin. Can be multiple, familial or associated with radiation treatment.
- Vein of Galen malformation: arteriovenous fistula between the deep choroidal arteries and median prosencephalic vein, forming a large midline varix. Most commonly presents in newborn with heart failure.
- Dural arteriovenous fistula: multiple enlarged vascular channels within the wall of the dural venous sinus. The torcula is the most common location.
- Developmental venous anomaly: common, incidental finding. Small tuft of enlarged medullary veins, converge towards a larger central vein.

Management and prognosis

- Treatment may be required acutely if haemorrhage is large.
- Follow-up treatment is to reduce annual bleeding risk of 3%.
- Surgery, endovascular treatment most common methods of treatment.
- Radiosurgery can be used on single or small lesions, but takes years to reach effect.

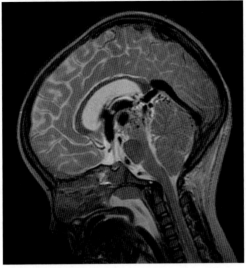

Fig. 8.26 Sagittal T2W MRI of a child with a large midbrain AVM.

Germinal matrix haemorrhage

The germinal matrix is a transient region of vessels, and migrating neurons. Premature infants may bleed in this region. After the age of 34 weeks, haemorrhage in this region—the caudo-thalamic groove—is very unlikely. The exact cause is unknown, but probably relates to perinatal hypoxia, stress, labile blood pressure, and poorly developed autoregulation of cerebral perfusion.

Clinical signs

Hypotonia, ↓haemoglobin, seizures, hyperreflexia.

Imaging

Ultrasound

- Acute haemorrhage is hyperechoic.
- Ependymal lining may become thick and hyperechoic.
- Ventriculomegaly.
- ▶Do not confuse with normal choroid plexus (which is also hyperechoic).

Grading

I: confined to the caudothalamic groove.
II: extends into ventricle.
III: fill and expands the ventricle.
IV: extension into the brain parenchyma.

Management and prognosis

- Grades I and II, good prognosis.
- Grades III and IV, variable long-term outlook, may have spastic diplegia, developmental delay, seizures.
- Some patients may require ventriculoperitoneal shunting, or 3rd ventriculostomies for hydrocephalus.

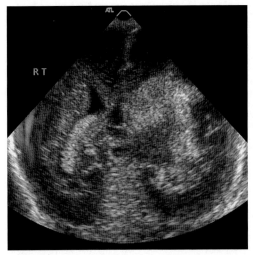

Fig. 8.27 Coronal cranial ultrasound image of a newborn premature baby with extensive intraventricular haemorrhage, extending in to the brain parenchyma on the left (grade IV IVH).

Hypoxic ischaemic encephalopathy (HIE)

Hypoxic ischaemic encephalopathy usually relates to perinatal birth asphyxia in children, but can occur at other times, for example as a consequence of major trauma. The pattern of brain damage depends on several factors:

- The age of the child. In neonates whether they are premature or born at term.
- Sudden or gradual onset.
- Duration of injury.
- Severity of brain hypoperfusion.

⚠There can be overlap between the patterns of injury, often a consequence of a varying pattern of hypoperfusion.

Patterns of brain damage seen in HIE

Periventricular

Seen in pre-term infants, secondary to mild–moderate hypoperfusion. This is also called periventricular leukomalacia (PVL), describing the white 'flare' appearance of the periventicular white matter seen acutely on ultrasound. Over time the white matter may become cystic. The cysts may decompress into the ventricles. Over time, the ventricles may become passively enlarged due to periventricular white matter loss. The corpus callosum often appears thinned. There may be evidence of periventricular gliosis, but this can be absent in children born very prematurely. PVL is often associated with spastic diplegia. Germinal matrix haemorrhage may accompany PVL.

Parasagittal watershed injury

This pattern occurs in mild–moderate hypoperfusion in term infants, and older children. Damage in this region occurs when hypoxia is of less sudden onset and less severe, allowing blood flow to be redirected to the basal ganglia, brainstem and cerebellum. Long-term morbidity can still be severe as the cerebral cortex can be severely affected.

Ventrolateral thalami and basal ganglia

Damage to the central grey matter occurs when hypoxia is of sudden onset and very severe. In term neonates this tends to affect the posterior putamen and vetrolateral thalami. Often damage extends into the periro-landic cortex.

Radiological findings

Ultrasound

Periventricular leukomalacia.

CT

Can be very subtle initially. Low attenuation areas develop over time.

MRI

- Changes can initially be very subtle:
  - Grey/white matter junction may be ill-defined.
  - Gyri swollen, cisterns and sulci compressed.

- Cortex ↑T2 signal.
- Cortex may be ↑T1 signal due to pseudolaminar necrosis.

▶Diffusion-weighted imaging very helpful to diagnose acute ischaemia/infarction: ↑signal on diffusion imaging, ↓signal on ADC map.

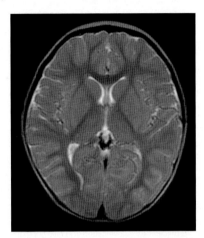

Fig. 8.28 Axial T2W MRI of a child who had suffered an acute profound hypoxic event. The occipital cortex is seen to be slightly bright and swollen.

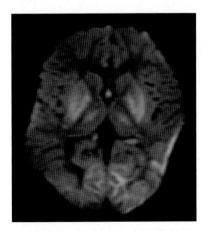

Fig. 8.29 Diffusion-weighted imaging of the same child highlights areas of damage (areas that are bright). The extent of damage to the occipital cortex, basal ganglia and thalami is much clearer on this image.

Medulloblastoma (posterior fossa PNET)

This highly cellular, dense tumour arises from the roof of the 4th ventricle. It usually presents before the age of 5. The clinical history is usually short (<1mth). Typical symptoms include nausea and vomiting, and ataxia. It is slightly more common in boys. It is the most common posterior fossa tumour in childhood (30–40%).

Imaging findings

CT

- Hyperdense on pre-contrast images is characteristic.
- 20% calcify.
- Usually midline tumour, filling the 4th ventricle.
- Lateral location is more common in older patients.
- 90% enhance post-contrast.

MRI

▶Important to give contrast and scan spine, as up to 33% present with metastatic disease.

- Restricted diffusion (as a very cellular tumour).
- 90% enhance post-contrast: often heterogenous pattern.

Differential diagnosis

Differentiation from other tumours can be very difficult.

- Ependymoma: often extrude though foramina, but medulloblastoma may also show this feature. Calcification and haemorrhage more common.
- Pilocytic astrocytoma: typically cystic with enhancing nodule.
- Atypical teratoid/rhabdoid tumour: usually younger children.

Management and prognosis

- Surgery and chemotherapy +/– radiotherapy.
- Patients with no metastatic disease, total resection and favourable histology have an excellent prognosis (100% 5-yr survival).
- Patients with gross residual tumour post surgery, and metastatic disease have a 5-yr survival rate of about 20%.

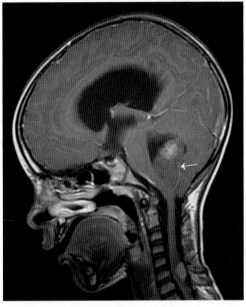

Fig. 8.30 Post-contrast MRI of a child with a medullobastoma (white arrow) filling the 4th ventricle. There is an enhancing spinal drop metastasis (black arrow).

Ependymoma

This slow-growing posterior fossa tumour usually arises within the 4th ventricle. Clinical symptoms can range from headaches, nausea, to ataxia, neck pain and torticollis. These tumours usually affect 1–5-year-olds (there is a second peak in young adults).

Imaging findings

CT
- Midline posterior fossa tumour.
- Calcification and hydrocephalus is common.
- Contrast enhancement is variable.

MRI
- Heterogenous tumour, calcification and haemorrhage common.
- Tends to exude from the 4th ventricle, through the foramen of Lushka, magendie and magnum.
- Contrast enhancement is variable.
- Can metastasise to CSF, and spine, but less frequently at presentation than medulloblastoma.

Differential diagnosis
- Medulloblastoma: hyperdense on non-contrast CT, arises from the roof (rather than the floor) of the 4th ventricle.
- Astrocytoma: cyst with enhancing solid component.
- Atypical teratoid/rhabdoid: young patients, variable enhancement.

Management and prognosis
- Surgical resection, radiation +/− chemotherapy.
- Prognosis dependent on total resection: this is often difficult due to the adherent, extruding characteristics of the tumour.

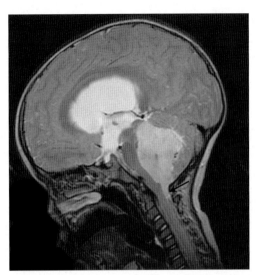

Fig. 8.31 Sagittal T2W MRI of a child with an ependymoma filling the 4th ventricle. This is causing hydrocephalus: the third ventricle is dilated. The tumour extends though the foramen magnum posterior to the cervical spinal cord.

Craniopharyngioma

This partly solid, partly cystic tumour arises from Rathkes' pouch epithelium. Hence these tumours lie in a suprasellar location. These tumours are slow-growing. Patients present with visual field defects, headaches, and short stature.

Imaging findings

CT
▶ Calcification present in the majority.
- The solid component usually enhances.

MRI
- T1WI: cystic component may have ↑signal. The fluid found at surgery is often like 'machine oil'.
- T2WI: there is usually a cystic component, calcified areas are variable in appearance.
- FLAIR: cyst usually ↑signal.
- T2* gradient: calcified areas dark due to susceptibility artefact.
- Post-contrast: solid component and cyst wall usually enhances brightly.
- Circle of Willis vessels are usually displaced, by the central tumour.

Differential diagnosis
- Rathke's cleft cyst: usually not calcified.
- Pituitary adenoma.
- Suprasellar arachnoid cyst: no calcification or enhancement.
- Hypothalamic astrocytoma.

Management and prognosis
- Surgery, cyst aspiration, radiotherapy.
- This slow growing tumour usually has a good prognosis.
- Recurrence rate >5cm 80%, <5cm 20%.
- Complications of treatment: pituitary/hypothalamic dysfunction.

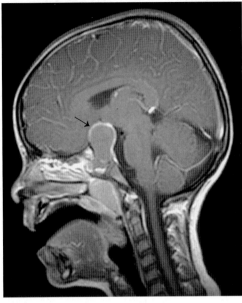

Fig. 8.32 Sagittal post-contrast MRI of a child with a suprasellar, rim enhancing mass (black arrow), due to craniopharyngioma.

Desmoplastic neuroepithelial tumour (DNET)

DNETs are benign cortical masses, associated with an area of cortical dysplasia. They are a cause of partial complex seizures in children and young adults. They do not grow, or show very slow growth over time.

Imaging findings

CT
- Cortically based low attenuation lesion.
- May scallop the inner table of the skull vault.
- Calcification in 20–40%.
- Nodular or patchy enhancement in 20%.

MRI
▶ 'Bubbly' mass, ↑↑T2 signal, ↓T1 signal.
- No surrounding oedema.
- Bleeding into the tumour is rare.
- Diffusion-weighted imaging: usually not restricted.
- Usually does not enhance, but faint enhancement in 20%.

Differential diagnosis
- Taylor's dysplasia: single tuberous sclerosis lesion.
- Glioma.
- Ganglioglioma: calcification common.
- Pleomorphic xanthoastrocytoma: usually enhancing dural tail.

Management and prognosis
- Can cause seizures which are difficult to control medically.
- Surgical excision may be required.
- Recurrence is rare.

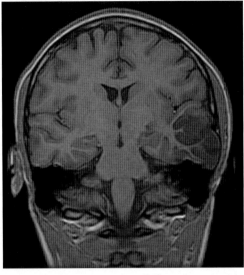

Fig. 8.33 Coronal T1 gradient MRI of a patient with a left temporal DNET. It has the typical appearance: a cortically based lesion with a 'bubbly' appearance.

Index